T5-AQF-484

Cardiovascular Trials Review

Third Edition

Edited by:

Robert A. Kloner, MD, PhD
Yochai Birnbaum, MD

Studies Compiled By:

Robert A. Kloner, MD, PhD
Yochai Birnbaum, MD

Robert A. Kloner, MD, PhD
Director of Research,
Heart Institute,
Good Samaritan Hospital,
Professor of Medicine,
University of Southern California,
Los Angeles, CA

Yochai Birnbaum, MD
Department of Cardiology
Rabin Medical Center
Beilinson Campus
Petah-Tikvah, Israel
Lecturer
Sackler Faculty of Medicine
Tel Aviv University
Tel Aviv, Israel

Dedicated to the memory of Philip Kloner
1925–1997

Copyright 1998 by Le Jacq Communications, Inc.
All rights reserved.

Reproduction or translation of any part of this work without permission of
the copyright owner is unlawful. Requests for permission or further information should be addressed to the Permissions Department, Le Jacq
Communications, Inc., 777 West Putnam Avenue, Greenwich, CT 06830

ISBN 0-9626020-7-8

Printed in the United States of America.

Table of Contents

b. PTCA Vs Stenting Vs Thrombolytic Therapy

c. Anticoagulation/Antiplatelet

d. Early Vs Late Intervention After Acute Myocardial Infarction

e. Remodeling After Infarction

f. Miscellaneous and Adjunctive Therapy

g. Thrombolytic Misc.

2. Unstable Angina/ Non Q Wave Infarction

3. Stable Angina Pectoris and Silent Ischemia-Medical Therapy

4. Interventional Cardiology
a. PTCA or CABG Vs Medical Therapy

b. PTCA Vs CABG

c. PTCA Vs Stenting Vs Other Percutaneous Devices

5. Hypertension

6. Congestive Heart Failure

7. Lipid Lowering Studies

8. Arrhythmia

Introduction

The purpose of *Cardiovascular Trials Review Third Edtion* is to review those trials which have made a major impact on the practice of clinical cardiology within the last 8 years. We have included only studies that were published in English and concentrated mainly on publications that have appeared since 1990 and have studied either pharmacological or device therapy. The text is divided into major headings of diseases such as myocardial infarction and unstable angina. In general, we gave priority to prospective randomized trials with preference to multicenter studies and those that included several hundred patients. In this third edition we have added over 150 new entries and concentrated on trials from 1997-1998.

We truly have been amazed by the increasing number of new, large clinical trials in the literature. Since the early '90's there has been a virtual explosive growth in the number of these trials.

Unfortunately, we were not able to include all studies. There are many other excellent studies which may not appear in this review. However, a review of the trials included in this book should give the reader a flavor of the types and designs of major clinical trials that have influenced the practice of clinical cardiology.

We have tried to use only a minimal amount of abbreviations in the text: CI- confidence interval; ECG- electrocardiogram; and RR- relative risk; PTCA- percutaneous transluminal coronary angioplasty; CABG- coronary artery bypass graft; MI - myocardial infarction; LV- left ventricle; LDL- low density lipoprotein (cholesterol); HDL- high density lipoprotein (cholesterol).

The drugs, indications for drugs, and drug dosages may or may not be approved for general use by the Food and Drug Administration (FDA). Physicians should consult the package inserts and/or Physicians' Desk Reference for drug indications, contraindications, side effects, and dosages as recommended. We thank Sharon L. Hale for her help with this manuscript.

Robert A. Kloner, MD, PhD
Yochai Birnbaum, MD
Los Angeles, CA
October, 1998.

1. Acute Myocardial Infarction
a. Thrombolytic Therapy

GISSI

*Gruppo Italiano per lo Studio della Streptochinasi
nell'Infarto miocardico*

Title	a. Effectiveness of intravenous thrombolytic treatment in acute myocardial infarction.
	b. Long-term effects of intravenous thrombolysis in acute myocardial infarction: final report of the GISSI study.
Authors	GISSI
Reference	a. Lancet 1986;I:397-401.
	b. Lancet 1987;II:871-874.
Disease	Acute myocardial infarction.
Purpose	To evaluate the efficacy of intravenous streptokinase to reduce in-hospital and 1-year mortality in patients with acute myocardial infarction, and to define the time interval from onset of symptoms to therapy and that therapy is still effective.
Design	Randomized, open label, multicenter.
Patients	11,712 patients with suspected acute myocardial infarction ≤12 h of onset of symptoms, with ≥1 mm ST elevation or depression in any limb lead or ≥2 mm in any precordial lead. No age restriction.
Follow-up	1 year.
Treatment regimen	Streptokinase 1.5 million U IV over 1 h, or no treatment.
Additional therapy	According to normal practice. No restrictions.

GISSI

Gruppo Italiano per lo Studio della Streptochinasi nell'Infarto miocardico

(continued)

Results
a. 21 day course: Overall mortality was 13.0% in the control and 10.7% in the treated group (relative risk 0.81, 95% CI 0.72-0.90, p=0.0002). In patients treated within 3 h from onset of symptoms mortality was 12.0% and 9.2% for the control and streptokinase groups (RR 0.74, 95% CI 0.63-0.87, p=0.0005), while for those treated 3-6 h the mortality was 14.1% and 11.7%, respectively (RR 0.80, 95% CI 0.66-0.98, p=0.03). Treatment beyond 6 h did not result in a significant difference in mortality between the groups (14.1% vs 12.6%, p=NS, RR 0.87 for those treated 6-9 h; and 13.6% vs 15.8%, p=NS, RR 1.19 for those treated 9-12 h after onset of symptoms). Subgroup analysis revealed beneficial effects for streptokinase in patients with anterior and multi-site infarction. However, patients with lateral infarctions or ST depression had a trend towards worse outcome with streptokinase than without (although without statistical significance). The incidence of anaphylactic shock and bleeding attributed to streptokinase were low.
b. After 1 year, mortality was 17.2% in the streptokinase and 19.0% in the control group (RR 0.90, 95% CI 0.84-0.97, p=0.008). The difference in mortality was seen only in those treated within 6 h of onset of symptoms.

Conclusions
a. Streptokinase is a safe and effective therapy for patients with acute myocardial infarction treated within 6 h of onset of symptoms.
b. The beneficial effects of streptokinase were still apparent after 1 year.

TIMI-1

Thrombolysis in Myocardial Infarction Trial (phase 1)

Title	Thrombolysis in Myocardial Infarction (TIMI) Trial, phase I: a comparison between intravenous tissue plasminogen activator and intravenous streptokinase. Clinical findings through hospital discharge.
Authors	Chesbero JH, Knatterud G, Roberts R, et al.
Reference	Circulation 1987;76:142-154.
Disease	Acute myocardial infarction.
Purpose	To compare two regimens of intravenous thrombolytic therapy: rt-PA and streptokinase.
Design	Randomized, double blind, multicenter.
Patients	290 patients with acute myocardial infarction <75 years old < 7 hours from onset of symptoms with chest pain >30 min and ST elevation $\geq$0.1 mV in $\geq$2 contiguous leads. Patients with cardiogenic shock were excluded.
Follow-up	Coronary angiography before and 10, 20, 30, 45, 60, 75, 90 min, after onset of thrombolytic therapy and predischarge. Clinical visits at 6 weeks and 6 months.
Treatment regimen	Streptokinase 1.5 million units or placebo IV over 1 h, and rt-PA or placebo over 3 h (40, 20, and 20 mg in the 1st, 2nd and 3rd hours).
Additional therapy	Lidocaine (1-1.5 mg/kg bolus + infusion 2-4 µg/min) for >24 h; intracoronary nitroglycerin 200 µg; heparin 5000 U bolus and infusion 1000 U/h for 8-10 days. Aspirin 325 mg X3/d and dipyridamole 75 mg X3/d after heparin was stopped.

Results	At 30 min after initiation of therapy 24% and 8% of the rt-PA and streptokinase-treated patients achieved TIMI grade flow of 2 or 3 (P<0.001). At 90 min after initiation of therapy, 62% of the rt-PA and 31% of the streptokinase-treated patients achieved TIMI grade flow of 2 or 3 (P<0.001). 44% and 22% of the rt-PA and streptokinase-treated patients had patent arteries upon discharge (p<0.001). There was no difference in global or regional left ventricular function either in the pre-treatment or predischarge study. Fever or chills occurred in 4% and 15% of the rt-PA and streptokinase groups (p<0.01). Death within 21 days occurred in 4% and 5% of the rt-PA and streptokinase groups. The reduction in circulating fibrinogen and plasminogen and the increase in plasma fibrin split products at 3 and 24 h were significantly more pronounced in the streptokinase treated patients (p<0.001). The occurrence of bleeding was comparable in the 2 groups (66% and 67% of the rt-PA and streptokinase, respectively).
Conclusions	Treatment with rt-PA resulted in more rapid reperfusion than streptokinase. However, there was no difference in either mortality, bleeding complications, or left ventricular function between the groups.

ISIS-2

International Study of Infarct Survival 2

Title	Randomized trial of intravenous streptokinase, oral aspirin, both, or neither among 17,187 cases of suspected acute myocardial infarction: ISIS-2.
Authors	ISIS-2 Collaborative Group.
Reference	Lancet 1988;II:349-360.
Disease	Acute myocardial infarction.
Purpose	To assess the efficacy of oral aspirin, streptokinase infusion, and their combination in the treatment of acute myocardial infarction.
Design	Randomized, double blind, 2X2 factorial, placebo-controlled, multicenter.
Patients	17,187 patients with suspected acute myocardial infarction <24 h of onset of symptoms.
Follow-up	Maximum 34 months, median 15 months.
Treatment regimen	1. Streptokinase 1.5 million U over 1 h IV. 2. Aspirin 162.5 mg/d for 1 month. 3. Streptokinase 1.5 million U over 1 h IV + Aspirin 162.5 mg/d for 1 month. 4. Neither.
Additional therapy	No restrictions.

ISIS-2

International Study of Infarct Survival 2

(continued)

Results

5-week vascular mortality among the streptokinase and placebo treated patients was 9.2% and 12.0%, respectively (odds reduction: 25%, 95% CI 18-32%, p<0.00001). 5-week vascular mortality among the aspirin treated was 9.4% and for the placebo 11.8% (odds reduction: 23%, 95% CI 15-30%, p<0.00001). The combination of aspirin and streptokinase was better than either agent alone. 5-week vascular mortality among the streptokinase and aspirin treated patients was 8.0%, while it was 13.2% among those allocated to neither treatment (odds reduction: 42%, 95% CI: 34-50%). The odds reductions at treatment 0-4, 5-12, and 13-24 h after onset of symptoms were 35%, 16%, and 21% for streptokinase alone; 25%, 21%, and 21% for aspirin alone; and 53%, 32%, and 38% for the combination. Streptokinase was associated with excess bleeding requiring transfusion (0.5% vs 0.2%, p<0.001) and of cerebral hemorrhage (0.1% vs 0.0%, p<0.02). However, total strokes were similar (0.7% vs 0.8%). Aspirin reduced the rates of nonfatal reinfarction (1.0% vs 2.0%, p<0.00001) and nonfatal stroke (0.3% vs 0.6%, p<0.01) and was not associated with increased risk of cerebral or noncranial hemorrhages. Patients allocated to the combination therapy had fewer reinfarctions (1.8% vs 2.9%), strokes (0.6% vs 1.1%), and deaths (8.0% vs 13.2%) than those allocated to neither therapy. The difference in mortality produced by either aspirin, streptokinase, or their combination remained significant after 15 months of follow-up.

Conclusions

Aspirin and streptokinase independently reduced mortality in patients with acute myocardial infarction. The combination of the 2 drugs has a synergistic effect on mortality without increasing the rates of stroke.

AIMS

APSAC Intervention Mortality Study

Title	a. Effect of intravenous APSAC on mortality after acute myocardial infarction: preliminary report of a placebo-controlled clinical trial. b. Long-term effects of intravenous anistreplase in acute myocardial infarction: final report of the AIMS study.
Authors	AIMS Trial Study Group.
Reference	a. Lancet 1988;I;545-549. b. Lancet 1990;335:427-431.
Disease	Acute myocardial infarction.
Purpose	To compare survival up to 1 year in patients with acute myocardial infarction randomized to APSAC (anisoylated plasminogen streptokinase activator complex) or placebo.
Design	Randomized, double blind, placebo-controlled, multicenter.
Patients	a. 1004 patients, age ≤70 years with acute myocardial infarction, ≥30 min pain, <6 h of onset of symptoms, ≥1 mm ST elevation in ≥2 limb leads or >2 mm in >2 precordial leads. b. 1258 patients, same criteria, including the first 1004 patients.
Follow-up	1 year.
Treatment regimen	APSAC 30 U or placebo IV over 5 min.

APSAC Intervention Mortality Study

(continued)

Additional therapy	IV heparin started 6 h after initiation of therapy, warfarin for ≥3 months. Other medications according to common practice. Timolol 10 mg/d for 1 year if not contraindicated.
Results	a. 30-day mortality was 12.2% on placebo and 6.4% on APSAC (47% reduction of mortality, 95% CI 21-65%, p=0.0016). Percentage reduction of mortality with APSAC was similar whether therapy was started 0-4 or 4-6 h after onset of symptoms.
	b. 30-day mortality was 12.1% on placebo and 6.4% on APSAC (50.5% reduction of mortality, 95% CI 26-67%, p=0.0006). 1 year mortality was 17.8% on placebo and 11.1% on APSAC (42.7% reduction of mortality, 95% CI 21-59%, p=0.0007). Major cardiovascular complications (shock, cardiac arrest, rupture, ventricular septal defect, and ventricular fibrillation) occurred in 12.3% and 16.7% of the APSAC and placebo groups, respectively (p=0.03).
Conclusions	Intravenous APSAC within 6 h of onset of symptoms reduced mortality in acute myocardial infarction.

ASSET

Anglo-Scandinavian Study of Early Thrombolysis

Title	a. Trial of tissue plasminogen activator for mortality reduction in acute myocardial infarction. Anglo-Scandinavian Study of early Thrombolysis (ASSET). b. Effects of alteplase in acute myocardial infarction: 6-month results from the ASSET study.
Authors	Wilcox RG, von der Lippe G, Olsson CG, et al.
Reference	a. Lancet 1988;II:525-530. b. Lancet 1990;335:1175-1178.
Disease	Acute myocardial infarction.
Purpose	To evaluate the efficacy of tissue plasminogen activator versus placebo in reduction of mortality in acute myocardial infarction.
Design	Randomized, double blind, placebo-controlled, multicenter.
Patients	a. 5009 patients, b. 5013 patients, age 18-75 years, with suspected acute myocardial infarction within 5 h of onset of symptoms. No ECG criteria were required.
Follow-up	6 months.
Treatment regimen	Tissue plasminogen activator (t-PA) or placebo 10 mg IV bolus, 50 mg infusion over 1 h, and then 40 mg over 2 h.
Additional therapy	IV heparin 5000 U bolus, and infusion of 1000 U/h for 21 h.

ASSET

Anglo-Scandinavian Study of Early Thrombolysis

(continued)

Results
a. One month mortality was 7.2% and 9.8%, in the t-PA and placebo groups (a relative reduction of 26%, 95% CI 11-39%, p=0.0011). Bleeding (major+minor) and major bleeding occurred in 6.3% and 1.4% of the t-PA, and 0.8% and 0.4% of the placebo groups, respectively. The incidence of stroke was similar (1.1% and 1.0%). There was no difference in recurrent infarction or development of heart failure rates. In those with abnormal ECG on entry, t-PA was associated with 24.5% relative reduction in 1 month mortality (8.5% vs 11.2%, 95% CI 9-37%).

b. 6 month mortality rate was 10.4% in the t-PA and 13.1% in the placebo group (relative reduction of risk 21%, 95% CI 8-32%, p=0.0026). 6 month mortality for patients with proven infarction was 12.6% and 17.1%, respectively (relative reduction of risk 26.3%, 95% CI 14-38%). The effect was similar for anterior and inferior infarctions. However, t-PA did not reduce cardiac readmissions, reinfarctions, development of heart failure, angina, or death beyond 1 month. 12 month mortality (for 4230 patients) was 13.2% and 15.1% for t-PA and placebo group (p<0.05).

Conclusions
t-PA therapy within 5 h of onset of symptoms, compared to placebo, reduced mortality sustained to 1 year, but not the rates of recurrent infarction, angina, or development of heart failure.

GISSI-2

*Gruppo Italiano per lo Studio della Streptochinasi
nell'Infarto miocardico 2*

Title	a. GISSI-2: A factorial randomized trial of alteplase versus streptokinase and heparin versus no heparin among 12,490 patients with acute myocardial infarction. b. In-hospital mortality and clinical course of 20,891 patients with suspected acute myocardial infarction randomized between alteplase and streptokinase with or without heparin.
Authors	a. GISSI b. The International Study Group.
Reference	a. Lancet 1990;336:65-71. b. Lancet 1990;336:71-75.
Disease	Acute myocardial infarction.
Purpose	To compare the efficacy of intravenous streptokinase and tissue plasminogen activator (t-PA) for the treatment of acute myocardial infarction, and to evaluate the effects of adding heparin therapy to aspirin on the incidence of recurrent ischemia.
Design	Randomized, open label, 2X2 factorial, multicenter.
Patients	a. 12,381 patients. b. 20,768 patients (including 12,490 from the GISSI-2). All patients had chest pain + ST elevation $\geq$1mm in any limb lead and/or ST$\geq$2 mm in any precordial lead, within 6 h of onset of symptoms. No age limit.
Follow-up	In-hospital course, predischarge echocardiography.

GISSI-2

Gruppo Italiano per lo Studio della Streptochinasi nell'Infarto miocardico 2

(continued)

Treatment regimen	a. Streptokinase 1.5 million U over 30-60 min + heparin SC 12,500 UX2/d, starting 12 h after initiation of thrombolytic infusion and continued until discharge. b. t-PA 10 mg bolus, 50 mg over 1 h, and 40 mg over 2 h + heparin SC 12,500 UX2/d, starting 12 h after initiation of thrombolytic infusion and continued until discharge. c. Streptokinase 1.5 million U over 30-60 min without heparin. d. t-PA 10 mg bolus, 50 mg over 1 h, and 40 mg over 2 h without heparin.
Additional therapy	Oral aspirin 300-325 mg/d. Atenolol 5-10 mg IV.
Results	a. The t-PA and streptokinase groups did not differ in mortality (9.0% and 8.6%), clinical heart failure (7.7% and 8.1%), or occurrence of left ventricular ejection fraction ≤35% (2.5% and 2.2%). Combined end points occurred in 23.1% and 22.5%, respectively. The rates of recurrent infarction, post-infarction angina, stroke, and bleeding were not different between the t-PA and streptokinase groups. Allergic reactions and hypotension were more common in the streptokinase than t-PA treated patients. There was no differences regarding mortality (8.3% vs 9.3%), heart failure (8.0% vs 7.8%), or ejection fraction ≤35% (2.3% vs 2.4%) between the heparin and no-heparin groups. There was no difference in reinfarction, post-infarction angina, and stroke between the 2 groups. Major bleeding was more common in the heparin treated patients (1.0% vs 0.6%, RR 1.64, 95% CI 1.09-2.45). b. In-hospital mortality was 8.9% for t-PA, 8.5% for streptokinase (RR 1.05, 95% CI 0.96-1.16), and 8.5% for heparin versus 8.9% without heparin. More strokes occurred with t-PA (1.3%) than with streptokinase (0.9%), while major bleeding occurred in 0.6% and 0.9% of the t-PA and streptokinase treated patients.
Conclusions	Streptokinase and t-PA appear equally effective and safe. Adding heparin subcutaneously to thrombolysis and aspirin did not alter prognosis, except for an increase in major bleeding.

MITI-1

Myocardial Infarction Triage and Intervention

Title	a. Myocardial infarction triage and intervention project-phase I: patient characteristics and feasibility of prehospital initiation of thrombolytic therapy. b. Prehospital-initiated vs hospital-initiated thrombolytic therapy. The myocardial infarction triage and intervention trial.
Authors	a. Weaver WD, Eisenberg MS, Martin JS, et al. b. Weaver WD, Cerqueira M, Hallstrom AD.
Reference	a. J Am Coll Cardiol 1990;15:925-931. b. JAMA 1993; 270:1211-1216.
Disease	Acute myocardial infarction.
Purpose	a. To assess the feasibility and the time saving, of the strategy of prehospital initiation of thrombolytic therapy by paramedics. b. To determine the effect of prehospital initiated treatment of acute myocardial infarction vs hospital-initiated therapy.
Design	a. Patients with chest pain were evaluated by paramedics by obtaining history, physical examination, and electrocardiogram that was transmitted to a base station physician. The physician determined whether the patient met the criteria for prehospital thrombolysis. b. Randomized, controlled trial.
Patients	a. 2472 patients, <75 years old, with chest pain ≥15 min and <6 h, who called 911. b. 360 patients with symptoms of acute myocardial infarction for 6 or fewer hours. Patients had to have ST-segment elevation and no risk factors for serious bleeding.

Follow-up	a. 9 months. b. In-hospital - 30 days.
Treatment regimen	b. Patients received aspirin and alteplase either before or after hospital arrival. Once in the hospital, both groups received heparin.
Results	a. 677 patients (27%) had suitable clinical findings consistent with possible acute myocardial infarction and no apparent risk for thrombolytic therapy. Electrocardiograms of 522 of the 677 patients were transmitted to the base station. Only 107 (21%) of these tracings demonstrated ST elevation. 453 patients developed acute myocardial infarction in hospital. 163 (36%) of the 453 patients met the screening history and examination criteria and 105 (23.9%) had ST elevation. The average time from onset of symptoms to prehospital diagnosis was 72±52 min (median 52 min). This was 73±44 min (median 62 min) earlier than the actual time when thrombolytic therapy was started in hospital. b. More patients whose therapy was started before hospital arrival had resolution of pain by admission, 23% vs 7%, (p<.001). There was no difference in composite score of combined death, stroke, serious bleeding, and infarct size between groups. Secondary analysis of time to treatment and outcomes showed that treating within 70 min of symptoms resulted in better outcome, that is lower composite score, p=.009. Early therapy was associated with lower mortality (1.2%) compared to late mortality (8.7%, p=0.04) and infarct size and ejection fraction were improved with early therapy.
Conclusions	a. Paramedic selection of patients for potential prehospital initiation of thrombolytic therapy is feasible and may shorten the time to initiation of thrombolytic therapy. b. Initiating treatment before hospital arrival did not improve outcome. However, therapy started within 70 min of symptom onset, whether in the hospital or outside of the hospital, was associated with the better outcome.

TEAM-2

The Second Thrombolytic Trial of Eminase in Acute Myocardial Infarction

Title	Multicenter patency trial of intravenous anistreplase compared with streptokinase in acute myocardial infarction.
Authors	Anderson JL, Sorensen SG, Moreno FL, et al.
Reference	Circulation 1991;83;126-140.
Disease	Acute myocardial infarction.
Purpose	To compare the efficacy of anistreplase (APSAC) and streptokinase on early patency and reocclusion rates.
Design	Randomized, double blind, multicenter.
Patients	370 patients, aged <76 years, with chest pain of >30 min, ≤4 h of onset of symptoms, and ST elevation of ≥1 mm in ≥1 limb lead or ≥2 mm in ≥1 precordial lead. Patients in cardiogenic shock, previous coronary artery bypass grafting, balloon angioplasty within 1 month, blood pressure >200/120 mmHg, or contraindications to thrombolytic therapy were excluded.
Follow-up	90-240 min coronary angiography. Patients with TIMI flow 0 or 1 were allowed to undergo angioplasty. Patients with initial TIMI flow 2-3, who did not undergo mechanical intervention, were catheterized again 18-48 h after initiation of protocol.
Treatment regimen	1. Anistreplase 30 U over 2-5 min IV and streptokinase placebo. 2. Placebo and Streptokinase 1.5 million U over 60 min.

TEAM-2

The Second Thrombolytic Trial of Eminase in Acute Myocardial Infarction
(continued)

Additional therapy	Heparin 5000-10,000 U bolus at the start of catheterization. IV infusion 1000 U/h was commenced after the angiography for >24 h. Diphenhydramine 25-50 mg IV was recommended.
Results	Early (mean 140 min) patency rate (TIMI flow 2-3) was 72% with APSAC and 73% with streptokinase. However, TIMI flow 3 was seen in 83% and 72%, respectively (p=0.03). Mean residual coronary artery stenosis was 74% vs 77.2%, respectively (p=0.02), in those who achieved TIMI flow 2-3. Reocclusion risk within 1-2 days was found in 1.0% and 2.1% of the APSAC and streptokinase patients. Enzymatic and electrocardiographic evolution was similar. In-hospital mortality was 5.9% vs 7.1% (p=0.61). Bleeding complications, stroke, allergic reactions, and cardiovascular complications were similar.
Conclusions	Streptokinase and APSAC were equally effective and safe as thrombolytic therapy within 4 h of onset of acute myocardial infarction.

TAMI-5

Thrombolysis and Angioplasty in Myocardial Infarction- 5

Title	a. Evaluation of combination thrombolytic therapy and timing of cardiac catheterization in acute myocardial infarction. Results of Thrombolysis and Angioplasty in Myocardial Infarction-phase 5 randomized trial. b. Effects of thrombolytic regimen, early catheterization, and predischarge angiographic variables on 6-week left ventricular function.
Authors	a. Califf RM, Topol EJ, Stack RS, et al. b. Ward SR, Sutton JM, Pieper KS, et al.
Reference	a. Circulation 1991;83:1543-1556. b. Am J Cardiol 1997;79:539-544.
Disease	Acute myocardial infarction.
Purpose	To evaluate 3 thrombolytic regimens (tissue-type plasminogen activator (t-PA), urokinase, or both) and 2 strategies (immediate vs predischarge catheterization).
Design	Randomized, open label, 3X2 factorial, multicenter.
Patients	575 patients, age <76 years, with suspected acute myocardial infarction (chest pain ≤6 h; ST elevation ≥1 mm in ≥2 leads).
Follow-up	a. 5-10 days (contrast ventriculogram and clinical evaluation). b. Predischarge and 6 week radionuclide ventriculography (MUGA).
Treatment regimen	1. Urokinase 1.5 million U bolus +1.5 million U infusion over 90 min. 2. t-PA 6 mg bolus, 54 mg over the first h, and 40 mg over 2 h. 3. Urokinase 1.5 million U over 60 min with 1mg/kg t-PA over 60 min (10% given as a bolus, maximal dose 90 mg). The early invasive strategy consisted of coronary angiography after 90 min of initiation of therapy with rescue angioplasty when indicated. The deferred strategy required coronary angiography 5-10 days after admission.
Additional therapy	Aspirin 325 mg/d. Heparin was started at the end of thrombolytic infusion at a dose of 1000 IU/h for >48 h. In the aggressive strategy additional 5000 IU heparin was given. Additional heparin was given during rescue angioplasty. Prophylactic lidocaine was used in most patients. Diltiazem 30-60 mgX3/d.

Results

a. Early patency rates were greater with the combination regimen (76%) vs 62% and 71% in the urokinase and t-PA arms (p=0.14). However, predischarge patency rates were similar. 5-10 days left ventricular ejection fraction was comparable among the three regimens and between the two strategies. Combination thrombolytic therapy was associated with less complicated clinical course and lower rate of reocclusion (2%) vs 7% and 11%, in the urokinase and t-PA regimens (p=0.04), and a lower rate of recurrent ischemia (25% vs 35% and 31%, respectively). Combination therapy was associated with the lower rates of the combined end point of death, stroke, reinfarction, reocclusion, heart failure, or recurrent ischemia (32% vs 45% and 40% for urokinase, and t-PA, respectively, p=0.04). Bleeding complications were comparable among the groups. Predischarge patency rates were 94% and 90% in the early invasive and early conservative strategies (p=0.065). Predischarge regional wall motion in the infarct zone was improved more with the early aggressive approach (-2.16 SDs/chord vs -2.49 SDs/chord, p=0.004). More patients in the early invasive strategy were free from adverse outcomes (67% vs 55%, p=0.004).

b. 219 patients underwent paired MUGA scan before discharge and at 6 weeks. Predischarge median left ventricular ejection fraction (25th, 75th percentile) was 58 (51, 63), 55 (46, 65), and 57 (48, 63) in the t-PA, urokinase, and combination groups, respectively (p=0.29). Predischarge ejection fraction was unaffected by the early catheterization strategy (p=0.75). The type of thrombolytic regimen (p=0.331, p=0.645) and the catheterization strategy (p=0.60, p=0.256)) had no effect on either rest or exercise global left ventricular ejection fraction 6 weeks after enrollment. The type of thrombolytic regimen (p=0.59) and the catheterization strategy (p=0.36) had no effect on regional wall motion score at the infarct zone. Rescue PTCA was associated with worse 6-week regional wall motion (p=0.002) in the early catheterization group (univariate analysis). After adjustment for predischarge infarct-zone wall motion score, rescue PTCA was still predictive of worse regional function at 6 weeks (p=0.007).

TAMI-5

Thrombolysis and Angioplasty in Myocardial Infarction- 5

(continued)

Conclusions	Combination thrombolytic therapy is more effective than single agent therapy for achievement of early and sustained reperfusion and for reducing the incidence of in-hospital complications. The early intervention strategy may result in better clinical outcome. The early beneficial effect of early catheterization on regional function was not sustained, and both global and regional function was comparable among the 3 thrombolytic regimens and between the early and deferred coronary angiography groups.

TAMI-7

Thrombolysis and Angioplasty in Myocardial Infarction VII

Title	Accelerated plasminogen activator dose regimens for coronary thrombolysis.
Authors	Wall TC, Califf RM, George BS, et al.
Reference	J Am Coll Cardiol 1992;19:482-489.
Disease	Acute myocardial infarction.
Purpose	To evaluate the efficacy of 5 different regimens of tissue plasminogen activator (t-PA) administration in acute myocardial infarction.
Design	Randomized, multicenter.
Patients	219 patients, >18 and <76 years old, with suspected acute myocardial infarction >30 min pain unresponsive to sublingual nitrate, ≤6 h from onset of symptoms, ≥1 mm ST elevation in ≥2 leads or ST depression in V1-V4.
Follow-up	In-hospital events, pre-treatment, and 5-10 days coronary angiography.
Treatment regimen	1. t-PA 1mg/kg over 30min (10% bolus), 0.25mg/kg over 30min. Max. dose 120mg. 2. t-PA 1.25mg/kg over 90min (20 mg bolus). Max. dose 120mg. 3. t-PA 0.75mg/kg over 30min (10% bolus), 0.50mg/kg over 60min. Max. dose 120mg. 4. t-PA 20mg bolus, 30min wait, 80mg over 120min. Max. dose 100mg. 5. t-PA 1mg/kg over 30min + urokinase 1.5 million U over 1h. Max. dose 90mg.

Thrombolysis and Angioplasty in Myocardial Infarction VII
(continued)

Additional therapy	Standard care including lidocaine, oxygen, morphine, and nitrates. Aspirin 325 mg/d. Heparin infusion 1,000 U/h started at the end of thrombolytic infusion and continued for 5-10 days. Metoprolol IV 15 mg if no contraindication existed.
Results	90 min patency rates were 63%, 61%, 83%, 67%, and 72% for protocols 1-5, respectively. Reocclusion occurred in 11%, 3%, 4%, 14%, and 3%, respectively. Protocol 3 achieved the highest rate of reperfusion and a low rate of reocclusion. Predischarge left ventricular ejection fraction was not statistically different among the groups. There was no difference in bleeding complications among the groups. Death, reocclusion, restenosis, and reinfarction tended to be less frequent in protocol 3, however, without statistical significance.
Conclusions	Accelerated t-PA administration according to protocol 3 is a relatively safe strategy achieving high 90 min patency rate and low reocclusion and complication rates.

ISIS-3

International Study of Infarct Survival 3

Title	ISIS-3: a randomized comparison of streptokinase vs tissue plasminogen activator vs anistreplase and of aspirin plus heparin vs aspirin alone among 41299 cases of suspected acute myocardial infarction.
Authors	ISIS-3 Collaborative Group.
Reference	Lancet 1992;339:753-770.
Disease	Acute myocardial infarction.
Purpose	1. To compare 3 thrombolytic agents: tissue plasminogen activator (t-PA), streptokinase, and anisoylated plasminogen streptokinase activator complex (APSAC). 2. To compare treatment with heparin + aspirin with aspirin.
Design	Randomized, double blind (for thrombolytic agents) and open label (for heparin), 3X2 factorial, multicenter.
Patients	41,299 patients with suspected acute myocardial infarction within 24 h of onset of symptoms. No ECG criteria were used.
Follow-up	6 months.
Treatment regimen	1. Streptokinase 1.5 million U over 1 h. 2. t-PA 0.04 MU/kg as a bolus, and 0.36 MU/kg over 1 h, and then 0.067 MU/kg/h for 3 h. 3. APSAC 30 U over 3 min. Half of the patients received heparin subcutaneous 12,500 U X2/d for 1 week started 4h after initiation of thrombolytic therapy.
Additional therapy	162 mg chewed aspirin on admission and then 162 mg/d.

ISIS-3

International Study of Infarct Survival 3

(continued)

Results

Addition of heparin SC to aspirin resulted in excess of major noncerebral hemorrhages (1.0% vs 0.8%, p<0.01) and of cerebral hemorrhages (0.56% vs 0.40%, p<0.05). However, total stroke occurred equally (1.28% vs 1.18%). Recurrent infarction occurred less in the heparin treated patients (3.16% vs 3.47%, p=0.09), especially during the scheduled heparin treatment. During the scheduled heparin treatment (0-7 days) mortality was 7.4% and 7.9% in the heparin and no heparin groups (p=0.06). However, 35-day and 6 months mortality were comparable.

APSAC was associated with more allergic reaction and noncerebral bleeding and a trend towards more strokes than streptokinase. Reinfarction and 35-day mortality were comparable (3.47% and 10.6% vs 3.55% and 10.5% in the streptokinase and APSAC groups, respectively). There was no difference in 6-month survival between the groups. t-PA was associated with less allergic reactions than streptokinase, but with higher rates of noncerebral bleeding. Stroke occurred in 1.04% of the streptokinase and 1.39% of the t-PA groups (p<0.01). t-PA was associated with less reinfarction (2.93% vs 3.47% in the t-PA and streptokinase groups, p<0.02). However, 35-day mortality was comparable (10.3% vs 10.6%, respectively). 6-month survival was similar.

Conclusions

It might be that heparin may produce at least a small improvement in survival and will reduce reinfarction, especially during the treatment period. There was no advantage of APSAC over streptokinase. The excess strokes observed with t-PA overshadows the reduction in reinfarction rate. t-PA is not better than streptokinase.

LATE

Late Assessment of Thrombolytic Efficacy

Title	Late assessment of thrombolytic efficacy (LATE) study with alteplase 6-24 h after onset of acute myocardial infarction.
Authors	Late Study Group.
Reference	Lancet 1993;342:759-766.
Disease	Acute myocardial infarction.
Purpose	To assess the efficacy of intravenous thrombolytic therapy beginning more than 6 h after the onset of symptoms.
Design	Randomized, double blind, placebo controlled, multicenter.
Patients	5711 patients with acute myocardial infarction >18 years old, 6-24 h from onset of symptoms.
Follow-up	Clinical follow-up for 6 months (73% were followed up for 1 year).
Treatment regimen	Intravenous alteplase (r-tPA) 10 mg bolus, 50 mg infusion over 1 h, and 20 mg/hour for 2 h or matching placebo.
Additional therapy	Aspirin 75-360 mg/d. IV heparin for 48 h was recommended.

LATE

Late Assessment of Thrombolytic Efficacy

(continued)

Results	35-day mortality for patients treated 6-12 h after onset of symptoms was 8.9% vs 12.0% in the alteplase and placebo groups, respectively (95% CI 6.3-45.0%, p=0.02). 35-day mortality for patients treated >12 h after onset of symptoms was 8.7% vs 9.2% in the alteplase and placebo groups, respectively (p=0.14).
Conclusions	Thrombolytic therapy reduces 35-day mortality even if given up to 12 h after onset of symptoms.

EMERAS

Estudio Multicèntrico Estreptoquinasa Reùblicas de Amèrica del Sur

Title	Randomized trial of late thrombolysis in patients with suspected acute myocardial infarction.
Authors	EMERAS Collaborative Group.
Reference	Lancet 1993;342:767-772.
Disease	Acute myocardial infarction.
Purpose	To evaluate the efficacy of late treatment (6-24 h) with intravenous streptokinase for acute myocardial infarction.
Design	Randomized, double blind, placebo control, multicenter.
Patients	4534 patients with acute myocardial infarction > 6h and ≤24 h of onset of symptoms. ECG criteria were not required.
Follow-up	1 year.
Treatment regimen	Streptokinase 1.5 million U or placebo infused over 1 h.
Additional therapy	Aspirin 160 mg/d.

EMERAS

Estudio Multicèntrico Estreptoquinasa Reùblicas de Amèrica del Sur

(continued)

Results   Side effects such as hypotension, allergic reactions, and bleeding were more common with streptokinase therapy. There was no difference between in-hospital mortality, the streptokinase (11.9%), and placebo (12.4%) groups. Among the 2080 patients presenting 7-12 h from onset of symptoms there was a nonsignificant trend towards less mortality with streptokinase (11.7% vs. 13.2%), whereas the mortality difference among the 1791 patients presenting 13-24 h after onset of symptoms was small (11.4% vs 10.7%). One year mortality was comparable between the streptokinase and placebo group.

Conclusions   Streptokinase therapy 7-24 h after onset of symptoms did not show clear benefit. A modest reduction in mortality among patients treated 6-12 h after onset of symptoms is possible.

GUSTO-1

Global Utilization of Streptokinase and Tissue Plasminogen Activator for Occluded Coronary Arteries

Title	a. An international randomized trial comparing 4 thrombolytic strategies for acute myocardial infarction. b. Risk factors for in-hospital nonhemorrhagic stroke in patients with acute myocardial infarction treated with thrombolysis. Results from GUSTO-1. c. Impact of an aggressive invasive catheterization and revascularization strategy on mortality on patients with cardiogenic shock in the global utilization of streptokinase and tissue plasminogen activator for occluded coronary arteries. (GUSTO - 1) Trial. An observational study.
Authors	a. The GUSTO Investigators. b. Mahaffey KW, Granger CB, Sloan MA, et al. c. Berger PB, Holmes DR, Stebbins AL, et al.
Reference	a. N Engl J Med 1993;329:673-682. b. Circulation 1998; 97:757-764. c. Circulation 1997; 96:122-127.
Disease	a. + b. Acute myocardial infarction. c. Coronary artery disease, acute myocardial infarction, cardiogenic shock.
Purpose	a. To compare the effects of 4 thrombolytic strategies on outcome. b. To determine the risk factors that result in nonhemorrhagic stroke in patients with acute myocardial infarction. c. To determine the influence of an aggressive interventional strategy of early percutaneous transluminal coronary angioplasty and coronary bypass surgery on survival in patients with acute myocardial infarction with cardiogenic shock who survived $\geq$ h after shock from the GUSTO-1 study.
Design	a. Randomized, open label, multicenter. b. Assessment of univariable and multivariable risk factors for nonhemorrhagic stroke and creating a scoring normogram. c. Observational study. In GUSTO - 1 angiography and revascularization were not protocol - mandated but were selected by some physicians.

GUSTO-1

Global Utilization of Streptokinase and Tissue Plasminogen Activator for Occluded Coronary Arteries

(continued)

Patients	a. 41,021 patients with acute myocardial infarction < 6 h from onset of symptoms with chest pain>20 min and ST segment elevation $\geq$0.1 mV in $\geq$2 limb leads , or $\geq$0.2 mV in $\geq$2 precordial leads. b. 247 patients with nonhemorrhagic stroke from the GUSTO 1 trial. c. 2200 patients with cardiogenic shock defined as systolic blood pressure <90 mmHg for $\geq$1 h not responsive to fluids or the need for positive inotropic agents to maintain systolic blood pressure >90 mmHg. Of these, 406 patients received early coronary angiography and 1794 did not.
Follow-up	a. 30 days clinical follow-up. b. Focuses on in-hospital - 30 day. c. 30 days.
Treatment regimen	a. 1. intravenous streptokinase 1.5 million U over 60 min with subcutaneous heparin 12,500 U BID; 2. streptokinase 1.5 million U over 60 min with intravenous heparin (5000 U bolus and 1000U/h); 3. accelerated t-PA (15 mg bolus, 0.75 mg/kg over 30 min, and 0.5 mg/kg over 60 min) with intravenous heparin (5000 U bolus and 1000U/h); and 4. the combination of intravenous t-PA (1.0 mg/kg over 60 min, with 10% given as a bolus) and streptokinase (1.0 million U over 60 min) with intravenous heparin (5000 U bolus and 1000U/h). b. As per GUSTO 1. c. Early coronary angiography within 24 h of shock onset and coronary angioplasty or bypass surgery vs no early angiography and interventional procedure.
Additional therapy	a. Chewable aspirin 160 mg on admission and 160-325 mg/d thereafter. IV 5 mg atenolol in 2 divided doses, followed by 50-100 mg/d PO was recommended if no contraindications existed.

GUSTO-1

*Global Utilization of Streptokinase and Tissue Plasminogen
Activator for Occluded Coronary Arteries*
(continued)

Results   a. 30-day mortality was 7.2% for the streptokinase with SC heparin group; 7.4% for the streptokinase and IV heparin group, 6.3% for the accelerated t-PA and IV heparin group; and 7.0% for the combination group. Thus, 14% reduction (95% CI 5.9-21.3%) in 30-day mortality for accelerated t-PA as compared with the two groups of streptokinase therapy. Hemorrhagic stroke occurred in 0.49%, 0.54%, 0.72%, and 0.94% in the 4 groups, respectively (p=0.03 for the difference between t-PA and streptokinase; p<0.001 for the combination therapy compared to streptokinase-only). A combined end point of death or disabling stroke was lower in the t-PA treated patients (6.9%) than in patients receiving the streptokinase-only regimens (7.8%) (p=0.006).

b. 42 (17%) died and 98 (40%) of the 247 nonhemorrhagic stroke patients were disabled at 30-day follow-up. Baseline clinical predictors of nonhemorrhagic stroke included older age, higher heart rate, history of stroke or transient ischemic attack, diabetes, prior angina, hypertension. Other factors included worse killip class, coronary angiography, coronary artery bypass surgery, and atrial fibrillation/flutter.

c. 30 day mortality was 38% in patients with early angiography and revascularization where appropriate vs 62% in patients who did not receive this strategy (p=.0001). There were important differences in baseline characteristics: the aggressive strategy group tended to be younger, had less prior infarction and a shorter time to thrombolytic therapy. After adjusting for baseline differences the aggressive strategy still was associated with reduced 30 day mortality (odds ratio 0.43, CI =0.34 - 0.54, p=.0001).

Conclusions   a. The mortality of patients with acute myocardial infarction treated with accelerated t-PA and intravenous heparin is lower than those receiving streptokinase with either subcutaneous or intravenous heparin.

b. A normogram can predict the risk of nonhemorrhagic stroke based on clinical characteristics.

c. Early angiography and revascularization when appropriate is associated with lower 30 day mortality in patients with acute myocardial infarction and cardiogenic shock.

GUSTO-1 (angiographic substudy)

Global Utilization of Streptokinase and Tissue Plasminogen Activator for Occluded Coronary Arteries

Title	a. The effects of tissue plasminogen activator, streptokinase, or both on coronary-artery patency, ventricular function, and survival after acute myocardial infarction. b. Non Q wave vs Q wave myocardial infarction after thrombolytic therapy. Angiographic and prognostic insights from the Global Utilization of Streptokinase and Tissue Plasminogen Activator for Occluded Coronary Arteries - I Angiographic Substudy. c. Extended mortality benefit of early postinfarction reperfusion.
Authors	a. The GUSTO Angiographic Investigators. b. Goodman SG, Langer A, Ross AM, et al. c. Ross AM, Coyne KD, Moregra E, et al.
Reference	a. N Engl J Med 1993;329:1615–1622. b. Circulation 1998;97:444–450. c. Circulation 1998;97:1549–1556.
Disease	a. Acute myocardial infarction. b. Coronary artery disease, myocardial infarction. c. Coronary artery disease, myocardial infarction.
Purpose	a. To compare the speed of reperfusion and the effect on left ventricular function and outcome of tissue plasminogen activator and streptokinase. b. To obtain further insight into the pathophysiology and prognosis of non Q wave infarctions in the thrombolytic era and compare their outcomes to Q wave infarction. c. To describe the effect of early and complete reperfusion on left ventricular function and long-term (2-year) mortality.

GUSTO-1 (angiographic substudy)

Global Utilization of Streptokinase and Tissue Plasminogen Activator for Occluded Coronary Arteries

(continued)

Design	a. Randomized, open label, multicenter. b. Examination of ECG, coronary anatomy, LV function, mortality among patients with ST elevation infarction in GUSTO - 1 angiographic subset in non Q wave vs Q wave infarcts. c. As per GUSTO - 1. Follow-up extended to 2 years.
Patients	a. 2431 patients with acute myocardial infarction < 6 hours from onset of symptoms with chest pain>20 min and ST segment elevation ≥0.1 mV in ≥2 limb leads, or ≥0.2 mV in ≥2 precordial leads. b. 2046 patients with acute myocardial infarction. 409 non Q wave patients; 1637 Q wave patients c. 2375 patients that were part of the angiography substudy.
Follow-up	a. Patients were randomized to cardiac catheterization at 90 min, 180 min, 24 h or 5-7 days. The group that underwent coronary angiography at 90 min underwent it again after 5-7 days. 30 days clinical follow-up. b. 2 years. c. 2 years.
Treatment regimen	a. 1. intravenous streptokinase 1.5 million U over 60 min with subcutaneous heparin 12,500 U BID; 2. streptokinase 1.5 million U over 60 min with intravenous heparin (5000 U bolus and 1000 U/hour); 3. accelerated t-PA (15 mg bolus, 0.75 mg/kg over 30 min, and 0.5 mg/kg over 60 min) with intravenous heparin (5000 U bolus and 1000 U/hour); and 4. the combination of intravenous t-PA (1.0 mg/kg over 60 min, with 10% given as a bolus) and streptokinase (1.0 million U over 60 min) with intravenous heparin (5000 U bolus and 1000 U/hour). b. As per GUSTO 1. c. As per GUSTO 1.

GUSTO-1 (angiographic substudy)

Global Utilization of Streptokinase and Tissue Plasminogen Activator for Occluded Coronary Arteries

(continued)

Additional therapy	a. Chewable aspirin 160 mg on admission and 160-325 mg/d thereafter. IV 5 mg atenolol in 2 divided doses, followed by 50-100 mg/d PO was recommended if no contraindications existed.
Results	a. 90 min patency rate was 54% in the streptokinase + heparin SC, 60% in the streptokinase+ heparin IV, 81% in the t-PA, and 73% in the combination therapy (p<0.001 for t-PA vs the 2 streptokinase groups). However, at 180 min the difference disappeared. TIMI flow III at 90 min was achieved by 29%, 32%, 54%, and 38%, respectively (p<0.001 for t-PA vs the 2 streptokinase groups). There was no significant differences among the groups in the rate of reocclusion. Regional wall motion was better in the t-PA than the other 3 groups. 30-day mortality was 6.5%, 7.5%, 5.3%, and 7.8%, respectively. Mortality was correlated with lack of patency at 90 min (8.9% in patients with TIMI flow grade 0-1 at 90 min vs 4.4% in patients with TIMI flow grade 3, p=0.009).
	b. Non Q wave patients were more likely to have an infarct-related artery that was nonanterior 67% vs 58% for Q wave patients (p=.012). Non Q wave infarcts were less likely to have a proximal occlusion (33%) compared to patients with a Q wave infarct (39%; p=.021). Non Q wave patients had a lesser degree of ST elevation in a nonanterior location. Infarct-related patency occurred earlier and was more complete in non Q wave infarcts. Global ejection fraction was 66% in non Q wave vs 57% in Q-wave infarcts (p<.0001) and regional left ventricular function was also better. Two-year mortality was 6.3% in non Q waves vs 10.1% in Q Wave infarcts (p=0.02). Rates of in-hospital coronary revascularization procedures were similar in non Q (42%) and Q wave patients (44%).
	c. There was a significant survival benefit and preservation of left ventricular ejection fraction for early complete reperfusion assessed by angiography, that occurred beyond 30 days. Early TIMI 3 flow resulted in a 3 patient per 100 mortality reduction during the first 30 days; and an additional 5 lives per 100 from 30 days to 2 years.

GUSTO-1 (angiographic substudy)

Global Utilization of Streptokinase and Tissue Plasminogen Activator for Occluded Coronary Arteries

(continued)

Conclusions
a. Accelerated t-PA regimen achieved faster and more complete reperfusion and was associated with better regional wall motion and outcome.
b. Patients who developed non Q wave infarcts after thrombolysis had a better prognosis than Q wave patients probably related to earlier and more complete infarct related artery patency with better left ventricular function.
c. Early and successful reperfusion provide mortality benefits that are amplified beyond the first month after reperfusion and extend into at least 2 years.

Update
A one year follow-up study [Califf RM, et al. Circ. 1996;94:1233-1238] showed that one year mortality rates remained in favor of t-PA (9.1%) vs streptokinase with subcutaneous heparin (10.1%, p=0.01), vs steptokinase with IV heparin (10.1%, p=.009). Combination of IV t-PA and streptokinase had an intermediate outcome (9.9%).

GUSTO II a

Intravenous Heparin Vs Recombinant Hirudin for Acute Coronary Syndromes

Reference	Circulation 1994;90:1631-1637.
Disease	Acute myocardial infarction, unstable angina pectoris.
Purpose	To compare the efficacy and safety of recombinant hirudin with heparin in acute coronary syndromes.
Design	Randomized, double blind, multicenter.
Patients	Adult patients, with chest discomfort and ECG changes, within 12 h of onset of symptoms, and no contraindications to thrombolytic therapy or heparin.
Follow-up	30 day clinical follow-up.
Treatment regimen	Thrombolytic therapy with either tissue plasminogen activator or streptokinase for patients with ST segment elevation. Patients were randomized to heparin or hirudin infusion for 72-120 h.
Remarks	GUSTO-2A was terminated prematurely after 2564 patients were enrolled due to higher rates of hemorrhagic stroke in the hirudin treated patients. GUSTO 2B was continued with lower doses of hirudin. Preliminary data presented at the American College of Cardiology meeting 1996 suggested that hirudin had no major treatment benefit over heparin on 30 day mortality but a small reduction in recurrent myocardial infarction rate.

GUSTO II b

The Global Use of Strategies to Open Occluded Coronary Arteries (GUSTO) IIb

Title	A comparison of recombinant hirudin with heparin for the treatment of acute coronary syndromes.
Author	GUSTO IIb Investigators.
Reference	N Engl J Med 1996; 335:775-782.
Disease	Acute myocardial infarction.
Purpose	To compare the direct thrombin inhibitor, recombinant hirudin, to heparin in patients with unstable angina or acute myocardial infarction.
Design	Randomized, multicenter.
Patients	12,142 patients with unstable angina or non Q wave myocardial infarction.
Follow-up	30 days.
Treatment regimen	Infusion of hirudin or heparin for 3-5 days. Hirudin initially given in a bolus dose of 0.1 mg /kg IV followed by a continuous infusion of 0.1mg/kg/hr. Heparin was given as a bolus of 5000 U followed by a continuous infusion of 1000 U per h.

GUSTO II b

The Global Use of Strategies to Open Occluded Coronary Arteries (GUSTO) IIb

(continued)

Results   At 24 h, death or myocardial infarction was lower in hirudin group compared to heparin group (1.3% vs 2.1%, p =0.001). At 30 days the primary end point of death or nonfatal myocardial infarction or reinfarction occurred in 8.9% in the hirudin group vs 9.8% in the heparin group (p = 0.06). Hirudin's benefits mainly were related to reducing myocardial infarction or reinfarction. The incidence of serious or life - threatening bleeding was similar in the 2 groups; hirudin was associated with higher incidence of moderate bleeding.

Conclusions   Hirudin had a small advantage over heparin, primarily related to reducing the risk of nonfatal myocardial infarction. The benefit was most pronounced at 24 h but dissipated over time.

GUSTO IIb (angioplasty substudy)

The Global Use of Strategies to Open Occluded Coronary Arteries in Acute Coronary Syndromes (GUSTO IIb) Angioplasty Substudy Investigators

Title	A clinical trial comparing primary coronary angioplasty with tissue plasminogen activator for acute myocardial infarction.
Author	The Global Use of Strategies to Open Occluded Coronary Arteries in Acute Coronary Syndromes (GUSTO IIb) Angioplasty Substudy Investigators.
Reference	N Engl J Med 1997; 336:1621-1628.
Disease	Acute myocardial infarction.
Purpose	To compare primary percutaneous transluminal coronary angioplasty to thrombolytic therapy for acute myocardial infarction.
Design	Randomized, multicenter.
Patients	1138 patients with acute myocardial infarction.
Follow-up	30 days - 6 mon.
Treatment regimen	Primary angioplasty or accelerated thrombolytic therapy with recombinant tissue plasminogen activator.
Results	At 30 days the primary composite end point of death, non-fatal reinfarction, and nonfatal disabling stroke occurred in 9.6% of the angioplasty patients and 13.7% of the t-PA patients (odds ratio 0.67; 95% CI = 0.47 - 0.97, p = 0.033). At 6 mon the incidence of the composite endpoint was not significantly different between the 2 groups (14.1% for angioplasty vs 16.1% for t-PA, p = NS).
Conclusions	Primary angioplasty for acute myocardial infarction is an "excellent alternative" for myocardial reperfusion and has a "small-to-moderate short term clinical advantage over thrombolytic therapy with t-PA."

GUSTO III

The Global Use of Strategies to Open Occluded Coronary Arteries (GUSTO III)

Title	A comparison of reteplase with alteplase for acute myocardial infarction.
Author	The Global Use of Strategies to Open Occluded Coronary Arteries (GUSTO III) Investigators.
Reference	N Engl J Med 1997; 337:1118-1123.
Disease	Acute myocardial infarction.
Purpose	To compare the efficacy and safety of reteplase, which is a mutant of alteplase that has a longer half life than alteplase, to alteplase in patients with acute myocardial infarction.
Design	Randomized, multicenter, open-label.
Patients	15,059 patients with acute myocardial infarction. Patients had to present within 6 h after onset of symptoms with ST elevation or bundle-branch block.
Follow-up	30 days.
Treatment regimen	Patients randomly assigned on a 2:1 ratio to receive a 10 MU reteplase bolus followed by a second bolus 30 min later or an accelerated infusion of alteplase, up to 100 mg over 90 min. Alteplase was given as a 15mg bolus followed by infusion of 0.75mg/kg of body weight over 30 min (not to exceed 50 mg) and then 0.5mg/kg (up to 35 mg) over the next 60 minutes. Aspirin and heparin were given to all patients.

GUSTO III

The Global Use of Strategies to Open Occluded
Coronary Arteries (GUSTO III)
(continued)

Results
: 30 day mortality was 7.47% for reteplase and 7.24% for alteplase (p=NS). Stroke occurred in 1.64% of patients on reteplase and 1.79% of patients on alteplase (p=NS). Combined endpoint of death or nonfatal, disabling stroke were similar at 7.89% and 7.91% for reteplase and alteplase, respectively.

Conclusions
: Although reteplase is easier to administer than alteplase it did not provide improved survival benefit and had the same rate of stroke.

EMIP

The European Myocardial Infarction Project Group

Authors	The European Myocardial Infarction Project Group
Title	Prehospital thrombolytic therapy in patients with suspected acute myocardial infarction.
Reference	N Engl J Med 1993;329:383-389.
Disease	Acute myocardial infarction.
Purpose	To compare the efficacy and safety of prehospital vs in-hospital administration of thrombolytic therapy for patients with suspected acute myocardial infarction.
Study Design	Randomized, double blind, multicenter.
Follow-up	30 day clinical follow-up.
Treatment regimen	Patients were randomized to 30 U of anistreplase IV over 4-5 min given by the emergency medical personnel outside the hospital, followed by placebo after hospitalization, or to placebo outside the hospital followed by 30 units of anistreplase after admission.
Concomitant therapy.	Concomitant No limitations, except for anticoagulant therapy
Patients	5469 patients with chest pain of $\geq$30 min, or pain unresponsive to nitrates, $\leq$6 h of onset of symptoms. Patients on oral anticoagulants, with a history of stroke, major trauma, or bleeding diathesis were excluded. Patients were stratified according to the presence of ST segment elevation on the qualifying ECG.

EMIP

The European Myocardial Infarction Project Group

(continued)

Results   The patients in the prehospital therapy group received thrombolytic therapy 55 min earlier than those in the hospital therapy group. 30 day mortality was 9.7% vs 11.1% in the prehospital and hospital groups (risk reduction 13%, 95% CI -1 to 26%, p=0.08). Cardiac mortality was 8.3% vs 9.8%, respectively (risk reduction 16%, 95% CI 0 to 29%, p=0.049). There was no obvious correlation between the reduction in 30 day mortality and the time interval between the onset of symptoms and the first injection. During the preadmission period there were more patients with ventricular fibrillation (2.5% vs 1.6%, p=0.02), shock (6.3% vs 3.9%, p<0.001), and stroke (0.1% vs 0, p=0.09) in the prehospital therapy than the in-hospital group. However, there was no differences between the groups in the incidence of bleeding, the overall incidence of stroke, ventricular fibrillation, and shock during the hospital period.

Conclusions   Prehospital administration of thrombolytic therapy for patients with suspected acute myocardial infarction is feasible and safe. Although overall mortality was not reduced, cardiac mortality was significantly reduced.

MITI-2

The Myocardial Infarction Triage and Intervention Trial

Authors	Weaver DW, Cerqueira M, Hallstrom AP, et al.
Title	Prehospital-initiated vs hospital-initiated thrombolytic therapy. The myocardial infarction triage and intervention trial.
Reference	JAMA 1993;270:1211-1216.
Disease	Acute myocardial infarction.
Purpose	To evaluate the effect of prehospital vs in-hospital administration of thrombolytic therapy for suspected acute myocardial infarction.
Study Design	Randomized, controlled, multicenter.
Follow-up	In-hospital clinical events. Estimation of final infarct size by thallium single photon emission tomography and left ventricular function by radionuclide ventriculography at 30 days.
Treatment regimen	Patients were randomized to either prehospital or in-hospital initiation of IV aspirin 325 mg and alteplase 100 mg infusion over 3 h. No placebo was given in the field to the hospital treated group.
Concomitant therapy	Standard care: oxygen, morphine, lidocaine, atropine, vasopressors or diuretics when indicated. IV heparin 5000 U bolus followed by continuous infusion for ≥48 h was started upon admission.
Patients	360 patients, ≤75 years old, with suspected acute myocardial infarction, within 6 h of onset of symptoms. Patients with risk factors for bleeding were excluded.

MITI-2

The Myocardial Infarction Triage and Intervention Trial

(continued)

Results
98% of the patients had subsequent evidence of acute myocardial infarction. Initiation of therapy before admission shortened the time interval from onset of symptoms to therapy from 110 to 77 min (p<0.001). 23% of the prehospital group vs 7% of the in-hospital group had resolution of pain upon admission (p<0.001). However, there was no difference between the groups in the composite score of death, stroke, serious bleeding, infarct size (406.4 vs 400.4 for the prehospital vs in-hospital groups, p=0.64), total mortality (5.7% vs 8.1%, p=0.49), infarct size (6.1% vs 6.5%, p=0.72), or ejection fraction (53% vs 54%, p=0.34). A secondary analysis of the time to therapy and outcome demonstrated that treatment initiated within 70 min of onset of symptoms was associated with better outcome (composite score, p=0.009; mortality 1.2% vs 8.7%, p=0.04; infarct size 4.9% vs 11.2%, p<0.001; and ejection fraction 53% vs 49%, p=0.03) than later treatment. Identification of patients eligible for thrombolytic therapy by paramedics reduced the time interval from hospitalization to therapy from 60 min (for nonrandomized patients) to 20 min (for the in-hospital therapy allocated group).

Conclusions
There was no improvement in outcome associated with prehospital administration of thrombolytic therapy. However, treatment within 70 min of onset of symptoms was associated with better outcome. Prehospital identification of patients eligible for thrombolytic therapy was associated with shortening of the time interval to therapy.

TIMI-4

Thrombolysis in Myocardial Infarction 4 Trial

Title	a. Comparison of front-loaded recombinant tissue-type plasminogen activator, anistreplase, and combination thrombolytic therapy for acute myocardial infarction: Results of the Thrombolysis in Myocardial Infarction (TIMI) 4 trial. b. Rescue angioplasty in the thrombolysis in myocardial infarction (TIMI) 4 trial.
Authors	a. Cannon CP, McCabe CH, Diver DJ, et al. b. Gibson CM, Cannon CP, Greene RM et al.
Reference	a. J Am Coll Cardiol 1994;24:1602-1610. b. Am J Cardiol 1997; 8:21-26.
Disease	a. Acute myocardial infarction.
Purpose	a. To compare 3 regimens of thrombolytic therapy: anistreplase (APSAC), front-loaded recombinant tissue-type plasminogen activator (rt-PA), or combination of the 2 agents. b. To determine the angiographic and clinical outcomes of patients with a patent coronary artery 90 min after thrombolysis compared to those that had an occluded infarct artery at this time treated with either rescue or no-rescue angioplasty.
Design	a. Randomized, double blind, multicenter study.
Patients	a. 382 patients with acute myocardial infarction <80 years old < 6 h from onset of symptoms with chest pain>30 min and ST segment elevation ≥ 0.1 mV in ≥ 2 contiguous leads or with new left bundle branch block.
Follow-up	a. 90 min and 18-36 h coronary angiography. Predischarge technetium-99m sestamibi scan. 6 week and 1 year follow-up.

TIMI-4

Thrombolysis in Myocardial Infarction 4 Trial

(continued)

Treatment regimen	a. Front-loaded rt-PA; APSAC (Eminase); or a combination of rt-PA and APSAC.
Additional therapy	a. Heparin (5000 U bolus and infusion) and aspirin 325 mg/d. Intravenous and oral metoprolol.
Results	a. At 90 min, the incidence of TIMI grade 3 flow was 60.2%, 42.9%, and 44.8% of the rt-PA, APSAC, and combination-treated patients (rt-PA vs. APSAC, p<0.01; rt-PA vs combination, p=0.02). The incidence of unsatisfactory outcome (death, severe heart failure, LVEF<40%, reinfarction, TIMI grade flow<2 at 90 min or 18-36 h, reocclusion, major hemorrhage, or severe anaphylaxis) was 41.3%, 49%, and 53.6% for the rt-PA, APSAC, and combination therapy (rt-PA vs. APSAC, p=0.19; rt-PA vs combination, p=0.06). 6 week mortality was 2.2%, 8.8%, and 7.2%, respectively (rt-PA vs APSAC, p=0.02; rt-PA vs combination, p=0.06). b. The incidence of TIMI 3 flow was higher after successful rescue angioplasty (87%) than after successful thrombolysis (65%; p = 0.002) and the number of frames needed to opacify standard landmarks was lower (that is flow was faster) with PTCA compared to thrombolysis. In-hospital adverse events occurred in 29% of successful rescue PTCA patients and 83% of failed rescue PTCAs (p=0.01). Among patients in whom rescue PTCA was performed (including successes and failures) 35% experienced an adverse event, which was the same as 35% incidence in patients not undergoing rescue PTCA. These values tended to be higher than 23% incidence of adverse events in patients with patent arteries following thrombolysis (p=0.07).
Conclusions	a. Front-loaded rt-PA is associated with higher rates of early reperfusion and trends toward better clinical outcome and survival than either APSAC or a combination of rt-PA and APSAC. b. While restoration of flow at 90 min with rescue PTCA was superior to successful thrombolysis, the incidence of adverse events for strategy of rescue PTCA was not improved over no rescue PTCA.

INJECT

International Joint Efficacy Comparison of Thrombolytics

Title	Randomized, double blind comparison of reteplase double bolus administration with streptokinase in acute myocardial infarction (INJECT): trial to investigate equivalence.
Authors	International Joint Efficacy Comparison of Thrombolytics.
Reference	Lancet 1995;346:329-336.
Disease	Acute myocardial infarction.
Purpose	To compare the effect of reteplase and streptokinase in acute myocardial infarction.
Design	Randomized, double blind, multicenter.
Patients	6010 patients, $\geq$18 years old, with chest pain of $\geq$30 min, within 12 h of onset of symptoms, ST elevation $\geq$1 mm in $\geq$2 limb leads, or $\geq$2 mm in $\geq$2 precordial leads, or bundle branch block.
Follow-up	6 months clinical follow-up.
Treatment regimen	Two boluses of 10 MU reteplase given 30 min apart +1 h infusion of placebo streptokinase, or 2 retaplase placebo boluses and 1.5 MU IV streptokinase.
Additional therapy	Aspirin 250-320 mg initially, then 75-150 mg/d. IV heparin 5000 U before infusion of thrombolytics, and heparin infusion 1000 U/h 60 min after trial infusion for >24 h.

Results	35 day mortality was 9.02% vs 9.53% in the reteplase and streptokinase groups (a difference of -0.51%, 95% CI -1.98% to 0.96%). 6 month mortality was 11.02% vs 12.05%, respectively (a difference of -1.03%, 95% CI -2.65% to 0.59%, p=0.217). There was a nonsignificant excess of in-hospital strokes in the reteplase patients (1.23% vs 1.00%). Bleeding events were similar (total: 15.0% vs 15.3%, requiring transfusion: 0.7% vs 1.0%, respectively). Hypotension during hospitalization was more common with streptokinase (17.6% vs 15.5%, p<0.05). Allergic reactions occurred more often with streptokinase (1.8% vs 1.1%, p<0.05).
Conclusions	Reteplase is a safe and an effective thrombolytic agent.

RAPID

Reteplase vs Alteplase Infusion in Acute Myocardial Infarction

Title	More rapid, complete, and stable coronary thrombolysis with bolus administration of reteplase compared with alteplase infusion in acute myocardial infarction.
Authors	Smalling RW, Bode C, Kalbfleisch J, et al.
Reference	Circulation 1995;91:2725-2732.
Disease	Acute myocardial infarction.
Purpose	To compare the 90 min coronary patency rates of bolus administration of reteplase (r-PA) and standard-dose alteplase (tPA).
Design	Randomized, open label, multicenter.
Patients	606 patients, age 18-75 years, with ≥30 min chest pain and ST elevation of ≥1 mm in the limb leads and ≥2 mm in the precordial leads, within 6 h of onset of symptoms. Patients with left bundle branch block, prior coronary artery bypass surgery, previous Q wave infarction in the same territory, previous angioplasty within 2 weeks, previous cerebral vascular event, or severe hypertension were excluded.
Follow-up	30 min, 60 min, 90 min and 5-14 days coronary angiography.
Treatment regimen	1. 15 MU r-PA as a single bolus. 2. 10 MU r-PA bolus followed by 5 MU 30 min later. 3. 10 MU r-PA bolus followed by 10 MU 30 min later. 4. TPA 60 mg over 1 h (6-10 mg as an initial bolus) followed by 40 mg over 2 h.
Additional therapy	Soluble aspirin 200-325 mg/d. IV heparin 5000 U bolus before thrombolytic therapy, followed by 1000 U/h for ≥24 h.

RAPID

Reteplase vs Alteplase Infusion in Acute Myocardial Infarction
(continued)

Results   60 min patency (TIMI flow grade II and III) were 67.0%, 72.1%, 77.6%, and 66.3% in groups 1-4 (r-PA 10+10 vs TPA p=0.079). At 90 min, patency rates were 62.8%, 66.7%, 85.2%, and 77.2%, respectively (r-PA 10+10 vs TPA p=0.084). Late patency was 85.5%, 80.5%, 95.1%, and 87.8% (r-PA 10+10 vs TPA p=0.04). TIMI flow III was higher in the r-PA 10+10 than TPA at 60 min (51.0% vs 32.7%, p=0.009), at 90 min (62.7% vs 49.0%, p=0.019), and at discharge (87.8% vs 70.7%, p<0.001). Global left ventricular function at 90 min was similar in the TPA and r-PA 10+10 groups. However, at discharge ejection fraction was higher in the r-PA 10+10 (53±1.3% vs 49±1.3%, p=0.034). Regional wall motion improved in the r-PA 10+10 from 90 min to pre-discharge, while in the TPA group there was no improvement. There was a trend towards less rescue angioplasty in the r-PA 10+10 than TPA group (p=0.11). The need for blood transfusion was similar (4.5% in the TPA vs 3.9% in the r-PA 10+10), while intracranial bleeding occurred in 2.6% vs 0%, respectively. Reocclusion occurred in 7.8% of the TPA vs 2.9% in the r-PA 10+10 (p=NS). The 30-day mortality was 3.9% vs 1.9%, respectively. Reinfarction rate and the incidence of heart failure were similar between the groups.

Conclusions r-PA given as a double bolus of 10 MU+ 10 MU 30 min apart resulted in more rapid and complete reperfusion than standard-dose TPA and was associated with improved global and regional left ventricular function at discharge.

RAPID II

Reteplase vs Alteplase Infusion in Acute Myocardial Infarction II

Title	Randomized comparison of coronary thrombolysis achieved with double bolus reteplase (recombinant plasminogen activator) and front-loaded, accelerated alteplase (recombinant tissue plasminogen activator) in patients with acute myocardial infarction
Authors	Bode C, Smalling RW, Berg G, et al.
Reference	Circulation 1996;94:891-898.
Disease	Acute myocardial infarction.
Purpose	To assess whether a double bolus regimen of reteplase, a deletion mutant of wild-type tissue plasminogen activator, results in better 90 min coronary artery patency rates compared with accelerated front-loaded infusion of alteplase (tissue plasminogen activator).
Design	Randomized, open label, parallel group, multicenter.
Patients	324 patients, >18 years old with ≥30 min of chest pain that was not relieved by nitroglycerin, ≤12 h from onset of pain, and ST segment elevation of ≥0.1 mV in limb leads or ≥0.2 mV in precordial leads, or left bundle branch block. Patients with prior coronary artery bypass surgery, previous stroke or known intracranial structural abnormalities, PTCA within 2 weeks, previous Q wave myocardial infarction in the same territory, severe hypertension, use of oral anticoagulants, recent (<3 months) major surgery or active or potential internal bleeding were excluded.
Follow-up	Coronary angiography at 30, 60, 90 min, and 5-14 days after initiation of therapy, clinical follow-up for 35 days.

RAPID II

Reteplase vs Alteplase Infusion in Acute Myocardial Infarction II

(continued)

Treatment regimen	Randomization to a bolus of reteplase (10 MU given over 2-3 min) at the start of therapy and after 30 min, or to alteplase 15 mg bolus, 0.75 mg/kg over 30 min (maximum 50 mg), 0.5 mg/kg over 60 min (maximum 35 mg).
Additional Therapy	Aspirin 160 to 350 mg/d. Intravenous heparin, 5000 IU bolus followed by 1000 IU/h for ≥24 h. Target aPTT 2.0 times the control value.
Results	90 min following initiation of therapy, infarct related coronary artery patency (TIMI flow grade 2 or 3) was higher in the reteplase group (83.4% vs 73.3%, p=0.031). TIMI flow grade 3 was achieved in 59.9% vs 45.2%, respectively (p=0.011). At 60 min, TIMI flow grade 2 or 3 was found in 81.8% of the reteplase group vs 66.1% in the alteplase group (p=0.032), and TIMI flow grade 3 was found in 51.2% vs 37.4%, respectively (p=0.006). Follow-up angiograms were available in 75.7% and 72.9% of the reteplase and alteplase-treated patients. Late overall and TIMI flow grade 3 patency were comparable between the groups. Patients treated with reteplase had better patency in all time-to-treatment categories. Additional interventions to restore flow in the infarct related artery during the first 6 h was lower in the reteplase group (13.6% vs 26.5%; p=0.004). The incidence of reocclusion during hospitalization was comparable (9.0% vs 7.0% for reteplase and alteplase, respectively, p=0.61). 35-day mortality was 4.1% vs 8.4%, respectively (p=0.11). The incidence of stroke (1.8% vs 2.6%) was similar. The composite end point of unsatisfactory outcome at 35 days (death, reinfarction, congestive heart failure or shock, or an ejection fraction of <40%) was comparable (21.3% vs 22.6% in the reteplase and alteplase groups). 12.4% vs 9.7% of the patients, respectively, required transfusion (p=0.43). There was no difference in global or infarct zone left ventricular function between the groups.
Conclusions	Double bolus dose of reteplase was associated with higher rates of reperfusion at 60 and 90min after initiation of therapy than front-loaded alteplase infusion, without an increase in the risk of complications.

COBALT

The Continuous Infusion vs Double Bolus Administration of Alteplase (COBALT) Investigators

Title	A comparison of continuous infusion alteplase with double bolus administration for acute myocardial infarction.
Author	The Continuous Infusion Vs Double Bolus Administration of Alteplase (COBALT) Investigators.
Reference	N Eng J Med 1997; 337:1124-1130.
Disease	Acute myocardial infarction.
Purpose	To determine whether there are advantages of double bolus alteplase over accelerated infusion of alteplase.
Design	Randomized, multicenter, open design.
Patients	7169 patients with acute myocardial infarction.
Follow-up	30 days.
Treatment regimen	Weight-adjusted, accelerated infusion of 100 mg alteplase or a bolus of 50 mg alteplase over a period of 1-3 min followed by a second bolus 30 min later of 50 mg (or 40 mg for patients weighing less than 60 kg).
Results	The study was stopped early because of concern about the safety of double bolus therapy. 30-day mortality was higher in the double bolus group at 7.98% vs the accelerated infusion group at 7.53%. Stroke incidence was 1.92% with double bolus alteplase vs 1.53% with accelerated infusion of alteplase (p=0.24) and hemorrhagic stroke was 1.12% and .81% respectively (p=0.23).

COBALT

The Continuous Infusion vs Double-Bolus Administration of Alteplase (COBALT) Investigators

(continued)

Conclusions   Double bolus alteplase was not equivalent to accelerated infusion alteplase, according to prespecified criteria. Accelerated infusion of alteplase over a period of 90 min remains the preferred regimen.

COMPASS

The Comparison Trial of Saruplase and Streptokinase

Title	Randomized, double blind study comparing saruplase with streptokinase therapy in acute myocardial infarction: the COMPASS equivalence trial.
Authors	Tebbe U, Michels R, Adgey J, et al.
Reference	J Am Coll Cardiol 1998;31:487-493.
Disease	Acute myocardial infarction.
Purpose	To compare the efficacy and safety of saruplase, a recombinant unglycosylated human single-chain urokinase-type plasminogen activator, and streptokinase in patients with acute myocardial infarction.
Design	Randomized, double blind, multicenter.
Patients	3089 patients, >20 years old, with chest pain and ECG changes compatible with acute myocardial infarction, within 6 h of onset of symptoms. Patients with severe hypertension, high risk of bleeding, major trauma or surgery within 1 month, hypersensitivity to streptokinase or previous exposure to streptokinase within 1 year were excluded.
Follow-up	30 days and 1 year clinical follow-up.
Treatment regimen	Patients were randomized to 1. heparin 5000 IU bolus, saruplase 20 mg bolus, and saruplase 60 mg infusion over 1 hour and streptokinase-placebo infusion over 1 hour; or 2. placebo-heparin, streptokinase 1.5 MU infusion over 60 min, and saruplase-placebo infusion.

COMPASS

The Comparison Trial of Saruplase and Streptokinase

(continued)

Additional therapy	Oral or intravenous aspirin 200-400 mg on admission followed by ≥75 mg/d. Heparin infusion, started 30 min after the end of the thrombolytic infusion and continued for ≥24 hours. The use of intravenous nitrates was recommended
Results	Total mortality at 30 days was 5.7% in the saruplase group vs 6.7% in the streptokinase group (odds ratio 0.84; p=0.242). One year mortality was 8.2% and 9.6%, respectively (p=0.193). Death from ventricular rupture/tamponade (21.6% vs 6.7%, of all mortality cases respectively; p=0.003) and fatal stroke (11.4% vs 4.8%; p=0.092) were more common in the saruplase group. In contrast, hypotension (31.4% vs 38.1%; p=0.001) and cardiogenic shock (3.3% vs 4.6%; p=0.067) occurred less frequently in the saruplase group. The incidence of arrhythmia and angina was similar in the 2 groups. Bleeding rates were comparable between the groups (mild in 10.4% of the saruplase group and 10.9% in the streptokinase group; moderate in 6.9% and 7.0%; and severe in 2.1% and 2.5%, respectively). The incidence of stroke was 1.4% in both groups. Hemorrhagic strokes occurred more frequently in the saruplase group (0.9%) than the streptokinase group (0.3%)(p=0.038), whereas thromboembolic strokes were more common in the streptokinase group (1.0% vs 0.5%; p=0.145). Allergic reactions were noted in 1.6% of the saruplase group and in 4.1% of the streptokinase group (p<0.001).
Conclusions	Saruplase was comparable to streptokinase in terms of total mortality. Saruplase was associated with more hemorrhagic strokes, but less thromboembolic strokes and less allergic reactions.

SESAM

Study in Europe with Saruplase and Alteplase in Myocardial Infarction

Title	Comparison of saruplase and alteplase in acute myocardial infarction.
Authors	Bar FW, Meyer J, Vermeer F, et al.
Reference	Am J Cardiol 1997;79:727-732.
Disease	Acute myocardial infarction.
Purpose	To compare the speed of reperfusion, 60 min and 90 min patency rates, and coronary reocclusion rates following thrombolytic therapy with alteplase (tPA) and saruplase unglycosylated recombinant single-chain urokinase-type plasminogen activator in acute myocardial infarction.
Design	Randomized, double blind multicenter.
Patients	473 patients, ≤70 years old, with suspected acute myocardial infarction, within 6 h of onset of symptoms. Patients with nondiagnostic ECG, cardiogenic shock, previous coronary artery bypass surgery, use of oral anticoagulants, chronic concomitant disease, or an increased risk of bleeding were excluded.
Follow-up	Coronary angiography 45 min and 60 min after initiation of the thrombolytic therapy. If coronary flow was <TIMI grade III 60 min after initiation of thrombolytic therapy, an angiography was repeated at 90 min. Coronary angiography was repeated at 24-40 hours.

SESAM

Study in Europe with Saruplase and Alteplase in Myocardial Infarction
(continued)

Treatment regimen	Randomization to: 1. intravenous saruplase 20 mg bolus, followed by an infusion of 60 mg over 1 h; or 2. intravenous alteplase 10 mg bolus, followed by an infusion of 50 mg over 1 h and then 40 mg over the next 2 h. Patients with TIMI grade flow 0 to 1 at 90 min could undergo balloon angioplasty.
Additional therapy	Intravenous bolus heparin 5000 U before the thrombolytic agent and another 5000 U bolus before coronary angiography. Heparin infusion, started after the first bolus and continued until the second coronary angiography. Intravenous aspirin 300 mg before the study medication. If coronary flow was <TIMI grade III 60 min after initiation of thrombolytic therapy, repeated angiography at 90 min.
Results	82% of the patients underwent angiography at 45 min, 94.7% at 60 min, and 91.8% at 24-40 hours. At 45 min, 74.6% of the saruplase group vs 68.9% of the alteplase group had TIMI grade flow II or III (p=0.22). At 60 min 79.9% vs 75.3% of the saruplase and alteplase groups had TIMI grade II or III (p=0.26). Patency rates (excluding patients who underwent rescue angioplasty) were 79.9% vs 81.4% (p=0.72), respectively at 90 min and 99% vs 98% at 24-40 h. At 24-40 h, patency rates for all patients (including those who underwent intervention) were 94.0% vs 93.6%. Reocclusion within 24-40 h occurred in 1.2% of the saruplase group vs 2.4% of the alteplase group (p=0.68). Reocclusion after rescue angioplasty occurred in 22% of the saruplase vs 15% of the alteplase treated patients. In-hospital mortality was 4.7% in the saruplase group and 3.8% in the alteplase group. Reinfarction occurred in 4.2% in both groups, severe bleeding in 9.3% of the saruplase group and 8.4% of the alteplase group, hemorrhagic stroke in 0.8% in both groups, and embolic stroke in 0.8% and 1.3%, respectively.
Conclusions	Alteplase in a 3 h infusion regimen and saruplase had a similar safety profile. Early patency rates were high with both agents and reocclusion rates were similarly low.

TIMI 10A

Thrombolysis in Myocardial Infarction 10A

Title	TNK - Tissue plasminogen activator in acute myocardial infarction. of the thrombolysis in myocardial infarction (TIMI) 10A dose - ranging trial.
Author	Cannon CP, McCabe CH, Gibson M, et al.
Reference	Circulation 1997; 95:351-356
Disease	Coronary artery disease, acute myocardial infarction.
Purpose	To evaluate the pharmacokinetics, safety, and efficacy of TNK-TPA (TNK-tissue plasminogen activator), a genetically engineered variant of TPA which has slower plasma clearance, greater fibrin specificity, and is more resistant to plasminogen activator inhibitor.
Design	Phase 1, dose-ranging pilot trial.
Patients	113 patients with acute ST-segment elevation myocardial infarction who presented within 12 h of chest pain.
Follow-up	360 min.
Treatment regimen	Single bolus of TNK-TPA over 5 - 10 sec with doses of 5 to 50 mg. All patients received aspirin and heparin.

Results
The plasma clearance of TNK-TPA was 125 - 216 ml/min across 5 - 50 mg doses, about one third of that previously reported for wild-type TPA. Plasma half life ranged from 11 - 20 min (while previous reports with TPA report 3.5 min). There was a dose dependent increase in systemic plasmin generation but only a 3% reduction in fibrinogen and a 13% reduction in plasminogen. The frequency of TIMI grade 3 of the infarct vessel, documented by 90 min angiography was 59% at 30 mg and 64% at 50 mg (p=.032). TIMI grade 2 or 3 flow (defined as patency) was 85% overall and did not differ by dose. Rescue angioplasty was performed in 16 of 17 patients with TIMI grade 0 or 1 flow. 6.2% of patients developed hemorrhage, which occurred mainly at vascular access sites.

Conclusions
TNK-TPA unlike the TPA has a long half-life which allows it to be delivered as a single bolus. TNK-TPA is very fibrin specific and appears to have an encouraging initial patency rate.

1. Acute Myocardial Infarction

b. PTCA Vs Stenting Vs Thrombolytic Therapy

PAMI-1

Primary Angioplasty in Myocardial Infarction 1

Title	a. A comparison of immediate angioplasty with thrombolytic therapy for acute myocardial infarction. b. Predictors of in-hospital and 6 month outcome after acute myocardial infarction in the reperfusion era: the primary angioplasty in myocardial infarction (PAMI) trial.
Authors	a. Grines CL, Browne KF, Marco J, et al. b. Stone GW, Grines CL, Browne KF, et al.
Reference	a. N Engl J Med 1993;328:673-679. b. J Am Coll Cardiol 1995;25:370-377.
Disease	Acute myocardial infarction.
Purpose	To compare the results of primary coronary angioplasty with intravenous tissue plasminogen activator for acute myocardial infarction.
Design	Randomized, open label, multicenter.
Patients	395 patients within 12 h of onset of chest pain with ≥1 mm ST elevation in ≥2 adjacent leads. No age limit.
Follow-up	a. Clinical follow-up at 6 months. Radionuclide ventriculography within 24 h and at 6 weeks. Exercise thallium scan predischarge. b. 6 month clinical follow-up.
Treatment regimen	1. Tissue plasminogen activator (t-PA) 100 mg over 3 h. 2. Immediate coronary angiography and angioplasty if suitable.

PAMI-1

Primary Angioplasty in Myocardial Infarction 1

(continued)

Additional therapy	Intravenous nitroglycerin for ≥24 h, chewed aspirin 325 mg and 325 mg/d thereafter and 10,000 U bolus heparin started before randomization. Intravenous heparin infusion was continued for 3-5 days. Diltiazem 30-60 mg X4/d.
Results	a. 90% of the patients assigned to angioplasty underwent the procedure. The success rate was 97%. In-hospital mortality was 6.5% and 2.6% in the t-PA and angioplasty groups, respectively (p=0.06). Reinfarction or death occurred in 12.0% and 5.1%, respectively (p=0.02). Intracranial hemorrhage occurred in 2.0% and 0, respectively (p=0.05). The mean length of the hospital stay was shorter in the angioplasty group (7.5±3.3 vs 8.4±4.6 days, p=0.03). The mean ejection fraction at rest and during exercise were similar at 6 weeks. By 6 months, death in 7.9% and 3.7% (p=0.08) and recurrent infarction or death had occurred in 16.8% and 8.5% (p=0.02) of the t-PA and angioplasty groups, respectively.
	b. By 6 months, cumulative mortality and reinfarction rate was 8.2% and 17.0% in the angioplasty and t-PA groups (p=0.02). By multiple logistic regression analysis only advanced age, prior heart failure, and treatment with t-PA vs angioplasty were independently associated with increased in-hospital mortality.
Conclusions	Primary angioplasty resulted in lower occurrence of non-fatal recurrent infarction or death and lower rates of intracranial hemorrhage than t-PA.

A Comparison of Immediate Coronary Angioplasty with Intravenous Streptokinase in Acute Myocardial Infarction

Title	A comparison of immediate coronary angioplasty with intravenous streptokinase in acute myocardial infarction.
Authors	Zijlstra F, de Boer MJ, Hoorntje JCA, et al.
Reference	N Engl J Med 1993;328:680-684.
Disease	Acute myocardial infarction.
Purpose	To compare the results of immediate coronary angioplasty with intravenous streptokinase infusion for acute myocardial infarction.
Design	Randomized, open labeled, one center.
Patients	142 patients, age <76 years, with acute myocardial infarction (symptoms ≥ 30 min; < 6 h from onset of symptoms, or 6-24 h if there was evidence of continuing ischemia; ST elevation >1 mm in ≥2 leads).
Follow-up	In-hospital recurrent ischemia, predischarge symptom-limited exercise test, radionuclide ventriculography, and coronary angiography.
Treatment regimen	1. Streptokinase 1.5 million U over 1 h. 2. Immediate coronary angiography and angioplasty.
Additional therapy	Aspirin 300 mg IV, and then 300 mg/d orally. Intravenous nitroglycerin and intravenous heparin for >48 h.

Results
Death occurred in 4 (6%) of the 72 patients that received streptokinase, but in none of the 70 patients assigned to angioplasty (p=0.13). Recurrent infarction occurred in 9 (13%) patients that received streptokinase, but in none of the patients assigned to angioplasty (p=0.003). Post infarction angina developed in 14 (19%) and 4 (6%) patients in the streptokinase and angioplasty groups (p=0.02). Mean left ventricular ejection fraction before discharge was $45\pm12\%$ in the streptokinase group, and $51\pm11\%$ in the angioplasty group (p=0.004). The infarct related artery was patent in 68% and 91%, respectively (p=0.001). Residual stenosis was $76\pm19\%$ and $36\pm20\%$, respectively (p<0.001). There was no difference in the complication rate between the groups. Ischemic ST segment depression during the exercise test developed in 41% and 21% of the streptokinase and angioplasty groups (p=0.01). Left ventricular ejection fraction during exercise was $46\pm15\%$ and $52\pm14\%$, respectively (p=0.02).

Conclusions
Immediate angioplasty was associated with higher rates of patency, lower grade of residual stenosis, better left ventricular function, and less recurrent ischemia and infarction than intravenous streptokinase therapy.

Immediate Angioplasty Compared With the Administration of a Thrombolytic Agent

Title	Immediate angioplasty compared with the administration of a thrombolytic agent followed by conservative treatment for myocardial infarction.
Authors	Gibbons AJ, Holmes DR, Reeder GS, et al.
Reference	N Engl J Med 1993;328:685-691.
Disease	Acute myocardial infarction.
Purpose	To compare direct angioplasty with administration of thrombolytic agent followed by conservative approach in the management of acute myocardial infarction.
Design	Randomized, open labeled, one center.
Patients	103 patients, age <80 years, with acute myocardial infarction (pain ≥30 min, ≤12 h from onset of symptoms, ST elevation of ≥1 mm in ≥2 adjacent leads, or new ST depression of ≥2 mm in ≥2 precordial leads. Patients with contraindication to thrombolytic therapy or in cardiogenic shock were excluded.
Follow-up	Technetium 99m sestamibi scan before therapy, and 6-14 days later, radionuclide ventriculography at rest predischarge and at 6 weeks.
Treatment regimen	1. Double chain tissue plasminogen activator (duteplase) 0.6 million U/kg over 4 h. Heparin 5000 U bolus and infusion for 5 days, and then subcutaneous 12,500 U X2/d. 2. Heparin 5,000 +10,000 U bolus, coronary angioplasty. Intravenous heparin infusion for 5 days.
Additional therapy	162.5 mg of chewable aspirin, and 162.5 mg/d thereafter. ß blockers if not contraindicated.

(continued)

Results   56 patients received t-PA (time from onset of symptoms to start of infusion 232±174 min), and 47 underwent angioplasty (first balloon inflation 277±144 min after onset of symptoms). Mortality was similar (2 in each group). Myocardial salvage for anterior infarction, as assessed by the difference between the pre-treatment to predischarge MIBI defect size, was 27±21% and 31±21% of the left ventricle, in the t-PA and angioplasty groups, respectively. For nonanterior infarctions salvage was 7±13% and 5±10%, respectively. There was no difference in ejection fraction between the groups at discharge or after 6 weeks.

Conclusions   There was no difference in myocardial salvage between immediate angioplasty and intravenous thrombolytic therapy followed by conservative therapy.

DANAMI

DANish Trial in Acute Myocardial Infarction

Title	Danish multicenter randomized study of invasive vs conservative treatment in patients with inducible ischemia after thrombolysis in acute myocardial infarction (DANAMI).
Author	Madsen JK, Grande P, Saunamaki K, et al.
Reference	Circulation 1997; 96:748-755.
Disease	Coronary artery disease, inducible myocardial ischemia post infarction.
Purpose	To compare invasive therapy (PTCA or CABG) with conservative therapy in patients with inducible myocardial ischemia after a first myocardial infarction treated with thrombolytic therapy.
Design	Randomized, multicenter.
Patients	1008 patients ≤69 years old with a definite acute myocardial infarction and thrombolytic therapy begun within 12 h of symptom onset. Patients had to have either symptomatic angina pectoris >36 hours after admission or a positive pre-discharge exercise tolerance test.
Follow-up	Median 2.4 years (range 1 - 4 years).
Treatment regimen	Patients were randomized to conservative therapy (nitrates, beta blockers, calcium channel blockers) vs invasive therapy (PTCA or CABG) within 2 - 5 weeks of randomization. All patients received aspirin.

DANAMI

DANish Trial in Acute Myocardial Infarction

(continued)

Results   505 patients were randomized to conservative therapy;
            503 to invasive. At 2.4 years mortality was 3.6% with inva-
            sive therapy vs 4.4% with conservative therapy (p=NS).
            The invasive strategy was associated with a lower inci-
            dence of recurrent acute myocardial infarction compared
            to conservative therapy (5.6% vs 10.5%; p = .0038); and
            lower incidence of admission for unstable angina (17.9%
            vs 29.5%, p<.00001). The primary endpoint was the com-
            posite of death, reinfarction, or unstable angina, and
            occurred at lower rates with invasive therapy at 1, 2, and
            3 years (15.4%, 23.5%, 31.7%) than conservative therapy
            (29.5%, 36.6%, and 44.0% p≤ .00001).

Conclusions Patients with inducible ischemia before discharge from
            acute myocardial infarction treated with thrombolysis
            should receive coronary arteriography and revasculariza-
            tion procedure.

Title	Effects of coronary stenting on restenosis and occlusion after angioplasty of the culprit vessel in patients with recent myocardial infarction.
Author	Bauters C, Lablanche J-M, Belle EV, et al.
Reference	Circulation 1997; 96:2854-2858.
Disease	Coronary artery disease, myocardial infarction.
Purpose	To determine the long-term effect of coronary stenting of infarct-related coronary lesions vs percutaneous transluminal coronary angioplasty (PTCA) alone.
Design	Comparison of consecutive patients undergoing stent implanation of infarct artery to matched patients who underwent PTCA without stenting within 24 h to 30 days after an acute myocardial infarction. Patients were matched for a number of clinical variables. 6 month angiograms were analyzed by quantitiative angiography.
Patients	200 acute myocardial infraction patients average age 57±11 years; 89% men.
Follow-up	6 months.
Treatment regimen	Coronary stenting (including bailout implantation, implantation of stent for suboptimal result after PTCA, or elective stent implantation) compared to PTCA.

***Effects of coronary stenting on restenosis and
occlusion after angioplasty of the culprit vessel in
patients with recent myocardial infarction.***

(continued)

Results
Immediately after the procedure there was a larger acute gain in the stent group (p<.0001), with a mean minimal lumen diameter of 2.58 ± 0.44 mm in the stent group vs the balloon group (1.97 ± 0.43 mm, p<.0001). At 6 months, patients in the stent group had a larger net gain (1.02 ± 0.79 vs 0.56 ± 0.68 mm, p<.0001), and a larger minimal lumen diameter (1.72 ± 0.69 vs 1.23 ± 0.72mm, p<.0001). By categorical analysis 27% of the stent group had restenosis compared to 52% of the PTCA group (p<.005). At 6 months, total occlusion at the dilated site occurred in 1% of the stent group and 14% of the PTCA group (p<.005).

Conclusions
Coronary stenting of the infarct-related artery was associated with less restenosis at 6 months compared to PTCA alone. Whether this translates to improvement in left ventricular function or clinical outcome remains to be determined.

PAMI-2

Primary Angioplasty in Myocardial Infarction-2

Title	a. A prospective, randomized trial evaluating early discharge (day 3) without noninvasive risk stratification in low risk patients with acute myocardial infarction: PAMI-2 b. A prospective, randomized evaluation of prophylactic intraaortic balloon counterpulsation in high risk patients with acute myocardial infarction treated with primary angioplasty.
Authors	a. Brodie B, Grines CL, Spain S, et al. b. Stone GW, Marsalese D, Brodie BR, et al.
Reference	a. J Am Coll Cardiol 1995;25 (Suppl A:430A). b. J Am Coll Cardiol 1997;29:1459-1467.
Disease	Acute myocardial infarction
Purpose	To evaluate the effectiveness of both early discharge (third day) in low-risk patients and prophylactic intra-aortic balloon pumping (IABP) in high-risk patients with acute myocardial infarction undergoing primary angioplasty.
Design	Randomized, multicenter.
Patients	1,100 patients with ongoing chest pain ≤12 h after symptom onset, with ST elevation ≥1 mm in ≥2 contiguous leads. Patients with ST depression, LBBB, or nondiagnostic ECG were included if acute catheterization demonstrated an occluded coronary artery with regional LV dysfunction. Patients with cardiogenic shock, bleeding diathesis, and those who had received thrombolytic therapy were excluded.
Treatment regimen	Chewable aspirin 324 mg and intravenous heparin 5000-10000 U, nitroglycerin and beta-blockers. Coronary angiography with left ventriculography, and then, primary PTCA or emergent CABG (for unprotected left main coronary artery stenosis >60%, severe 3 vessel disease with a patent infarct related artery, or features precluding PTCA). High risk patients (age >70 years, 3 vessel disease, LVEF ≤45%, vein graft occlusion, persistent malignant ventricular arrhythmias or suboptimal PTCA result) were randomized to prophylactic IABP for 36-48 h unless an IABP was contraindicated or conservative treatment (no-IABP). Low risk patients were randomized into accelerated discharge (day 3) and traditional care (discharge at 5-7 days) groups.

PAMI-2

Primary Angioplasty in Myocardial Infarction-2
(continued)

Additional therapy	Stenting and atherectomy were rarely used during the study. Intravenous heparin for ≥72 h, nitroglycerin infusion for 24 h, and oral aspirin 325 mg/d were used.
Results	After PTCA 437 patients were considered high risk and 471 patients as low risk. Among the low risk patients in-hospital and postdischarge outcomes were similar in the early discharge and traditional care groups. High risk patients were randomized to IABP (n=211) or conservative therapy (no-IABP)(n=226). In only 182 patients (86.3%) of the 211 patients IABP was successfully inserted. IABP was inserted in 26 (11.5%) of patients assigned to no-IABP. In an intention to treat analysis, in-hospital death occurred in 4.3% of the IABP and 3.1% of the non-IABP (p=0.52). IABP did not prevent reinfarction (6.2% vs 8.0%, in the IABP and no-IABP, respectively (p=0.46)); reocclusion of the infarct related artery (6.7% vs 5.5% (p=0.64)); heart failure or hypotension (19.9% vs 23.0% (p=0.43)); or the combined end-point of death, reinfarction, reocclusion, stroke, hypotension, or new-onset heart failure (28.9% vs 29.2% (p=0.95)). IABP was associated with increased risk of stroke (2.4% vs 0.0% (p=0.03)). The findings were similar when only the 382 randomized patients who received their assigned therapy were included. However, IABP was associated with modest reduction of recurrent ischemia (13.3% vs 19.6% (p=0.08)) and need for repeated catheterization (7.6% vs 13.3% (p=0.05)), but an increased bleeding complications (36.0% vs 27.4% (p=0.05)). Paired pre-PTCA and predischarge left ventriculography, performed in 217 patients, showed that there was no difference in improvement in global LVEF and infarct zone regional wall motion between the IABP and no-IABP groups.
Conclusions	A prophylactic insertion of IABP in high risk hemodynamically stable acute myocardial infarction after primary angioplasty did not decrease mortality, reocclusion of the infarct related artery, or reinfarction, and was associated with an increased rate of stroke. Among the low risk patients in-hospital and postdischarge outcomes were similar in the early discharge and traditional care groups.

PAMI Stent Pilot Trial

Title	Prospective, multicenter study of the safety and feasibility of primary stenting in acute myocardial infarction: in-hospital and 30-day results of the PAMI stent pilot trial.
Authors	Stone GW, Brodie BR, Griffin JJ, et al.
Reference	J Am Coll Cardiol 1998;31:23-30.
Disease	Acute myocardial infarction.
Purpose	To evaluate the feasibility and safety of a primary stenting strategy in patients with acute myocardial infarction.
Design	Multicenter.
Patients	312 patients with chest pain ≤12 h in duration with ECG changes compatible with acute myocardial infarction. Patients in cardiogenic shock and those with contraindications to heparin, aspirin or ticlopidine, increased risk for bleeding, and recent thrombolytic therapy were excluded. Only patients that actually underwent primary PTCA were included in the study.
Follow-up	6 months clinical follow-up.
Treatment regimen	Percutaneous transluminal coronary angioplasty (PTCA), unless TIMI grade flow 3 was present with an infarct related artery stenosis <70%, or if a very small vessel was occluded, or if the infarct related lesion could not be identified. Patients treated medically or surgically were excluded from the study. After PTCA, an attempt was made to insert a Johnson & Johnson Palmaz-Schatz stent.

PAMI Stent Pilot Trial

(continued)

Additional therapy	Upon enrollment, oral aspirin 324-500 mg, 250-500 mg ticlopidine, and 5000-10000 U bolus intravenous heparin. Intravenous beta-blockers were given unless contraindicated. 6 h after sheath removal, heparin infusion was given for 12 h. All patients received oral aspirin 325 mg/d, ticlopidine 250 mg BID, and beta-blockers. Angiotensin converting enzyme inhibitors were administered if hypertension, heart failure, or LV dysfunction was present.
Results	Primary angioplasty was performed in 312 patients; in 240 of them (77%) stenting was attempted. In 72 patients, stenting was not considered feasible. Stenting was performed more frequently in patients with 1 vessel disease, whereas it was attempted less often in patients with 3 vessel disease. In 236 (98%) of the 240 patients, stenting was successful. TIMI grade 3 flow was achieved in 94.4% of the stent group vs 87.3% of the PTCA only group (p=0.04). The mean residual stenosis was 12.1±16.2% in the stent group vs 33.3±14.3% in the PTCA-only group (p<0.0001). A <50% residual stenosis was obtained in 93.7% of the stent group vs 77.3% of the PTCA-only group (p<0.0001). In-hospital death occurred in 2 patients (0.8%), reinfarction in 4 patients (1.7%), and recurrent ischemia in 9 patients (3.8%) of the stent group. Only 3 patients (1.3%) needed target vessel revascularization for recurrent ischemia. None of the patients died or had reinfarction within 30 days after hospital discharge. Only 1 patient (0.4%) needed target vessel revascularization within 30 days after discharge.
Conclusions	Primary stenting is safe and feasible in most of the patients with acute myocardial infarction and is associated with good short-term results.

1. Acute Myocardial Infarction

c. Anticoagulation/ Antiplatelet

HART

Heparin-Aspirin Reperfusion Trial

Title	A comparison between heparin and low-dose aspirin as adjunctive therapy with tissue plasminogen activator for acute myocardial infarction.
Authors	Hsia J, Hamilton WP, Kleiman N, et al.
Reference	N Engl J Med 1990;323:1433-1437.
Disease	Acute myocardial infarction.
Purpose	To compare early intravenous heparin with oral aspirin as adjunctive therapy to tissue plasminogen activator for acute myocardial infarction.
Design	Randomized, open label, multicenter.
Patients	193 patients, age <76 years, with chest pain and ST elevation ≥ 1 mm in ≥ 2 contiguous leads, within 6 h from onset of symptoms.
Follow-up	7-24 h and 7 day cardiac catheterization. 7 day clinical course.
Treatment regimen	1. Oral aspirin 80 mg/d, started with the t-PA for 7 days. 2. IV heparin 5000 U bolus, followed by 1000 U/h, started with the t-PA for 7 days.
Additional therapy	Intravenous tissue plasminogen activator (t-PA) 6 mg bolus, 54 mg over the first h, 20 mg over the second h, and 20 mg over 4 h.

HART

Heparin-Aspirin Reperfusion Trial

(continued)

Results   At the time of the first angiogram, 82% and 52% of the infarct related arteries of the patients assigned to heparin and aspirin were patent (p<0.0001). Of the arteries that were initially patent, 88% and 95% in the heparin and aspirin groups remained patent after 7.4±2.4 days (p=0.17). The number of bleeding events and recurrent ischemia were similar between the groups. The mortality rate was 1.9% vs 4.0% in the heparin and aspirin groups, respectively (p=NS).

Conclusions   Coronary patency rate improved when heparin was added to t-PA compare to when aspirin was added.

TIMI-5

Thrombolysis in Myocardial Infarction 5 Trial

Title	A pilot trial of recombinant desulfatohirudin compared with heparin in conjunction with tissue-type plasminogen activator and aspirin for acute myocardial infarction: Results of the Thrombolysis in Myocardial Infarction (TIMI) 5 trial.
Authors	Cannon CP, McCabe CH, Henry TD, et al.
Reference	J Am Coll Cardiol 1994;23:993-1003.
Disease	Acute myocardial infarction.
Purpose	To compare the efficacy of recombinant desulfatohirudin (hirudin) to heparin as adjunctive therapy to thrombolysis in acute myocardial infarction.
Design	Randomized, multicenter, dose escalation trial.
Patients	246 patients with acute myocardial infarction < 6 hours from onset of symptoms with chest pain >30 min and ST segment elevation $\geq$0.1 mV in $\geq$2 contiguous leads or with new left bundle branch block.
Follow-up	90 min and 18-36 h coronary angiography. In-hospital clinical events.
Treatment regimen	Intravenous heparin or hirudin at 1 of 4 escalating doses (Bolus (mg/kg) and intravenous infusion mg/kg per h) of 0.15 and 0.05; 0.1 and 0.1; 0.3 and 0.1; and 0.6 and 0.2, respectively) for 5 days.
Additional therapy	Front-loaded tissue-type plasminogen activator and aspirin 160 mg/d. Intravenous and oral metoprolol.

TIMI-5

Thrombolysis in Myocardial Infarction 5 Trial

(continued)

Results

The primary efficacy end point (achievement of TIMI 3 flow at 90 min and 18-36 h without death or reinfarction before the second angiography) was achieved in 61.8% and 49.4% of the hirudin and heparin-treated patients, respectively (p=0.07). While 90 min patency of the infarct related artery was similar at 18-36 h, 97.8% and 89.2 % of the hirudin and heparin-treated patients had an open artery, respectively (p=0.01). In-hospital death or rein-farction occurred in 6.8% and 16.7% of the hirudin and heparin groups, respectively (p=0.02). Major hemorrhage occurred in 1.2% and 4.7% of the patients, respectively (p=0.09).

Conclusions

Hirudin is a relatively safe drug and has a several advantages over heparin, as an adjunctive to front-loaded tissue plasminogen activator therapy.

Title	Beneficial effects of RheothRx injection in patients receiving thrombolytic therapy for acute myocardial infarction. Results of a randomized, double blind, placebo-controlled trial.
Authors	Schaer GL, Spaccavento LJ, Browne KF, et al.
Reference	Circulation 1996;94:298-307.
Disease	Acute myocardial infarction.
Purpose	To evaluate the safety and efficacy of adjunctive therapy with RheothRx (poloxamer 188, a surfactanct with hemorheological and antithrombotic properties) in patients with acute myocardial infarction undergoing thrombolytic therapy.
Design	Randomized, double blind, placebo-controlled, multicenter.
Patients	114 patients, ≥18 years old, with suspected acute myocardial infarction (chest pain ≥30 min, ST elevation in ≥2 leads. All patients received thrombolytic therapy within 6 h of onset of symptoms. Patients with serum creatinine ≥3.0 mg/dL were excluded.
Follow-up	Clinical follow-up and 99mTc sestamibi tomographic imaging with radionuclide ventriculography before reperfusion and 5-7 days after infarction.
Treatment regimen	RheothRx (150 or 300 mg/kg over 1 h and then 15 or 30 mg/kg/h for 47 h) or placebo infusion was initiated immediately after initiation of thrombolytic therapy.
Additional therapy	Thrombolytic therapy (tPA or streptokinase). Chewable aspirin, nitrates, IV followed by oral β-blocker, and heparin for ≥48 h.

Results   75 patients were randomized to RheothRx and 39 to placebo. Baseline characteristics were not significantly different between the groups. RheothRx-treated patients had a 38% reduction in median infarct size (25th and 75th percentile) compared with placebo (16% (7,30) vs 26% (9,43); p=0.031), greater median myocardial salvage (13% (7,20) vs 4% (1,15); p=0.033), and higher ejection fraction (52% (43,60) vs 46% (35,60); p=0.02). RheothRx treated patients had lower rate of reinfarction (1% vs 13%, p=0.016). Therapy was well tolerated without adverse hemodynamic effects or bleeding.

Conclusions   Therapy with RheothRx was effective in reduction of infarct size and preservation of left ventricular function in patients undergoing thrombolytic therapy for acute myocardial infarction.

TIMI 9B

Thrombolysis and Thrombin Inhibition in Myocardial Infarction 9B

Title	a. Hirudin in acute myocardial infarction. Thrombolysis and thrombin inhibition in myocardial infarction (TIMI) 9B trial. b. Prospective temporal analysis of the outcome of preinfarction angina vs outcome. An ancillary study in TIMI-9B.
Authors	a. Antman EM, for the TIMI 9B Investigators. b. Kloner RA, Shook T, Antman E, et al.
Reference	a. Circulation 1996;94:911-921. b. Circulation 1998; 97:1042-1045.
Disease	Acute myocardial infarction.
Purpose	a. To compare the efficacy and safety of recombinant desulfatohirudin (Hirudin) with heparin as adjunctive therapy to thrombolysis and aspirin in acute myocardial infarction. b. To determine the importance of the time of onset of preinfarction angina in relationship to 30-day outcome in TIMI-9B.
Design	a. Randomized, double blind, multicenter. b. Standardized forms questioned patients regarding time of onset of angina in relationship to myocardial infarction.
Patients	a. 3002 Patients, ≥21 years old, with acute myocardial infarction with ≥1 mm ST segment elevation in ≥2 leads or new LBBB, within 12 h of onset of symptoms, and no contraindications to thrombolytic therapy. Patients with serum creatinine >2.0 mg/dl, cardiogenic shock, or receiving therapeutic doses of anticoagulants were excluded. b. 3002 patients with myocardial infarction.
Follow-up	a. 30 day clinical follow-up. b. 30 days.
Treatment regimen	a. Randomization to heparin or hirudin. Therapy started within 60 min after thrombolysis and continued for 96 h. Hirudin: bolus of 0.1 mg/kg (maximum 15 mg), followed by a continuous infusion of 0.1 mg/kg/h (maximum 15 mg/h). Heparin: a bolus of 5000 U, followed by continuous infusion of 1000 U/h. Target aPTT 55 to 85 sec. b. As per TIMI 9B.

TIMI 9B

Thrombolysis and Thrombin Inhibition in
Myocardial Infarction 9B
(continued)

Additional therapy	a. Intravenous thrombolytic therapy by the treating physician front loaded tPA (maximum 100 mg) over 90 min or streptokinase, 1.5 million U over 1 h. Aspirin 150 to 325 mg/d, β blockers, nitrates, calcium channel blockers, and other medications were permitted.
Results	a. The hirudin-treated patients were more likely to have an aPTT within the target range (p<0.0001). Only 15% of the hirudin group vs 34% of the heparin group had aPTT values <55 sec within the first 24 h of therapy. The primary end-point of death, recurrent myocardial infarction, severe heart failure, or cardiogenic shock by 30 days occurred in 11.9% of the heparin-treated group vs 12.9% of the hirudin-treated patients (p=NS). After adjustment for age, time to therapy, and type of thrombolytic therapy administered, there was no significant difference between the groups concerning occurrence of the primary end-point or in the occurrence of the individual elements of the composite end-point. Kaplan-Meier plots of the time to development of the composite endpoint and to the occurrence of death or reinfarction were comparable between the groups. Subgroup analyses could not identify a subgroup that clearly benefited from hirudin compared with heparin therapy. Major hemorrhage occurred in 5.3% of the heparin and 4.6% of the hirudin groups (p=NS), whereas intracranial hemorrhage in 0.9% vs 0.4%, respectively.
	b. Of 3002 patients, 425 reported angina before their myocardial infarction. Those patients with angina onset within 24 h of infarct onset had a lower 30 day cardiac event rate (mortality, recurrent myocardial infarction, heart failure, or shock) at 4% compared to those with onset of angina >24 h (17%, p = 0.03). Peak creatine kinase levels also were lower in patients with angina within 24 h of the infarction. Differences in baseline characteristics and use of antianginal drugs could not explain the difference.
Conclusions	a. Hirudin had no treatment benefit over heparin in patients with acute myocardial infarction that received intravenous thrombolytic therapy.
	b. Preinfarct angina was protective, only when it occurred within 24 h of the acute myocardial infarction. These temporal findings are consistent with the concept of preconditioning but do not rule out other mechanisms.

IMPACT-AMI

Integrelin to Manage Platelet Aggregation to Combat Thrombosis

Title	Combined accelerated tissue-plasminogen activator and platelet glycoprotein IIb/IIIa integrin receptor blockade with integrilin in acute myocardial infarction. Results of a randomized, placebo-controlled, dose-ranging trial.
Authors	Ohman EM, Kleiman NS, Gacioch G, et al.
Reference	Circulation 1997;95:846-854.
Disease	Acute myocardial infarction.
Purpose	To evaluate the effects of platelet inhibition by integrilin on reperfusion, bleeding, and clinical outcome of patients with acute myocardial infarction treated with accelerated alteplase (tPA), heparin, and aspirin.
Design	Placebo-controlled, dose-ranging, multicenter.
Patients	180 patients, 18 - 75 years old, within 6 h of onset of acute myocardial infarction. Patients >125 kg, bleeding diathesis, severe hypertension, prior stroke, current warfarin therapy, anemia, thrombocytopenia, renal failure, recent noncompressible vascular puncture, ≥10 min cardiopulmonary resuscitation within 2 weeks, severe trauma within 6 months, or vasculitis were excluded.
Follow-up	Continuous 12-lead digital ECG for the first 24 h. Coronary angiography at 90 min after initiation of thrombolytic therapy. Clinical follow-up for in-hospital events.
Treatment regimen	Patients were enrolled in 1 of 7 treatment groups of integrilin or placebo. Integrilin or placebo was administered within 10 min of initiation of alteplase.

IMPACT-AMI

Integrelin to Manage Platelet Aggregation to Combat Thrombosis
(continued)

Additional therapy	All patients received accelerated dose of alteplase IV (maximum dose 100 mg), and aspirin 325 mg/d. All but 2 groups received intravenous heparin. Target aPTT 2-2.5 times the control value.
Results	55 patients received placebo and 125 patients received integrilin. Of the 170 patients with adequate 90 min angiograms, patients allocated to the highest integrilin dose more often had complete reperfusion (TIMI flow grade III) than the placebo group (66% vs 39%, p=0.006). The rate of TIMI flow grade II or III was 87% vs 69%, respectively (p=0.01). The median time from initiation of thrombolytic therapy to steady-state recovery of ST segment deviation was 95 min for all integrilin-treated patients vs 116 min for the placebo-treated patients (p = 0.5). The duration was 65 min for the highest integrilin dose (p=0.05). 5.6% of the integrilin-treated patients vs 3.6% of the placebo-treated patients died (p=0.57). Death or reinfarction occured in 8.0% vs. 7.3%, respectively (p=0.87). The composite end-point of death, reinfarction, stroke, revascularization, or new in-hospital heart failure of pulmonary edema occurred in 45% of the integrilin (43% of the patients at the highest integrillin dose) vs 42% of the placebo-treated patients (p=0.71). Sustained hypotension occurred in 13% vs 16% respectively (p=0.53). Severe bleeding complications occurred in 2% of the integrilin-treated patients vs 5% of the placebo-treated patients, whereas moderate bleeding occurred in 14% vs 9% and mild bleeding in 63% vs 67% respectively.
Conclusions	Integrilin, when combined with alteplase, aspirin, and heparin, accelerated the speed of reperfusion. However, integrilin therapy was not associated with improved in-hospital outcome.

CARS

Coumadin Aspirin Reinfarction Study

Title	Randomized double blind trial of fixed low-dose warfarin with aspirin after myocardial infarction.
Authors	Coumadin Aspirin Reinfarction Study (CARS) Investigators.
Reference	Lancet 1997;350:389-396.
Disease	Acute myocardial infarction.
Purpose	To compare the efficacy and safety of low dose (80 mg/d) aspirin with low dose warfarin (1 or 3 mg/d) to that of aspirin (160 mg/d) in patients after acute myocardial infarction.
Design	Randomized, double blind, multicenter.
Patients	8803 men and postmenopausal women, 21-85 years of age, 3-21 days after an acute myocardial infarction. Patients with congestive heart failure, circulatory shock, rest angina unresponsive to medications, serious ventricular arrhythmias, history of bleeding or stroke, liver or renal disease, severe systemic disease, anemia, acute pericarditis during the index infarction, thyroid disorders, uncontrolled hypertension, hypersensitivity to warfarin, need for long term anticoagulation, or patients scheduled for CABG were excluded.
Follow-up	Maximum 33 months (median 14 months).
Treatment regimen	Randomization to 1. aspirin 160 mg/d; 2. warfarin 1 mg/d with aspirin 80 mg/d; and 3. warfarin 3 mg/d with aspirin 80 mg/d.

CARS

Coumadin Aspirin Reinfarction Study

(continued)

Results

The study was terminated prematurely by the data and safety monitoring committee based on similar efficacy of all 3 treatment arms. 3393 patients were randomized to aspirin 160 mg/d; 2028 to warfarin 1mg/d +aspirin; and 3382 to warfarin 3 mg/d + aspirin. 1 year life-table estimates for the primary event were 8.6% (95% CI 7.6 - 9.6%) for the aspirin 160 mg/d; 8.8% (95% CI 7.6 - 10.0%) for the warfarin 1mg/d + aspirin; and 8.4% (95% CI 7.4 - 9.4%) for the warfarin 3mg/d + aspirin. The relative risk of primary event (first occurrence of reinfarction, non-fatal ischemic stroke or cardiovascular mortality) in the aspirin 160 mg/d vs warfarin 3 mg/d + aspirin was 0.95 (95% CI 0.81-1.12; p=0.57). The relative risk of primary event in the aspirin 160 mg/d vs warfarin 1mg/d + aspirin was 1.03 (95% CI 0.87 - 1.22; p=0.74). The relative risk of primary event in the warfarin 1 mg/d + aspirin vs warfarin 3 mg/d + aspirin was 0.93 (95% CI 0.78 - 1.11; p=0.41). Life-table estimates for ischemic strokes in 1 year were the lowest in the aspirin 160 mg/d (0.58% (95% CI 0.29 - 0.87%)) than in the warfarin 1 mg/d + aspirin (1.1% (95% CI 0.64-1.5%; p vs aspirin alone = 0.05) and in the warfarin 3 mg/d + aspirin (0.80% (95% CI 0.47 - 1.1%; p vs aspirin alone = 0.16). 1 year life-table estimates for spontaneous major hemorrhage was higher in the warfarin 3 mg/d + aspirin (1.4% (95% CI 0.94 - 1.8%)) than in the aspirin 160 mg/d (0.74% (95% CI 0.43 - 1.1%; p=0.014)). Among patients assigned to warfarin 3 mg/d + aspirin, the median INR values were 1.51 at week 1, 1.27 at week 4, and 1.19 at month 6.

Conclusions

The combination therapy of warfarin at a dose of 1 or 3 mg/d and low dose aspirin (80 mg/d) had similar efficacy to that of aspirin 160 mg/d alone in patients after acute myocardial infarction.

FRAMI

The Fragmin in Acute Myocardial Infarction Study

Title	Randomized trial of low molecular weight heparin (dalteparin) in prevention of left ventricular thrombus formation and arterial embolism after anterior myocardial infarction: the fragmin in acute myocardial infarction (FRAMI) study.
Authors	Kontny F, Dale J, Abildgaard U, Pedersen TR, on the behalf of the FRAMI study group.
Reference	J Am Coll Cardiol 1997;30:962-969.
Disease	Acute myocardial infarction.
Purpose	To assess the role of dalteparin in prevention of left ventricular mural thrombus formation and arterial thromboembolism after an anterior wall acute myocardial infarction.
Design	Randomized, double blind, placebo controlled, multicenter.
Patients	776 patients with a first anterior acute myocardial infarction. Patients with previous myocardial infarction, non anterior myocardial infarction, time from onset of symptoms to randomization >15 h, ongoing treatment with or indication for heparin or oral anticoagulants, blood pressure over 210/115 mmHg, cerebrovascular event within 2 months, known allergy to trial medication, peptic ulcer, bleeding disorder, serious renal or liver failure, concomitant life threatening disease, alcohol abuse, or pregnancy were excluded.
Follow-up	Echocardiography on day 9±2, and clinical follow-up for 3 months (the present study reports only in-hospital course).

FRAMI

The Fragmin in Acute Myocardial Infarction Study

(continued)

Treatment regimen	Subcutaneous Dalteparin 150 IU/kg body weight BID or placebo for 9±2 days.
Additional therapy	Intravenous streptokinase, if no contraindications existed and symptoms ≤6 h. Aspirin 300 mg on admission and 160 mg/d thereafter. No other antithrombotic agents were permitted. High risk patients of thromboembolic events received warfarin at discharge.
Results	There were 388 patients in each treatment group. Thrombolytic therapy was administered to 91.5% of the patients and aspirin to 97.6%. After randomization, 137 patients were excluded from further participation in the study. Echocardiography was available for 517 patients (270 placebo, 247 dalteparin). LV thrombus was detected by echocardiography in 59 patients (21.9%) of the placebo group vs 34 patients (13.8%) in the dalteparin group (p=0.022). LV thrombus formation or arterial embolism occurred in 59 patients (21.9%) of the placebo vs only 35 patients (14.2%) of the dalteparin group (p=0.03). Mortality and reinfarction rates were comparable between the 2 groups. Major bleeding occurred more commonly in the dalteparin group (2.9%) than in the placebo (0.3%)(p=0.006). Minor bleeding occurred in 2.1% of the placebo and 13.4% of the dalteparin group. No allergic reactions were reported. Thrombocytopenia was detected in one dalteparin-treated patient.
Conclusions	Dalteparin was effective in preventing LV thrombus formation in patients with first anterior acute myocardial infarction, but was associated with increased risk for bleeding.

1. Acute Myocardial Infarction

d. Early Vs Late Intervention After Acute Myocardial Infarction

TAMI

Thrombolysis and Angioplasty in Myocardial Infarction

Title	A randomized trial of immediate vs delayed elective angioplasty after intravenous tissue plasminogen activator in acute myocardial infarction.
Authors	Topol EJ, Califf RM, George BS, et al.
Reference	N Engl J Med 1987;317:581-588.
Disease	Acute myocardial infarction.
Purpose	To compare the efficacy of immediate vs delayed (7-10 days) coronary angioplasty in patients with acute myocardial infarction treated with intravenous tissue plasminogen activator.
Design	Randomized, open label, multicenter.
Patients	386 patients, age ≤75 years, with acute myocardial infarction < 4h from onset of symptoms (<6 h if severe ongoing pain was present) with ST≥1 mm in ≥2 leads. Only patients with TIMI grade 2-3 and ≥50% residual stenosis suitable to angioplasty 90 min after initiation of thrombolytic therapy, without ≥50% left main stenosis or left main equivalent stenosis were included (n=197).
Follow-up	7 days.
Treatment regimen	Immediate angioplasty or deferred elective angioplasty 5-10 days later.
Additional therapy	Tissue plasminogen activator (t-PA) 150 mg over 6-8 h, 60-90 mg over the first h (10% of this as a bolus), heparin 5000 U IV and 500-1000 U/h ≥24 h, aspirin 325 mg/d, dipyridamole 75 mg X3/d, and diltiazem 30-60 mg X4/d.

Thrombolysis and Angioplasty in Myocardial Infarction

(continued)

Results   Bleeding complications were common (18% of patients needed transfusion). The incidence of reocclusion was similar in the immediate (11%) and delayed (13%) angioplasty. Global and regional left ventricular function were comparable. The mortality was higher in the immediate (4.0%) than delayed (1.0%) angioplasty (p=0.37). 7% and 2% of the immediate and elective angioplasty groups needed emergency CABG (p=0.17), while 5% and 16% needed emergency angioplasty, respectively (p=0.01).

Conclusions   In patients with acute myocardial infarction and initially successful thrombolysis, immediate angioplasty offers no advantage over delayed elective angioplasty.

TIMI 2-A

Thrombolysis in Myocardial Infarction Trial (phase 2A)

Title	a. Immediate vs delayed catheterization and angioplasty following thrombolytic therapy for acute myocardial infarction. TIMI II-A results. b. Comparison of immediate invasive, delayed invasive, and conservative strategies after tissue-type plasminogen activator. Results of the Thrombolysis in Myocardial Infarction (TIMI) phase II-A Trial.
Authors	a. The TIMI research group. b. Rogers WJ, Baim DS, Gore JM, et al.
Reference	JAMA 1988;260:2849-2858. Circulation 1990;81:1457-1476.
Disease	Acute myocardial infarction.
Purpose	To compare the results of 3 strategies of coronary angiography and angioplasty following intravenous thrombolytic therapy for acute myocardial infarction: immediate invasive, delayed invasive (18-48 h), and a conservative strategy.
Design	Randomized, open label, multicenter.
Patients	586 patients with acute myocardial infarction <76 years old < 4 hours from onset of symptoms with chest pain>30 min and ST elevation ≥0.1 mV in ≥2 contiguous leads.
Follow-up	Predischarge contrast ventriculography and coronary angiography. 1-year follow-up.

TIMI 2-A

Thrombolysis in Myocardial Infarction Trial (phase 2A)

(continued)

Treatment regimen	1. Coronary angiography within 2 h of rt-PA initiation. PTCA was attempted if coronary anatomy was suitable. 2. Coronary angiography within 18-48 h of rt-PA initiation. PTCA was attempted if coronary anatomy was suitable. 3 Conservative strategy: coronary angiography and intervention only in those who had either spontaneous recurrent ischemia or a positive exercise test.
Additional therapy	Intravenous rt-PA (150 mg over 6 h for the first 520 patients, and 100 mg in the remaining 2742 patients). Lidocaine (1-1.5 mg/kg bolus + infusion 2-4 mg/min) for >24 h; heparin 5000 U bolus and infusion 1000 U/h for 5 days, and then subcutaneous until discharge. Aspirin 81 mg/d for 6 days and then 325 mg/d. Nifedipine 10-20 mg X3/d was administrated for 96 h. Metoprolol was started before discharge for 1 year.
Results	Predischarge contrast left ventricular ejection fraction was similar among the 3 groups. The rates of patency of the infarct related artery at the time of predischarge were similar among groups. However, the mean residual stenosis was greater in the conservative therapy arm (67.2%) than in the immediate invasive (50.6%) and delayed invasive (47.8%) arms (p<0.001). Immediate invasive strategy led to a higher rate of coronary artery bypass graft surgery after angioplasty (7.7%) than in the delayed invasive (2.1%) and conservative (2.5%) arms (p<0.01). The need for blood transfusion was greater in the immediate invasive (13.8%) than in the delayed invasive (3.1%) and conservative (2.0%) groups (p<0.001). 1 year mortality and reinfarction rates were similar among the 3 groups.
Conclusions	Conservative strategy achieves equally good results with less morbidity compared to invasive strategies.

TIMI 2

Thrombolysis in Myocardial Infarction Trial (phase 2)

Title	a. Comparison of invasive and conservative strategies after treatment with intravenous tissue plasminogen activator in acute myocardial infarction. Results of the Thrombolysis in Myocardial Infarction (TIMI) Phase II Trial. b. 1-year results of the Thrombolysis in Myocardial Infarction investigation (TIMI) phase II trial.
Authors	a. The TIMI Study Group. b. Williams DO, Braunwald E, Knatterud G, et al.
Reference	a. N Engl J Med 1989;320:618-627. b. Circulation 1992;85:533-542.
Disease	Acute myocardial infarction.
Purpose	To compare an invasive strategy consisting of coronary angiography and angioplasty within 18-48 h of infarction and a conservative approach in which angiography was performed only in patients with spontaneous or exercise induced ischemia in patients with acute myocardial infarction treated with rt-PA.
Design	Randomized, open label, multicenter.
Patients	3262 patients with acute myocardial infarction <76 years old < 4 hours from onset of symptoms with chest pain>30 min and ST elevation ≥0.1 mV in ≥2 contiguous leads.
Follow-up	a. Predischarge radionuclide ventriculography at rest and during exercise. At 6 weeks clinical evaluation and maximal exercise test + radionuclide ventriculography. b. 1 year.

Treatment regimen	Coronary angiography and angioplasty (if arteriography demonstrated suitable anatomy) within 18-48 h of thrombolytic therapy vs coronary angiography only for patients who had either spontaneous recurrent ischemia or a positive exercise test (the conservative arm).
Additional therapy	Intravenous rt-PA (150 mg over 6 h for the first 520 patients, and 100 mg in the remaining 2742 patients). Lidocaine (1-1.5 mg/kg bolus + infusion 2-4 mg/min) for >24 h; heparin 5000 U bolus and infusion 1000 U/h for 5 days, and then subcutaneous until discharge. Aspirin 80 mg/d for 6 days and then 325 mg/d
Results	a. 53.7% and 13.3% of the invasive strategy and conservative groups underwent angioplasty within 14 days of admission. Reinfarction or death within 6 weeks occurred in 10.9% and 9.7% of the invasive and conservative group, respectively (p=0.25). Predischarge and 6-week left ventricular ejection fraction at either rest or during exercise were comparable. b. Death or nonfatal reinfarction within 1 year occurred in 14.7% and 15.2% of the invasive and conservative groups, respectively. There was no difference in death or recurrent infarction rates between the 2 groups. Anginal status at 1 year was comparable. Cardiac catheterization and angioplasty were performed more often in the invasive group (98% and 61.2%) vs the conservative group (45.2% and 20.5%). In patients with prior infarction, 6 weeks and 1 year mortality was lower in the invasive group (6.0% and 10.3%) than in the conservative group (11.5% and 17.0%), p= 0.04 and p=0.03, respectively.
Conclusions	In patients with acute myocardial infarction who are treated with rt-PA, heparin, and aspirin, the results of an invasive and conservative strategies are comparable.

SWIFT

Should We Intervene Following Thrombolysis?

Title	SWIFT trial of delayed elective intervention vs conservative treatment after thrombolysis with anistreplase in acute myocardial infarction.
Authors	SWIFT Trial Study Group.
Reference	Br Med J 1991;302:555-560.
Disease	Acute myocardial infarction.
Purpose	To compare a strategy of conservative management to early elective angiography and intervention following thrombolytic therapy for acute myocardial infarction.
Design	Randomized, open label, multicenter.
Patients	800 patients, <70 years of age, with clinical features of first acute myocardial infarction, ≤3 h from onset of symptoms, and ST elevation >1 mm in ≥2 limb leads or >2 mm in ≥2 precordial leads. Patients with cardiogenic shock, severe hypertension, or contraindication to thrombolytic therapy were excluded.
Follow-up	12 month clinical follow-up. Radionuclide left ventriculography 2-3 months (523 patients) and 12 months (492 patients) after randomization.
Treatment regimen	1. Coronary angiography within 48 h. Angioplasty was attempted for >50% residual stenosis. 2. Conservative management. Angiography was permitted for persisting or recurrent ischemia or after a positive exercise test.

Should We Intervene Following Thrombolysis?

(continued)

Additional therapy	Anistreplase 30 U IV over 5 min. Heparin infusion 1000 U/h was started 4-6 h later. Oral anticoagulation was optional. Oral ß blocker (timolol).
Results	43% of the early angiography group underwent angioplasty and 15% had coronary artery bypass grafting during the initial hospitalization. 3% of the conservative group had angioplasty and 2% bypass surgery. The median length of hospitalization was 11 and 10 days in the intervention and conservative groups (p<0.0001). 27% of the intervention group and 14% of the conservative group were in the hospital for >14 days. More patients in the conservative group underwent interventions during the 1 year follow-up. In-hospital mortality was 2.7% vs 3.3% in the conservative and intervention groups. 1 year mortality was 5.0% vs 5.8%, respectively (OR 1.18, 95% CI 0.64-2.10, p=0.64). In-hospital reinfarction occurred in 8.2% vs 12.1%, respectively, while reinfarction by 11 months was 15.1% vs 12.9% (OR 1.16, 95% CI 0.77-1.75, p=0.42). Angina at rest after 12 months occurred in 6.3% vs 3.4%, respectively (p=NS). The left ventricular ejection fraction at 2-3 and 12 months were comparable between the 2 groups.
Conclusions	There is no advantage for early routine intervention over a conservative approach following intravenous thrombolytic therapy for acute myocardial infarction.

1. Acute Myocardial Infarction

e. Remodeling After Infarction

SAVE

Survival and Ventricular Enlargement

Title	a. Rationale, design, and baseline characteristics of the survival and ventricular enlargement trial. b. Effect of captopril on mortality and morbidity in patients with left ventricular dysfunction after myocardial infarction. Results of the Survival and Ventricular Enlargement trial. c. Cardiovascular death and left ventricular remodeling 2 years after myocardial infarction. Baseline predictors and impact of long-term use of captopril: information from the survival and ventricular enlargement (SAVE) trial.
Authors	a. Moyé LA, Pfeffer MA, Braunwald E, et al. b. Pfeffer MA, Braunwald E, Moyé LA, et al. c. St. John Sutton M, Pfeffer MA, Moye L, et al.
Reference	a. Am J Cardiol 1991;68:70D-79D. b. N Engl J Med 1992;327:669-677. c. Circulation 1997; 96:3294-3299.
Disease	Acute myocardial infarction.
Purpose	To investigate whether captopril could reduce mortality and morbidity in patients with left ventricular dysfunction following myocardial infarction.
Design	Randomized, double blind, placebo-controlled, multicenter.
Patients	2231 patients, 21-80 years of age, 3-16 days after myocardial infarction with left ventricular ejection fraction ≤40%, but without active ischemia or overt heart failure.
Follow-up	Clinical follow-up for 24-60 months (average 42 months). Radionuclide ventriculogram at baseline and an average of 36 months later.

SAVE

Survival and Ventricular Enlargement

(continued)

Treatment regimen	Captopril (initial dose 12.5 mg, dose was increased gradually to 50 mg X3/d), or placebo.
Results	Total mortality was lower in the captopril group (20% vs 25%, risk reduction 19%, 95% CI 3-32%, p=0.019). The reduction of risk for cardiovascular mortality was 21% (95% CI 5-35%, p=0.014). The reduction in the risk of death from progressive heart failure was 36% (95% CI 4-58%, p=0.032). Progressive heart failure unresponsive to digitalis and diuretics developed in 11% of the captopril and 16% of the placebo patients (risk reduction 37%, 95% CI 20-50%, p<0.001). Recurrent myocardial infarction was experienced by 15.2% of the placebo and 11.9% of the captopril group (risk reduction 25%, 95% CI 5-40%, p=0.015). Deterioration of ≥9 U in left ventricular ejection fraction was detected in 16% of the placebo and 13% of the captopril group (p=0.17). c. A recent analysis obtained 2-D echocardiograms at 11 days and 1 and 2 years postinfarction. In 373 patients who had serial echocardiograms LV end-diastolic and end-systolic sizes increased from baseline to 2 years. While captopril reduced diastolic dilatation at 2 years (p=0.048) this effect was carried over from the first year of therapy. Increase in left ventricular size after 1 year were similar in captopril and placebo groups.
Conclusions	Long-term captopril therapy in patients with asymptomatic left ventricular dysfunction following acute myocardial infarction was associated with lower mortality and morbidity. These benefits were observed in patients who received thrombolytic therapy, aspirin, or ß blockers, as well as those who did not.

CONSENSUS II

Cooperative New Scandinavian Enalapril Survival Study II

Title	Effects of the early administration of enalapril on mortality in patients with acute myocardial infarction. Results of the Cooperative New Scandinavian Enalapril Survival Study II (CONSENSUS II).
Authors	Swedberg K, Held P, Kjekhus J, et al.
Reference	N Engl J Med 1992;327:678-684.
Disease	Acute myocardial infarction.
Purpose	To evaluate whether early administration of enalapril after acute myocardial infarction would reduce mortality during the 6 months follow-up.
Design	Randomized, double blind, placebo controlled, multicenter.
Patients	6090 patients within 24 h of onset of pain, with ST elevation in ≥ 2 leads, or new Q waves, or elevated levels of enzymes. Patients with supine blood pressure less than 105/65 mmHg were excluded.
Follow-up	41-180 days of follow-up.
Treatment regimen	IV infusion of 1mg enalapril at or placebo over 2h. If blood pressure declined <90/60 mmHg, the infusion was stopped temporarily. 6 h later, oral enalapril or placebo was started. The recommended starting dose was 2.5 mg X2/d with gradual increase up to 20 mg/d.
Additional therapy	Standard therapy including nitrates, ß blockers, calcium channel blockers, thrombolytic therapy, aspirin, anticoagulants, and diuretics, as indicated. If a patient needed angiotensin converting enzyme for heart failure, the patient was withdrawn from the study.

CONSENSUS II

Cooperative New Scandinavian Enalapril Survival Study II

(continued)

Results
The trial was terminated prematurely by the safety committee. By the end of the trial the mortality was 9.4% vs 10.2% in the placebo and enalapril groups (p=0.26). The mortality rates according to life-table analysis at 10 days and at 1, 3, and 6 months were 4.3% vs 4.6%, 6.3% vs 7.2%, 8.2% vs 9.1%, and 10.2% vs 11.0%, respectively (p=0.26). The relative risk associated with enalapril therapy was 1.10 (95% CI 0.93-1.29). Death due to progressive heart failure occurred in 3.4% and 4.3% of the placebo and enalapril groups, whereas there was no difference in sudden death; death due to myocardial rupture, or stroke. 30% of the placebo and 27% of the enalapril treated patients needed change of therapy due to heart failure (p<0.006). Reinfarction occurred in 9% of the patients in each group. Early hypotension (systolic blood pressure <90 mmHg, or diastolic blood pressure <50 mmHg) occurred in 3% of the control and 12% of the enalapril patients (p<0.001).

Conclusions
Enalapril therapy, started within 24 h of the onset of acute myocardial infarction, did not improve survival during the 180 days of follow-up.

AIRE

The Acute Infarction Ramipril Efficacy

Title	a. The acute infarction ramipril efficacy (AIRE) study: rationale, design, organization, and outcome definitions. b. Effect of ramipril on mortality and morbidity of survivors of acute myocardial infarction with clinical evidence of heart failure.
Authors	a. Hall AS, Winter C, Bogie SM, et al. b. The AIRE Study Investigators.
Reference	a. J Cardiovasc Pharmacol 1991;18(Suppl 2):S105-S109. b. Lancet 1993;342:821-828.
Disease	Acute myocardial infarction, heart failure.
Purpose	To determine whether early oral treatment with ramipril will reduce mortality in patients with heart failure complicating acute myocardial infarction.
Design	Randomized, double blind, placebo controlled, multicenter.
Patients	1986 patients, aged ≥18 years, with a definite myocardial infarction and signs of heart failure (even transient) in some period after the infarction. Patients with heart failure due to valvular heart disease, unstable angina, severe and resistant heart failure, or contraindications to angiotensin converting enzyme inhibition were excluded.
Follow-up	Clinical follow-up for >6 months (average 15 months).
Treatment regimen	3-10 days following infarction patients were randomized to receive ramipril 2.5 mg or placebo. The dose was increased to 5 mg X2/d (or 2.5 mg X2/d in case of intolerance).
Additional therapy	Patients could continue or begin any other medication except an angiotensin converting enzyme inhibitor.

The Acute Infarction Ramipril Efficacy

(continued)

Results	Total mortality was 17% in the ramipril and 23% in the placebo group (27% risk reduction, 95% CI 11%-40%, p=0.002). Separation of the survival curves occurred very early (within 30 days) and continued to diverge throughout the study. Severe heart failure developed in 14% vs 18%, respectively. There was no difference in the rates of stroke and reinfarction between the groups. Death, severe heart failure, myocardial infarction, or stroke developed in 28% vs 34% of the ramipril and placebo group (risk reduction 19%, 95% CI 5%-31%, p=0.008). Reported serious adverse events occurred in 58% of the ramipril vs 64% of the placebo. There was no difference in the occurrence of renal failure, angina, or syncope.
Conclusions	Ramipril therapy, started 3-10 days after infarction in patients with persistent or transient heart failure following infarction, resulted in reduction of mortality.

GISSI-3

Gruppo Italiano per lo Studio della Sopravvivenza nell'Infarto Miocardico III

Title	a. GISSI-3: effect of lisinopril and transdermal glyceryl trinitrate singly and together on 6 week mortality and ventricular function after acute myocardial infarction. b. 6 month effects of early treatment with lisinopril and transdermal glyceryl trinitrate singly and together withdrawn 6 weeks after acute myocardial infarction: the GISSI-3 trial. c. Effect of the ACE inhibitor lisinopril on mortality in diabetic patients with acute myocardial infarction. Data from the GISSI 3 study.
Authors	a. + b. GISSI. c. Zuanetti G, Latini R, Maggioni AP, et al.
Reference	a. Lancet 1994;343:1115-1122. b. J Am Coll Cardiol 1996;27:337-344. c. Circulation 1997; 96-4239-4245.
Disease	Acute myocardial infarction.
Purpose	To evaluate the efficacy of lisinopril, transdermal glyceryl trinitrate, and their combination on survival and left ventricular function following acute myocardial infarction.
Design	Randomized, open label, 2X2 factorial, multicenter.
Patients	18895 patients with chest pain, 24 h of onset of symptoms, and ST elevation or depression of ≥ 1 mm in ≥ 1 limb lead, or ≥ 2 mm in ≥ 1 precordial lead. Patients with severe heart failure, or contraindication to medications were excluded.
Follow-up	6 month clinical follow-up. Echocardiography at 6 weeks (14,209 patients).

GISSI-3

Treatment regimen	1. Oral lisinopril 5 mg at randomization and 10 mg/d for 6 weeks, or open control. 2. Glyceryl trinitrate (GTN) IV for 24 h, started at a rate of 5 µg/min and increased until systolic blood pressure fell by 10% or below 90 mmHg. >24 h transdermal GTN 10 mg/d for 14 h each day for 6 weeks, or placebo.
Additional therapy	Recommended therapy included thrombolysis (72% of the patients), oral aspirin (84%), and IV ß blockers (31%).
Results	a. + b. 13.3% of the control patients received non-study ACE inhibitors. The 6 week mortality was 6.3% and 7.1% in the lisinopril and control groups (OR 0.88, 95% CI 0.79-0.99, p=0.03). The survival curve separated on the first day and continued to diverge throughout the 6 weeks. The combined end point of mortality, heart failure beyond day 4 of infarction, left ventricular ejection fraction ≤35%, or ≥45% myocardial segments with abnormal motion occurred in 15.6% and 17.0% (OR 0.90, 95% CI 0.84-0.98, p=0.009). Rates of recurrent infarction, post-infarction angina, cardiogenic shock, and stroke were similar between the lisinopril and control groups. 57.1% of the patients that were not assigned to GTN received nitrates (11.3% for >5 days). GTN did not alter total mortality (6.5% vs 6.9%, p=0.28) or the combined end point (15.9% vs 16.7%, p=0.12). The GTN group had lower rate of post-infarction angina (20.0% vs 21.2%, OR 0.93, 95% CI 0.86-0.99, p=0.033), and cardiogenic shock (2.1.% vs 2.6%, OR 0.78, 95% CI 0.64-0.94, p=0.009). However, the rate of stroke was higher with GTN (0.9% vs 0.6%, p=0.027). After 6 months 18.1% vs 19.3% of the lisinopril and control groups developed severe left ventricular dysfunction or died (p=0.03), while 5.4% vs 5.8% developed clinical heart failure. No differences were found between patients with and without GTN, after 6 months. c. A recent retrospective analysis showed that in a subgroup of 2790 patients with diabetes that treatment with lisinopril decreased 6 week mortality (8.7% vs 12.4%) an effect that was greater (p=.025) than in nondiabetic patients. The effect was maintained at 6 months despite withdrawal from therapy at 6 weeks.

GISSI-3

Gruppo Italiano per lo Studio della Sopravvivenza nell'Infarto Miocardico III

(continued)

Conclusions   6 week lisinopril therapy reduced mortality and improved outcome after myocardial infarction. There is no evidence that GTN altered these outcomes significantly.
c. Early therapy with lisinopril in diabetic patients with acute myocardial infarction reduced 6-week mortality.

ISIS-4

International Study of Infarct Survival

Title	ISIS-4: a randomized factorial trial assessing early oral captopril, oral mononitrate, and intravenous magnesium sulphate in 58050 patients with suspected acute myocardial infarction.
Authors	ISIS-4 (4th International Study of Infarct Survival) Collaborative Group.
Reference	Lancet 1995;345:669-685.
Disease	Acute myocardial infarction.
Purpose	To assess the effects on major morbidity and 5-week mortality in patients with suspected acute myocardial infarction of early initiation of oral captopril, oral controlled-release mononitrate, and intravenous magnesium sulphate.
Design	Randomized double blind, placebo controlled (captopril and mononitrate); randomized (magnesium vs open control), multicenter.
Patients	58,050 patients with suspected infarction admitted within 24 h of onset of symptoms with no clear indications for, or contraindications to, the study medications. Patients that received nitrates for only a few days were included.
Follow-up	Clinical follow-up for 5 weeks (97% of the patients); 1 year (68% of the patients).

ISIS-4

International Study of Infarct Survival

(continued)

Treatment regimen	1. Patients were randomized to oral captopril or placebo (6.25 mg initially; 12.5 mg 2 h later; 25 mg 10-12 h later; and thereafter 50 mg BID for 28 days). 2. Patients received either oral mononitrate or placebo (30 mg upon randomization and after 10-12 h; 60 mg/d for 28 days). 3. Half the patients receive intravenous magnesium sulfate (8 mmol as a bolus over 15 min and then 72 mmol over 24 h).
Additional therapy	Antiplatelet therapy was recommended (received by 94% of patients). 70% of the patients received thrombolytic therapy.
Results	Analysis was by intention to treat. Captopril reduced 5-week mortality by 7% (95% CI of 13% - 1% reduction; p=0.02) (7.19% vs 7.69%, in the captopril and placebo groups, respectively). Mononitrate therapy did not alter 5-week mortality (7.34% vs 7.54% in the treated and control groups, respectively). Intravenous magnesium therapy did not reduce 5-week mortality (7.64% vs 7.24% in the magnesium and control groups, respectively).
Conclusions	Oral captopril, started early upon admission, reduces 5-week mortality in patients with suspected acute myocardial infarction. Oral mononitrate or intravenous magnesium sulfate did not reduce mortality.

SMILE

Survival of Myocardial Infarction Long-Term Evaluation

Title	The effect of the angiotensin-converting enzyme inhibitor zofenopril on mortality and morbidity after anterior myocardial infarction.
Authors	Ambrosioni E, Borghi C, Magnani B, for the Survival of Myocardial Infarction Long-Term Evaluation (SMILE) Study Investigators.
Reference	N Engl L Med 1995;332:80-85.
Disease	Anterior wall acute myocardial infarction.
Purpose	To evaluate whether 6 weeks of therapy with angiotensin-converting enzyme inhibitor zofenopril, started within 24 h after onset of infarction will improve short and long term outcome.
Design	Randomized, placebo-controlled, multicenter.
Patients	1556 patients with anterior wall acute myocardial infarction who did not receive reperfusion therapy (772 and 784 patients received zofenopril and placebo, respectively).
Follow-up	Clinical follow-up for 1-year.
Treatment regimen	Oral zofenopril 7.5 mg initially, and 12 h later. The dose was increased gradually to 30 mg BID if SBP>100 mmHg and there were no signs or symptoms of hypotension. Patients unable to tolerate the first dose were withdrawn from the study but included in the intention to treat analysis. Treatment was continued for 6 weeks.

SMILE

Survival of Myocardial Infarction Long-Term Evaluation

(continued)

Results
: 6 weeks after randomization, the zofenopril treated patients had a 46% reduction in the risk of severe congestive heart failure (95% CI 11-71%; p=0.018) and a 25% reduction in mortality rate (95% CI -11-60%; p=0.19). The incidence of severe heart failure and death were 4.1% and 6.5% for the placebo group and 2.2% and 4.9% for the zofenopril group, respectively. The 1 year mortality was lower in the zofenopril treated group (10.0%) than in the control (14.1%) (29% risk reduction; 95% CI 6-51%; p=0.011)

Conclusions
: 6 weeks of therapy with zofenopril, started within 24 h after onset of myocardial infarction, reduced 6 week and 1 year mortality and reduced the incidence of severe heart failure in patients with anterior wall acute myocardial infarction not receiving reperfusion therapy.

TRACE

Trandolapril Cardiac Evaluation

Title	A clinical trial of the angiotensin-converting enzyme inhibitor trandolapril in patients with left ventricular dysfunction after myocardial infarction.
Authors	Køber L, Torp-Pedersen C, Clarsen JE, et al.
Reference	N Engl J Med 1995;333:1670-1676.
Disease	Congestive heart failure, myocardial infarction.
Purpose	To determine whether patients with left ventricular dysfunction soon after myocardial infarction benefit from long-term oral ACE inhibition.
Design	Randomized, double blind, placebo-controlled, multicenter.
Patients	1749 patients, >18 years old, who survived acute myocardial infarction 2-6 days earlier. Only patients with echocardiographic proof of left ventricular dysfunction (wall-motion index ≤1.2) without contraindication or definite need for ACE inhibition were included.
Follow-up	24-50 months.
Treatment regimen	3-7 days after infarction patients were randomized to trandolapril 1 mg/d or placebo. The dose was gradually increased to 1-4 mg/d.
Additional therapy	Aspirin, ß blockers, calcium antagonists, diuretics, nitrates, and digoxin, as clinically indicated.

TRACE

Trandolapril Cardiac Evaluation

(continued)

Results   Total mortality after 4 years was 34.7% in the trandolapril group and 42.3% in the placebo group. The relative risk of death from any cause for the treated vs placebo groups was 0.78 (95% CI 0.67-0.91, p=0.001). The mortality curves diverged early and continued to diverge throughout the follow-up period. Cardiovascular death occurred in 25.8% and 33.0% of the trandolapril and placebo groups (RR 0.75, 95% CI 0.63-0.89, p=0.001). Trandolapril also reduced the rate of sudden death (RR 0.76, 95% CI 0.59-0.98, p=0.03) and the progression to severe heart failure (RR 0.71, 95% CI 0.56-0.89, p=0.003). There was a trend towards reduction of recurrent infarction with trandolapril (RR 0.86, 95% CI 0.66-1.13, p=0.29).

Conclusions   Long-term treatment with trandolapril in patients with left ventricular dysfunction soon after myocardial infarction reduces the rates of death, cardiovascular mortality, sudden death, and progression to severe heart failure.

CATS

Captopril And Thrombolysis Study

Title	a. Acute intervention with captopril during thrombolysis in patients with first anterior myocardial infarction. Results from the captopril and thrombolysis study (CATS). b. Which patient benefits from early angiotensin-converting enzyme inhibition after myocardial infarction? Results of 1 year serial echocardiographic follow-up from the captopril and thrombolysis study (CATS). c. Long-term anti-ischemic effects of angiotensin-converting enzyme inhibition in patients after myocardial infarction.
Authors	a. Kingma JH, van Gilst WH, Peels KH, et al. b. Van Gilst WH, Kingma H, Peels KH, et al. c. van den Heuvel, van Gilst, van Veldhuisen, et al.
Reference	a. Eur Heart J 1994;15:898-907. b. J Am Coll Cardiol 1996;28:114-121. c. J Am Coll Cardiol 1997;30:400-405.
Disease	Acute myocardial infarction.
Purpose	To evaluate the effects of early captopril therapy (within 6 h of onset of first anterior myocardial infarction) on left ventricular volume and clinical symptoms.
Design	Multicenter, randomized, double blind, placebo-controlled.
Patients	298 patients with first anterior acute myocardial infarction treated with streptokinase <6h of onset of symptoms. Patients with systolic blood pressure >200 or <100 mmHg or diastolic blood pressure >120 or <55 mmHg were excluded. Patients with renal insufficiency or intolerance to angiotensin-converting enzyme inhibitors, severe valvular heart disease, arrhythmias requiring antiarrhythmic therapy, serious systemic disease, AV conduction disturbances, or left bundle branch block were excluded.

CATS

Captopril And Thrombolysis Study
(continued)

Follow-up	12 months, clinical 24h ambulatory ECG monitoring, exercise test, and echocardiographic follow-up.
Treatment regimen	Immediately upon completion of streptokinase, captopril (6.25 mg) or placebo was given PO. The dose was repeated after 4 and 8h. Captopril 12.5 mg and 25 mg were given at 16h and 24h, respectively. If systolic blood pressure was <95 mmHg, the study medication was withheld until the next dosing time. The target dose was 25 mgX3/d.
Additional therapy	IV Streptokinase 1.5 million IU over 30 min. Aspirin, calcium antagonists and β-blockers were at the discretion of the local investigators.
Results	a+b. In the captopril group the number of patients with paired ventricular premature beats, accelerated idioventricular rhythm (AIVR) and nonsustained ventricular tachycardia (NSVT) were lower than in the placebo group. During the acute phase AIVR occurred in 33.8% vs 44.5%, in the captopril and placebo group (p<0.05), and NSVT in 31.7% vs 40.9%, respectively (p<0.05). Peak creatine kinase and cumulative α-hydroxybutyrate dehydrogenase release over 72h tended to be lower, and peak α-hydroxybutyrate dehydrogenase was lower in the captopril group than in the placebo group. A complete clinical follow-up over 1 year was obtained in 245 patients (82.2%). Analysis with the random coefficient model revealed no significant effect of captopril on changes in left ventricular volume over 12 months when compared with placebo. However, the occurrence of dilatation was lower in the captopril-treated group (p=0.018). Captopril was effective in reducing the occurrence of dilatation in medium size infarcts, tended to be effective in small infarcts, but was ineffective in large infarcts. The incidence of heart failure was lower in the captopril group (p<0.04). This effect was confined to patients with medium size infarctions.

Captopril And Thrombolysis Study
(continued)

Results	c. 244 patients underwent predischarge exercise test. After 3 months of therapy, exercise time increased equally in the placebo (86±13 s) and captopril group (69±12 s)(p=0.8). At 1 year exercise time increased further (by 13±11 s, and 33±13 s, respectively; p=0.7). Mean ST segment depression was comparable between the groups at 3 months and 12 months. During the 12 month treatment phase, 82 ischemic events were reported in the placebo group vs 52 in the captopril group (p=0.015). The number of ischemic events during the first 3 months of therapy were comparable, however, between 3 to 12 months 45 vs 21 events were detected in the placebo and captopril groups, respectively (p=0.009). Between 3-12 months 32% of the placebo vs 18% of the captopril treated patients experienced ischemic events (p=0.018). After 12 months, medications were withdrawn and both groups continued on single blind placebo for a month. During this month, 9 ischemic episodes were detected in the previous captopril treated group vs only 1 in the previous placebo group (p=0.006). 11 patients in the captopril vs only 1 in the placebo group needed antianginal medication after termination of the treatment phase (p=0.005).
Conclusions	Very early treatment with captopril reduces the occurrence of early dilatation and progression to heart failure, especially in patients with medium-size infarction. Captopril reduced the incidence of ischemia-related events after myocardial infarction. The effect became apparent only after 3 months of therapy. However, captopril did not alter exercise performance. After withdrawal from captopril therapy, a high incidence of ischemic events occurred.

AIREX

The Acute Infarction Ramipril Efficacy Extension Study

Title	Follow-up study of patients randomly allocated ramipril or placebo for heart failure after acute myocardial infarction: AIRE Extension (AIREX) Study.
Authors	Hall AS, Murray GD, Ball SG, on behalf of the AIREX Study Investigators.
Reference	Lancet 1997;349:1493-1497.
Disease	Acute myocardial infarction.
Purpose	To evaluate the long-term effects of ramipril therapy started early after acute myocardial infarction.
Design	Randomized, double blind, placebo-controlled, multicenter.
Patients	603 patients who participated in the AIRE study, aged ≥18 years, with a definite myocardial infarction and signs of heart failure (even transient) in some period after the infarction. Patients with heart failure due to valvular heart disease, unstable angina, severe and resistant heart failure, or contraindications to angiotensin-converting enzyme inhibition were excluded.
Follow-up	Follow-up for a minimum of 42 months and a mean of 59 months.

AIREX

The Acute Infarction Ramipril Efficacy Extension Study

(continued)

Treatment regimen	2-9 days following myocardial infarction patients were randomized to receive ramipril (n=302) 1.25 or 2.5 mg BID or placebo (n=301). The dose was increased to 5 mg BID (or 2.5 mg BID in case of intolerance). Randomized trial medications were given for an average of 13.4 months in the placebo group and 12.4 months in the ramipril group. Thereafter, trial medication was stopped in both groups and therapy with angiotensin-converting enzyme inhibitors was continued at the discretion of the attending physician.
Results	The average time from onset of myocardial infarction to therapy was 5 days in both groups. At hospital discharge 13.7% of the ramipril vs 5.3% of the placebo assigned patients were not receiving study medication. Withdrawal due to intolerance and refusal by the patients were more common in the ramipril group, whereas withdrawal because of severe heart failure was more common in the placebo group. All causes mortality was 38.9% in the placebo group and 27.5% in the ramipril group. The Kaplan-Meier survival curves separated early and continued to diverge over the first 2 years, and thereafter run parallel. The relative risk reduction 36% (95% CI 15-52%; p=0.002), and the absolute reduction in mortality was 11.4%.
Conclusions	The beneficial effects of ramipril started early after myocardial infarction in patients with heart failure were sustained over several years, despite discontinuation of the randomized study medication after approximately 1 year of therapy.

CCS-1

Chinese Cardiac Study

Title	Oral captopril vs placebo among 13634 patients with suspected acute myocardial infarction: interim report from the Chinese cardiac study (CCS-1).
Authors	Chinese Cardiac Study Collaborative Group.
Reference	Lancet 1995;345:686-687.
Disease	Acute myocardial infarction.
Purpose	To evaluate the effect of captopril therapy, started within 36 h of the onset of suspected acute myocardial infarction, on 4-week mortality.
Design	Randomized , placebo-controlled, multicenter.
Patients	13,634 patients with suspected acute myocardial infarction, within the first 36 h of onset of symptoms. Patients with hypotension or chronic use of large doses of diuretics were excluded.
Follow-up	4 weeks
Treatment regimen	Randomization to captopril (n=6814) or placebo (n=6820). Captopril was given at an initial dose of 6.25 mg, then 12.5 mg 2 h later, and then 12.5 mg TID
Additional therapy	Low dose aspirin was recommended.

Chinese Cardiac Study

(continued)

Results   88% of the captopril assigned and 91% of the placebo
               assigned patients completed the protocol or died earlier.
               Hypotension was the cause of discontinuation of treat-
               ment in 8.4% of the captopril and 4.9% of the placebo
               treated patients. Overall, 73% of the patients received
               aspirin, 27% thrombolytic therapy, 39% intravenous
               nitrates, and 20% diuretics. 4 week mortality was 9.05% in
               the captopril group vs 9.6% in the placebo group (p=NS).
               Persistent hypotension occurred in 16.3% and 10.8% of
               the captopril and placebo groups, respectively
               (p<0.0001). There was no difference in the rates of heart
               failure, ventricular fibrillation, other cardiac arrest, or
               advanced heart block. However, there was a nonsignifi-
               cant excess of cardiogenic shock with captopril (4.8% vs
               4.2%; p=NS). Among patients with admission systolic
               blood pressure <100 mmHg, 4 week mortality was 11.0%
               in the captopril group vs 10.0% in the placebo group.
               Among patients with systolic blood pressure 100-104
               mmHg, mortality was 11.4% vs 12.4%, respectively.

Conclusions   Captopril therapy, initiated within 36 h of onset of acute
               myocardial infarction, was associated with a non signifi-
               cant reduction in 4 week mortality and excess of hypoten-
               sion. Among patients with entry systolic blood pressure
               <100 mmHg captopril may be hazardous, but in those
               with mild hypotension and in normotensive patients early
               initiation of captopril may be relatively safe.

CEDIM

The L-Carnitine Echocardiografia Digitalizzata Infarto Miocardico

Title	Effects of L-carnitine administration on left ventricular remodeling after acute anterior myocardial infarction: The L-Carnitine Echocardiografia Digitalizzata Infarto Miocardico (CEDIM) trial.
Authors	Iliceto S, Scrutinio D, Bruzzi P, et al.
Reference	J Am Coll Cardiol 1995;26:380-387.
Disease	Acute myocardial infarction.
Purpose	To assess the effects of L-carnitine on left ventricular remodeling after anterior acute myocardial infarction.
Design	Randomized, double blind, placebo-controlled, multicenter.
Patients	472 patients, ≤80 years old, with a first anterior acute myocardial infarction, within 24 h of onset of infarction, and high quality 2-D echocardiograms. Patients with valvular, congenital heart disease, or cardiomyopathy were excluded.
Follow-up	12 months with repeated 2-D echocardiograms.
Treatment regimen	Randomization to L-carnitine (n=233) or placebo (n=239) within 24 h of onset of symptoms. L-carnitine was administered by continuous intravenous infusion at a dose of 9 g/d for the first 5 days and then 2 g TID orally for 12 months.

CEDIM

The L-Carnitine Echocardiografia Digitalizzata Infarto Miocardico

(continued)

Addtional therapy	Angiotensin-converting enzyme inhibitors were not recommended at the time of the study and were used by only 8% of patients. 78% of patients received thrombolytic therapy.
Results	348 patients had paired echocardiograms and were entered into the final analysis. Left ventricular end systolic and end diastolic volumes were significantly smaller at 3, 6, and 12 months after myocardial infarction in the L-carnitine treated patients than in the placebo group. On discharge, left ventricular end diastolic volume (LVEDV) was 90.9±2.33 ml in the L-carnitine group and 91.7±2.03 ml in the placebo group (p=0.15). After 12 months LVEDV was 99.3±2.06 ml and 105.4±2.37 ml, respectively (adjusted difference -7.23 ml; p=0.01). Discharge left ventricular end systolic volume (LVESV) was 47.8±1.16 ml and 48.8±1.53 ml, respectively (p=0.13). After the first year LVESV was 55.0±1.63 ml and 58.9±1.75 ml in the L-carnitine and placebo groups, respectively (adjusted difference -4.49 ml; p=0.03). Left ventricular ejection fraction at discharge was 48.1±0.47% and 48.1±0.52%, respectively (p=0.83). After 12 months it was 45.8±0.57% and 45.2±0.52% (adjusted difference +0.52%; p=0.46). In-hospital mortality was 4.7% in the L-carnitine group vs 5.9% in the placebo group (p=NS), whereas 1 year mortality was 4.3% vs 5.4%, respectively (p=NS). Heart failure during the first year developed in 1.7% of the L-carnitine group vs 4.2% in the placebo group (p=NS). However, there was no difference in the rates of unstable angina, reinfarction, coronary artery bypass surgery, or coronary angioplasty. In none of the patients, therapy was discontinued because of adverse events.
Conclusions	L-carnitine therapy for 12 months attenuated left ventricular remodeling and prevented dilatation in patients with first anterior acute myocardial infarction, without apparent adverse effects or increasing mortality and morbidity. However, no effect on left ventricular ejection fraction was detected.

Healing and Early Afterload Reducing Therapy

Title	Early vs delayed angiotensin-converting enzyme inhibition therapy in acute myocardial infarction. The Healing and Early Afterload Reducing Therapy Trial.
Author	Pfeffer MA, Greaves SC, Arnold JMO, et al.
Reference	Circulation 1997; 95:2643-2651.
Disease	Coronary artery disease, acute myocardial infarction.
Purpose	To determine the safety and efficacy of early (day 1) vs delayed (day 14) initiation of the angiotensin-converting enzyme inhibitor ramipril on echocardiographic measures of left ventricular dilatation and ejection fraction.
Design	Double blind, randomized, multicenter.
Patients	352 patients with anterior myocardial infarction.
Follow-up	14, 90 days.
Treatment regimen	Group 1 - early placebo, late full dose 10 mg ramipril; Group II - early low dose, late low dose [0.625 mg]; and Group III - early full dose and late full dose [10 mg]. Early treatment represented day 1-14; late 14-90 days.

Results	Early low dose did not alter clinical events. The risk of a systolic arterial pressure less than or equal to 90 mmHg during the first 14 days was greater in both ramipril groups. While LV ejection fraction increased in all groups during the early period, the full dose ramipril group had the greatest improvement in ejection fraction (+4.9% in full dose; 3.9% in low and, 2.4% in delayed, $p<.05$ for trend). The early full dose ramipril group was the only group that did not show an increase in LV diastolic area. At 6 months, only the group that received ramipril for the first time during the later period (placebo to full dose) showed improvement in wall motion. When all groups were on active therapy during the late phase, there was no further increase in diastolic area. Patients who were on placebo and then received full dose ramipril showed a trend toward decrease in LV end-systolic area and improvement in ejection fraction during the late phase.
Conclusions	In patients with acute anterior myocardial infarction early use of ramipril (titrated to 10 mg) attenuated LV remodeling and resulted in prompter recovery of LV ejection fraction.

1. Acute Myocardial Infarction

f. Miscellaneous and Adjunctive Therapy

TIMI 2-B

Thrombolysis in Myocardial Infarction Trial (phase 2B)

Title	a. Comparison of invasive and conservative strategies after treatment with intravenous tissue plasminogen activator in acute myocardial infarction. Results of the Thrombolysis in Myocardial Infarction (TIMI) Phase II Trial. b. Immediate vs deferred ß-blockade following thrombolytic therapy in patients with acute myocardial infarction. Results of the Thrombolysis in Myocardial Infarction (TIMI) II-B Study.
Authors	a. The TIMI Study Group. b. Roberts R, Rogers WJ, Mueller HS, et al.
Reference	a. N Engl J Med 1989;320:618-627. b. Circulation 1991;83:422-437.
Disease	Acute myocardial infarction.
Purpose	To compare the effects of immediate vs delayed (6 days) metoprolol therapy in patients with acute myocardial infarction treated with rt-PA (a substudy of the TIMI-2 Trial).
Design	Randomized, open label, multicenter study.
Patients	2948 patients with acute myocardial infarction <76 years old < 4 hours from onset of symptoms with chest pain>30 min and ST elevation ≥0.1 mV in ≥2 contiguous leads, of whom 1434 (49%) were eligible for ß-blocker therapy.
Follow-up	Predischarge radionuclide ventriculography at rest and during exercise. At 6 weeks clinical evaluation and maximal exercise test + radionuclide ventriculography. 1 year follow-up.

TIMI 2-B

Thrombolysis in Myocardial Infarction Trial (phase 2B)

(continued)

Treatment regimen	Immediate therapy: 3 IV injections of 5 mg metoprolol, and then 50 mg X2/d PO for 1 day and 100 mg X2/d thereafter. Delayed therapy: on day 6, 50 mg X2/d PO for 1 day and then 100 mg X2/d.
Additional therapy	Intravenous rt-PA (150 mg over 6 h for the first 520 patients, and 100 mg in the remaining 2742 patients). Lidocaine (1-1.5 mg/kg bolus + infusion 2-4 mg/min) for >24 h; heparin 5000 U bolus and infusion 1000 U/h for 5 days, and then subcutaneous until discharge. Aspirin 80 mg/d for 6 days and then 325 mg/d.
Results	The systolic blood pressure in the immediate group decreased during the first hour by 9.8% compared with 7.1% in the deferred therapy group (P<0.01). Mean heart rate decreased by 6% in the immediate group and increased in the deferred group (P<0.001). There was no difference in the occurrence of arrhythmias between the groups. Left ventricular ejection fraction was similar in both groups at predischarge (51.0% vs 50.1%) and at 6 weeks (50.4% and 50.8%, respectively). Regional ventricular function was also comparable. Overall, there was no difference in mortality between the groups. However, in the low risk patients 6 weeks mortality was 0 and 2.8% in the immediate and deferred ß-blocker therapy groups (p=0.007). Reinfarction was less common at 6 days and 6 weeks in the immediate treated group. However, there was no difference at 1 year.
Conclusions	ß-blockers are safe when given early after thrombolytic therapy to a selected population with acute myocardial infarction and are associated with lower risk of recurrent ischemia and reinfarction in the first week. However, long term prognosis and left ventricular function are similar to those who receive ß-blockers only after 6 days.

DAVIT II

The Danish Verapamil Infarction Trial II

Title	Effect of verapamil on mortality and major events after acute myocardial infarction (the Danish Verapamil Infarction Trial II- DAVIT II).
Authors	The Danish Study Group on Verapamil in Myocardial Infarction.
Reference	Am J Cardiol 1990;66:779-785.
Disease	Acute myocardial infarction.
Purpose	To assess whether long term therapy with verapamil, started from the second week after acute myocardial infarction will reduce mortality and morbidity compared with placebo.
Design	Randomized, double blind, placebo-controlled, multicenter.
Patients	1775 patients, <76 years old, 7-15 days after proven acute myocardial infarction. Patients with severe heart failure, hypotension, atrioventricular or sinoatrial blocks, or therapy with calcium channel or ß blockers due to angina, arrhythmia, or hypertension were excluded.
Follow-up	Clinical follow-up up to 18 months (mean 16 months).
Treatment regimen	Verapamil 120 mg X3/d (in cases of adverse drug reactions 120 mg X1-2/d was allowed) or placebo.
Additional therapy	Therapy with calcium channel blockers or ß blockers was not permitted. Nitrates were allowed.

DAVIT II

The Danish Verapamil Infarction Trial II

(continued)

Results
1 month after randomization 38.7% of the placebo and 33.2% of the verapamil group reported angina (p=0.02). However, after 12 months, the difference did not reach statistical significance (33.7% vs 28.6%).There was a trend towards reduction of total mortality (11.1% vs 13.8%, Hazard ratio (HR) 0.80, 95% CI 0.61-1.05, p=0.11), and a significant reduction of death or first reinfarction (18.0% vs 21.6%, HR 0.80, 95% CI 0.64-0.99, p=0.03) at 18 months with verapamil. In patients without heart failure during hospitalization, verapamil was associated with lower mortality (7.7% vs 11.8%, HR 0.64, 95% CI 0.44-0.94, p=0.02) and reinfarction (9.4% vs 12.7%, HR 0.67, 95% CI 0.46-0.97, p=0.02), while there was no difference in mortality (17.5% vs 17.9%) or reinfarction (14.3% vs 14.2%) between the groups in patients with heart failure during hospitalization.

Conclusions
Long-term verapamil therapy after an acute myocardial infarction resulted in reduction of mortality and reinfarction, but only in patients without heart failure.

Cardiac event rates after acute myocardial infarction in patients treated with verapamil and trandolapril vs trandolapril alone.

Title	Cardiac event rates after acute myocardial infarction in patients treated with verapamil and trandolapril vs trandolapril alone.
Author	Hansen JF, Hagerup L, Sigurd B, et al, for the Danish Verapamil Infarction Trial (DAVIT) Study Group.
Reference	Am J Cardiol 1997; 79: 738-741.
Disease	Acute myocardial infarction.
Purpose	To determine whether verapamil given to post-myocardial infarct patients with congestive heart failure, already on diuretics and angiotensin-converting enzyme inhibitor, would further reduce cardiac event rates.
Design	Randomized, double blind, multicenter study.
Patients	100 patients with acute myocardial infarction, congestive heart failure, on a diuretic.
Follow-up	3 months.
Treatment regimen	Patients were consecutively randomized to trandolapril 1 mg/day for 1 month and 2 mg/day for the following 2 months; or to trandolapril as above plus verapamil 240 mg/day for 1 month and 360 mg/day for 2 months. Trial medicines were begun 3 - 10 days after myocardial infarction.

Cardiac event rates after acute myocardial infarction in patients treated with verapamil and trandolapril vs trandolapril alone.

(continued)

Results
:   The primary combined end-point was of death, reinfarction, unstable angina, and readmission due to worsening congestive heart failure. 3 month event rates were 35% in the trandolapril group vs 14% in the trandolapril - verapamil group (hazard ratio 0.35; 95% CI = 0.15 -0.85, p = 0.015). Event rates of combined death, reinfarction, or unstable angina were 29% in the trandolapril group vs 10% in the trandolapril - verapamil group (hazard ratio 0.31; 95% CI - 0.11 - 0.86, p =0.018).

Conclusions
:   Verapamil reduced combined cardiac event rates when added to an ACE inhibitor in post-myocardial infarction patients with heart failure.

LIMIT-2

Leicester Intravenous Magnesium Intervention II Trial

Title	Intravenous magnesium sulphate in suspected acute myocardial infarction: results of the second Leicester Intravenous Magnesium Intervention Trial (LIMIT-2).
Authors	Woods KL, Fletcher S, Roffe C, Haider Y.
Reference	Lancet 1992;339:1553-1558.
Disease	Acute myocardial infarction.
Purpose	To evaluate the efficacy of intravenous magnesium sulphate infusion in reduction of early mortality following acute myocardial infarction.
Design	Randomized, double blind, placebo-controlled, unicenter.
Patients	2316 patients with suspected acute myocardial infarction (within 24 h of onset of symptoms). No electrocardiographic criteria were specified.
Follow-up	28 days clinical follow-up.
Treatment regimen	Saline or magnesium sulphate 8 mmol over 5 min followed by 65 mmol over 24 h.
Additional therapy	No restriction. Thrombolytic therapy was not required.

LIMIT-2

Leicester Intravenous Magnesium Intervention II Trial

(continued)

Results

Acute myocardial infarction was confirmed in 65% of the patients. 36% vs 35% of the magnesium and placebo patients received thrombolytic therapy, while 65% vs 66% received aspirin. 28 day mortality was 10.3% in the placebo and 7.8% in the magnesium group (odds ratio 0.74, 95% CI 0.55-1.00, p=0.04). Mortality odds ratios were 0.76 (95% CI 0.46-1.27) in the patients that received thrombolytic therapy and 0.72 (95% CI 0.49-0.99) for those who did not receive thrombolytic therapy. The incidence of clinical left ventricular failure was 11.2% in the magnesium and 14.9% in the placebo group (25% risk reduction, 95% CI 7%-39%, p=0.009). The prevalence of hypotension <100 mmHg for ≥1 h was similar. Sinus bradycardia was more common with magnesium (10.8% vs 8.0%, p=0.02). However, the incidence of AV block and tachyarrhythmias were similar.

Conclusions

Intravenous magnesium sulphate is a simple and safe therapy for acute myocardial infarction and was associated with reduction of mortality.

ESPRIM

European Study of Prevention of Infarct with Molsidomine.

Title	The ESPRIM trial: short-term treatment of acute myocardial infarction with molsidomine.
Authors	European Study of Prevention of Infarct with Molsidomine (ESPRIM) Group.
Reference	Lancet 1994;344:91-97.
Disease	Acute myocardial infarction.
Purpose	To compare the effects of molsidomine (a nitric oxide donor) with placebo in patients with acute myocardial infarction.
Design	Randomized, double blind, placebo-controlled, multicenter.
Patients	4017 patients with suspected acute myocardial infarction (chest pain >30 min, with onset <24 h). Patients in Killip class III or IV were excluded.
Follow-up	An average of 13 months clinical follow-up.
Treatment regimen	Molsidomine (IV linsidomine (the active metabolite of molsidomine) 1 mg/h for 48 h, followed by oral molsidomine 4 mg X4/d for 12 days. The control group received matching placebo.
Additional therapy	Non-study vasodilator therapy could be added by the physician. No limitation on additional therapy.

ESPRIM

European Study of Prevention of Infarct with Molsidomine.

(continued)

Results
48.5% of the molsidomine and 51.0% of the placebo received thrombolytic therapy before randomization, and 21.7% vs 20.0% after randomization. 35 day mortality was similar (8.4% vs 8.8% in the molsidomine and placebo groups, RR 0.96, 95% CI 0.78-1.17, p=0.66). There was no difference in long-term mortality 14.7% vs 14.2% in the molsidomine and placebo groups, respectively (p=0.67). The rates of the major and minor adverse events were similar, except for headache which was more common with the molsidomine group.

Conclusions
Nitric oxide donor was not effective in reduction of mortality following acute myocardial infarction.

TAMI-9

Thrombolysis and Angioplasty in Myocardial Infarction 9 Trial

Title	Intravenous fluosol in the treatment of acute myocardial infarction. Results of the thrombolysis and angioplasty in myocardial infarction 9 trial.
Authors	Wall TC, Califf RM, Blankenship J, et al.
Reference	Circulation 1994;90:114-120.
Disease	Acute myocardial infarction.
Purpose	To assess the efficacy of fluosol as an adjunctive therapy to reperfusion for acute myocardial infarction.
Design	Randomized, open label, multicenter.
Patients	430 patients, age >18 and <75 years, with suspected acute myocardial infarction <6 h of onset of symptoms, with ≥1 mm ST elevation in ≥2 leads.
Follow-up	Cardiac angiography and symptom-limited stress thallium scan 5-14 days after infarction. In-hospital clinical follow-up.
Treatment regimen	IV fluosol 1 ml/min, the rate was increased gradually to 20 ml/min. Total dose 15 ml/kg.
Additional therapy	Chewable aspirin 324 mg, IV heparin, and 100 mg tissue plasminogen activator over 3 h, 100% oxygen for 8 h. IV atenolol if no contraindications existed.

TAMI-9

Thrombolysis and Angioplasty in Myocardial Infarction 9 Trial

(continued)

Results	There was no significant difference between the control and fluosol groups in left ventricular ejection fraction (52% vs 51%), regional wall motion analysis (-2.2 SD/chord vs -2.4 SD/chord), or infarct size as measured by thallium scan. The analysis of anterior wall infarction yielded similar results. Patency rates of the infarct related arteries were similar. Rates of death (3.7% vs 5.6%) and stroke (0.9% vs 4.3%) were similar in the control and fluosol groups. However, the fluosol group experienced less recurrent infarction (4.2% vs 2.4%), but more heart failure and pulmonary edema (31% vs 45%; p=0.004). There was no difference in hemorrhagic complications.
Conclusions	Fluosol, as an adjunctive therapy to thrombolysis did not result in reduction of infarct size or improvement of left ventricular function and clinical outcome.

DIGAMI

Diabetes Mellitus Insulin-Glucose Infusion in Acute Myocardial Infarction

Title	a. Randomized trial of insulin-glucose infusion followed by subcutaneous insulin treatment in diabetic patients with acute myocardial infarction (DIGAMI study): effects on mortality at 1 year. b. Prospective randomized study of intensive insulin treatment on long-term survival after acute myocardial infarction in patients with diabetes mellitus.
Authors	a. Malmberg K, Rydén L, Efendic S, et al. b. Malmberg K for the DIGAMI Study Group.
Reference	a. J Am Coll Cardiol 1995;26:57-65. b. BMJ 1997;314:1512-1515.
Disease	Acute myocardial infarction, diabetes mellitus.
Purpose	a. To evaluate whether insulin-glucose infusion followed by multidose insulin therapy will decrease mortality in diabetic patients with acute myocardial infarction. b. To assess the long-term outcome of intensive insulin therapy begun at the time of an acute myocardial infarction in patients with diabetes mellitus.
Design	Randomized, open label, multicenter.
Patients	a. 620 patients with diabetes mellitus and a blood glucose level>11 mmol/l and with suspected acute myocardial infarction (chest pain of ≥15 min, ≤24 h of onset of symptoms).
Follow-up	a. 1 year. b. 3.4 years.

DIGAMI

Diabetes Mellitus Insulin-Glucose Infusion in Acute Myocardial Infarction

(continued)

Treatment regimen	Insulin-glucose or placebo infusion over ≥24 h, then SC insulin X4/d for ≥3 months.
Additional therapy	Thrombolytic therapy, if no contraindications existed and patients were admitted within 6 h of onset of symptoms. IV followed by oral metoprolol, if not contraindicated.
Results	a. Blood glucose decreased from 15.4±4.1–9.6±3.3 mmol/l in the infusion group over the first 24 h, and from 15.7±4.2–11.7±4.1 mmol/l among the control patients (p<0.0001). In-hospital mortality was 9.1% in the insulin vs 11.1% in the control group (p=NS). 1 year mortality was 18.6% vs 26.1%, respectively (relative risk reduction 29%, 95% CI 4%-51%, p=0.0273).The reduction in mortality was particularly evident in low risk patients and with no previous insulin therapy (3 month mortality 6.5% in the insulin vs 13.5% in the control, relative risk reduction 52%, p=0.046; 1 year mortality 8.6% vs 18.0%, respectively, relative risk reduction 52%, p=0.020). b.At 1 year fewer deaths (19%) occurred in the intensive insulin group vs the standard treatment group (26%; p =0.027). At 3.4 years the difference between groups persisted (33% vs 44%, p =0.011).
Conclusions	a. Insulin glucose infusion followed by a multidose insulin therapy improved 1 year survival in diabetic patients after acute myocardial infarction. b. Insulin-glucose infusion followed by 3 months of multiple dose insulin reduced mortality long-term in acute myocardial infarction patients with diabetes.

CRIS

Calcium antagonist Reinfarction Italian Study

Title	A controlled trial of verapamil in patients after acute myocardial infarction: results of the calcium antagonist reinfarction Italian study (CRIS).
Authors	Rengo F, Carbonin P, Pahor M, et al.
Reference	Am J Cardiol 1996;77:365-369.
Disease	Acute myocardial infarction.
Purpose	To evaluate the effects of verapamil on total mortality, cardiac mortality, reinfarction, and recurrent angina after an acute myocardial infarction.
Design	Randomized, double blind, placebo-controlled, multicenter.
Patients	1073 patients, age 30 - 75 years, who survived 5 days following an acute myocardial infarction. Patients with severe heart failure, Wolf-Parkinson-White syndrome, cardiac surgery, implanted pacemaker, right ventricular failure with pulmonary hypertension, concomitant severe disease, contraindication to verapamil, heart rate <50 beats/min, hypotension or hypertension, and chronic therapy with β blockers or calcium channel blockers were excluded.
Follow-up	mean follow-up 23.5 months.
Treatment regimen	7–21 days (mean 13.8 days) after myocardial infarction patients were randomized to placebo or verapamil retard 120 mgX3/d

CRIS

Calcium antagonist Reinfarction Italian Study

(continued)

Results

Study medication was discontinued before completion of follow-up in 36.9% of the placebo group and 35.6% of the verapamil group. Intention to treat analysis revealed no difference in mortality (5.4% vs 5.6%), cardiac mortality (4.1% vs 4.0%;), and sudden death (1.8% vs 2.1%), in the placebo and verapamil group, respectively. There was a trend toward less reinfarction in the verapamil group (7.3% vs 9.0%; relative risk (RR) 0.81; 95% CI 0.53-1.24). Verapamil therapy was also associated with a nonsignificant reduction in the rates of first major event (death or reinfarction, 9.0% vs 10.3%; RR 0.87; 95% CI 0.59-1.29), and first cardiac event (cardiac death, reinfarction, or hospital admission for chest pain, 15.4% vs 19.2%; RR 0.79; 95% CI 0.59-1.05). Less patients in the verapamil group developed angina (18.8% vs 24.3%; RR 0.8; 95% CI 0.5 to 0.9; p<0.05).

Conclusions

Verapamil therapy following myocardial infarction was not associated with reduced mortality. However, it was associated with less angina and a trend toward less reinfarction.

EMIAT

The European Myocardial Infarct Amiodarone Trial

Title	Randomised trial of effect of amiodarone on mortality in patients with left-ventricular dysfunction after recent myocardial infarction: EMIAT
Author	Julian DG, Camm AJ, Frangin G, et al.
Reference	Lancet 1997;349:667-674.
Disease	Acute myocardial infarction.
Purpose	To assess the efficacy of amiodarone on reduction of mortality of patients with left ventricular dysfunction following myocardial infarction.
Design	Randomized, double blind, placebo-controlled, multicenter.
Patients	1486 patients, 18-75 years old, 5-21 days (mean 15±3.9 days) after acute myocardial infarction with left ventricular ejection fraction <40%. Patients with contraindications to amiodarone, amiodarone therapy within 6 months, bradycardia <50 bpm, advanced atrioventricular block, hepatic disease, thyroid dysfunction, long QT syndrome, severe angina or heart failure, a likelihood of cardiac surgery, and those requiring active antiarrhythmic medications were excluded.
Follow-up	Clinical follow-up for 12 to 24 months (median 21 months). 24 h Holter ECG monitoring at baseline and after 2 weeks and 4 months.
Treatment regimen	Placebo or amiodarone (800 mg/d for 14 days, 400 mg/d for 14 weeks, and then 200 mg/d).
Additional therapy	β blockers and digoxin were permitted

EMIAT

The European Myocardial Infarct Amiodarone Trial

(continued)

Results

743 patients were included in each group. All cause mortality was similar (103 patients in the amiodarone group vs 103 in the placebo patients; risk ratio (RR) 0.99; 95% CI 0.76-1.31; p=0.96). Cardiac mortality was comparable (85 vs 89 patients, respectively; RR 0.94; 95% CI 0.70-1.26; p=0.67). However, arrhythmic deaths (33 vs 50 patients; RR 0.65; 95% CI 0.42-1.00; p=0.05) and arrhythmic death and resuscitated cardiac arrest (42 vs 61 patients; RR 0.68; 95% CI 0.46-1.00; p=0.05) were less common in the amiodarone than the placebo group. However, death from reinfarction occurred in 10 amiodarone treated patients vs only 3 of the placebo treated patients. Noncardiac mortality occurred in 18 of the amiodarone vs 13% of the placebo patients (RR 1.37; 95% CI 0.67-2.79). In intention-to-treat analysis of the 548 patients with arrhythmias at baseline, there was no statistically significant difference between the amiodarone and placebo groups concerning arrhythmic death, but there was reduction in the occurrence of the combined end-point of arrhythmic deaths and resuscitated cardiac deaths in the amiodarone group (p=0.048). During the trial, 38.5% of the amiodarone vs 21.4% of the placebo group discontinued the study medication. Clinical hypothyroidism occurred in 1.5% vs 0% of the amiodarone and placebo groups, whereas hyperthyroidism in 1.6% vs 0.5%, respectively. Pulmonary disorders occurred in 5.2% vs 4.0%, respectively.

Conclusions

Amiodarone therapy in survivors of myocardial infarction with left ventricular dysfunction was not associated with reduction of total mortality or cardiac mortality during a median follow-up of 21 months. However, the reduction in arrhythmic death and the apparent lack of proarrhythmic effect support the use of amiodarone in patients with ischemic heart disease and left ventricular dysfunction for whom antiarrhythmic therapy is indicated.

CAMIAT

Canadian Amiodarone Myocardial Infarction Arrhythmia Trial

Title	Randomized trial of outcome after myocardial infarction in patients with frequent or repetitive ventricular premature depolarisations: CAMIAT
Authors	Cairns JA, Connolly SJ, Roberts R, et al.
Reference	Lancet 1997;349:675-682.
Disease	Acute myocardial infarction.
Purpose	To assess the efficacy of amiodarone on reduction of the risk of resuscitated ventricular fibrillation or arrhythmic death among patients with left ventricular dysfunction following myocardial infarction with frequent or repetitive ventricular premature depolarizations.
Design	Randomized, double blind, placebo-controlled, multicenter.
Patients	1202 patients, >19 years old, 6-45 days after myocardial infarction, with a mean of 10 ventricular premature depolarizations per h or more by 24 h ambulatory ECG monitoring, or ≥1 run of ventricular tachycardia. Patients with contraindications to amiodarone; bradycardia (<50 bpm); atrioventricular block; QTc >480 ms; peripheral neuropathy; liver disease; pulmonary fibrosis; asthma; thyroid disease; need for antiarrhythmic therapy; therapy with tricyclic antidepressants, phenytoin, or sotalol; severe congestive heart failure; hypotension or angina; and patients with life expectancy of <2 years were excluded.
Follow-up	Repeated 24 h ambulatory ECG monitoring at baseline, 4, 8, 12 and 16 months. Clinical follow-up for 1 to 2 years (mean 1.79±0.44 years).
Treatment regimen	Placebo or amiodarone (a loading dose of 10 mg/kg in 2 divided daily doses for 2 weeks, then 400 mg/d. Patients older than 75 years and those who weighed <60 kg received 300 mg/d). If arrhythmia suppression was detected, the dose was reduced to 200-300 mg/d at month 4 and to 200 mg/d for 5-7 days/week at month 8.

CAMIAT

Canadian Amiodarone Myocardial Infarction Arrhythmia Trial (continued)

Results
There were 606 patients in the amiodarone group and 596 in the placebo group. 24 h ambulatory ECG monitoring at month 4 revealed arrhythmia suppression in 84% of the amiodarone group vs 35% of the placebo group, and at month 8 in 86% vs 39%, respectively. The mean percentage of the study drug being taken at each follow-up visit was 75% and 78% in the amiodarone and placebo groups. Only 6% of the patients in each group took <50% of the study medication. 221 (36.4%) patients of the amiodarone group vs 152 (25.5%) of the placebo group discontinued taking study medication for reasons other than outcome events (p<0.0005). Adverse effects resulting in discontinuation of study medication occurred in 159 (26.2%) patients of the amiodarone vs 82 (13.7%) patients in the placebo group (p<0.0005). Hypothyroidism was found in 3.3% vs 0.2%, respectively (p<0.0005). Proarrhythmia (0.3% vs 3.0%; p=0.002) and ventricular tachyarrhythmia (0.7% vs 2.0%; p=0.004) occurred less often in the amiodarone treated patients. Efficacy analysis revealed that the estimated risk of resuscitated ventricular fibrillation or arrhythmic death at 24 months was 1.77% per year for the amiodarone vs 3.38% per year for the placebo groups (48.5% relative-risk reduction; 95% CI 4.5 to 72.2%; p=0.018). 37 vs 50 patients of the amiodarone and placebo group died (rate per year for all-cause mortality 4.36% vs 5.42%; relative-risk reduction 21.2%; 95% CI -20.6% to 48.5%; p=0.136). 30 vs 44 patients of the amiodarone and placebo group died from cardiac causes (rate per year 3.53% vs 4.77%; relative-risk reduction 27.4%; 95% CI -15.5% to 54.4%; p=0.087). Intention-to-treat analysis revealed reduction in the risk for resuscitated ventricular fibrillation or arrhythmic death (relative-risk reduction 38.2%; 95% CI -2.1% to 62.6%; p=0.029); arrhythmic death (29.3%; 95% CI -19.6% to 58.2%; p=0.097); cardiac mortality (22.0%; 95% CI -15.9% to 47.6%; p=0.108); and total mortality (18.3%; 95% CI -16.1% to 42.6%; p=0.129). The cumulative rates of nonarrhythmic death were comparable (5.8% in the amiodarone group vs 6.2% in the placebo group; p=0.70).

Conclusions
Amiodarone therapy in survivors of myocardial infarction with frequent or repetitive ventricular premature depolarizations was associated with reduction of ventricular fibrillation or arrhythmic death. No proarrhythmic effect was observed. However, adverse effects mandating discontinuation of amiodarone were relatively common.

Beneficial effects of intravenous and oral carvedilol
treatment in acute myocardial infarction.
A placebo-controlled, randomized trial.

Title	Beneficial effects of intravenous and oral carvedilol treatment in acute myocardial infarction. A placebo-controlled, randomized trial.
Author	Basu, S. Senior R, Raval U, et al.
Reference	Circulation 1997; 96:183-191.
Disease	Coronary artery disease. Acute myocardial infarction.
Purpose	To determine the effects of acute and long-term treatment of acute myocardial infarction with the beta blocker carvedilol.
Design	Placebo-controlled, randomized, double blind, single center.
Patients	151 consecutive patients with acute myocardial infarction. Exclusion criteria included Killip Class IV heart failure, cardiogenic shock, bradycardia, hypotension, heart block, and insulin dependent diabetes.
Follow-up	6 months.
Treatment regimen	Initial therapy was 2.5 mg of carvedilol IV or placebo over 15 minutes, within 24 hours of chest pain, followed by 6.25 mg oral carvedilol or placebo twice-a-day for 2 days; then 12.5 mg to 25 mg x2/d for the duration of the study.

Beneficial effects of intravenous and oral carvedilol treatment in acute myocardial infarction. A placebo-controlled, randomized trial.

(continued)

Results   At 6 months carvedilol was associated with fewer cardiac events (cardiac death, reinfarction, unstable angina, heart failure, emergency revascularization, ventricular arrhythmia requiring therapy, stroke, additional cardiovascular therapy other than sublingual nitroglycerin, diuretics, hypertension, continuing ACE inhibitors, digitalis, or antiarrhythmics), at 18 compared to placebo at 31 (p<.02). After excluding end-points of revascularization and requirement for other cardiovascular medicine, there were 24 events in placebo vs 14 in carvedilol (p<.03). Among 54 patients with heart failure at study entry, 34 received carvedilol but did not exhibit adverse effects of carvedilol. As expected, carvedilol caused decreases in heart rate and blood pressure. Left ventricular ejection fraction was not significantly altered by carvedilol. In a subgroup of patient with LV ejection fraction <45%, carvedilol reduced LV remodeling.

Conclusions   Carvedilol was well tolerated following myocardial infarction, even in those with heart failure, and improved composite outcomes at 6 months.

CORE

Collaborative Organization for RheothRx Evaluation

Title	Effects of RheothRx on mortality, morbidity, left ventricular function, and infarct size in patients with acute myocardial infarction.
Author	Collaborative Organization for RheothRx Evaluation (CORE) Investigators.
Reference	Circulation 1997; 96:192-201.
Disease	Coronary artery disease, acute myocardial infarction.
Purpose	To determine the effect of various doses of RheothRx (poloxamer 188) on outcomes in patients with acute myocardial infarction.
Design	Randomized, multicenter. Several modifications of dosing regimens occurred throughout the initial phases of the study.
Patients	2948 patients with acute myocardial infarction.
Follow-up	6 months.
Treatment regimen	RheothRx vs control. Ultimately RheothRx was given as a h loading bolus plus 11-h infusion at low dose. Several dose modifications were made previous to this because of safety issues.

CORE

Collaborative Organization for RheothRx Evaluation

(continued)

Results   Initial high dose regimens of RheothRx were discontinued secondary to renal dysfunction (in 8.8% of patients). Lower dose regimens including boluses and infusions also were associated with renal dysfunction (2.7% - 4.1%) vs controls (1%). The composite endpoint of death, cardiogenic shock, and reinfarction at 35 days was 13.6% in all RheothRx patients vs 12.7% in controls. RheothRx was associated with a higher incidence of atrial arrhythmias and heart failure and a lower LV ejection fraction.

Conclusions   RheothRx had no effect on mortality, reinfarction, or cardiogenic shock in acute infarct patients. RheothRx had an adverse effect on renal function, heart failure, LV function, and atrial arrhythmias, and is not indicated in acute myocardial patients.

Elevated chlamydia pneumoniae antibodies,
cardiovascular events, and azithromycin in male survivors
of myocardial infarction.

Title	Elevated chlamydia pneumoniae antibodies, cardiovascular events, and azithromycin in male survivors of myocardial infarction.
Author	Gupta S, Leatham EW, Carrington D, et al.
Reference	Circulation 1997; 96:404-407.
Disease	Coronary artery disease, myocardial infarction.
Purpose	To determine the relationship between antibodies against chlamydia pneumonia (CP) and future cardiovascular events in male survivors of myocardial infarction (MI), and to determine the effect of azithromycin antibiotic therapy.
Design	Screening of 220 consecutive male survivors of myocardial infarction for anti-Cp antibodies. Patients with persisting seropositivity of ≥1/64 dilution were randomized to oral azithromycin or placebo. There was also a non-randomized untreated arm.
Patients	220 consecutive males survivors of myocardial infarction.
Follow-up	Mean follow up 18 months.
Treatment regimen	For patients with persistent seropositivity ≥1/64 received either oral azithromycin 500 mg/d for 3 days or 500 mg/d for 6 days or placebo.

Elevated chlamydia pneumoniae antibodies, cardiovascular events, and azithromycin in male survivors of myocardial infarction.

(continued)

Results

The occurrence of adverse cardiovascular events increased with increasing anti-Cp titre. Anti-Cp titres fell to ≤1/16 in 43% of patients receiving azithromycin vs only 10% taking placebo (p = .02). The azithromycin treated group had a 5 fold reduction in cardiovascular events compared to combined placebo and untreated nonrandomized group (odds ratio = 0.2; 95% C.I. = 0.05 to 0.8 p = 0.03). However the event rate was not significantly different between the azithromycin group and randomized placebo group alone.

Conclusions

Increased anti-Cp antibody titres may be a predictor for future cardiovascular events following myocardial infarctions. A short course of azithromyicn might lower this risk but larger studies are needed (and underway) to look at this issue.

***Short-acting nifedipine and diltiazem do not reduce
the incidence of cardiac events in patients with healed
myocardial infarctions.***

Title	Short-acting nifedipine and diltiazem do not reduce the incidence of cardiac events in patients with healed myocardial infarctions.
Author	Ishikowa K, Nakai S, Takenaka T, et al.
Reference	Circulation 1997; 95:2368-2373.
Disease	Coronary artery disease, healed myocardial infarction.
Purpose	To determine whether treatment with short-acting nifedipine or diltiazem reduces the likelihood of cardiac events.
Design	Open-trial, randomized (to control vs calcium channel antagonist).
Patients	1115 patients with "healed myocardial infarction." Inpatients began at 8 days after onset of infarction. Outpatients entered on first visit to the department. Average time interval from onset of myocardial infarction was 27 months.
Follow-up	Up to 100 months.
Treatment regimen	595 - no calcium blocker; 520 with calcium blocker. 341 received short-acting nifedipine 30 mg/d and 179 received short-acting diltiazem (90mg/d).

Short-acting nifedipine and diltiazem do not reduce the incidence of cardiac events in patients with healed myocardial infarctions.

(continued)

Results

Cardiac events (fatal or nonfatal recurrent myocardial infarction; death from congestive heart failure; sudden death; hospitalization because of worsening angina, congestive heart failure, or premature ventricular contraction) occurred in 51 patients (8.6%) not on calcium blockers and in 54 (10.4%) in the calcium-blocker group (odds ratio, 1.24; 95% CI 0.8 - 1.85).

Conclusions

Short-acting nifedipine and diltiazem conferred no protection in healed myocardial infarct patients.

SPRINT-2

The Secondary Prevention Reinfarction Israel Nifedipine Trial 2 Study

Title	Early administration of nifedipine in suspected acute myocardial infarction.
Authors	Goldbourt U, Behar S, Reicher-Reiss H, et al.
Reference	Arch Intern Med 1993;153:345-353.
Disease	Acute myocardial infarction.
Purpose	To assess the secondary prevention efficacy of nifidipine, administered early after admission for acute myocardial infarction.
Design	Randomized, double blind, placebo-controlled, multicenter.
Patients	1358 patients, 50-79 years old, with suspected acute myocardial infarction. Patients with hypotension, intolerance to nifedipine, heart disease other than coronary disease, previous cardiac surgery, LBBB or Wolff-Parkinson-White syndrome, or concomitant severe disease were excluded.
Follow-up	6 months.
Treatment regimen	Randomization to nifedipine or placebo, started within 48 h of admission. The nifedipine dose was titrated to 10 mg X 6/d by day 6. Patients with previous myocardial infarction, anginal syndrome before the index infarction, hypertension, NYHA class II-IV before admission, anterior myocardial infarction, maximal LDL levels >X3 the upper limit of normal could enter the long-term phase after discharge (nifedipine 15 mg QID or placebo for 6 months).

SPRINT-2

The Secondary Prevention Reinfarction Israel Nifedipine Trial 2 Study

(continued)

Results   The study was terminated prematurely by the Review Committee due to excess in early mortality in the nifedipine group. In 532 patients medication was discontinued during the titration phase. Therefore, 826 patients were included in the final group. Mortality during the first 6 days was higher in the nifedipine group (7.8%) than in the placebo group (5.5%)(adjusted odds ratio 1.60; 95% CI 0.86 to 3.00). Among the 826 patients who continued study medications during the long-term phase, mortality was 9.3% in the nifedipine group vs 9.5% in the placebo group. By intention-to-treat analysis, 6 month mortality in the 1358 randomized patients was 15.4% in the nifedipine group vs 13.3% in the placebo group (adjusted relative risk 1.33; 95% CI 0.98-1.80). Analysis according to the time of death for all randomized patients showed that the difference in mortality was mainly due to early (within 6 days) excess mortality in the nifedipine group. Recurrent nonfatal myocardial infarction among patients who participated in the long-term phase occurred in 5.1% of the nifedipine vs 4.2% of the placebo group. Chest pain was reported by 36.0% of the nifedipine group vs 34.8% of the placebo group. 7.5% of the nifedipine vs 7.0% of the placebo group needed rehospitalization because of unstable angina.

Conclusions   Nifedipine, started soon after admission, was associated with increased early mortality in patients with acute myocardial infarction. Long-term prophylactic therapy with nifedipine did not reduce mortality, recurrent myocardial infarction, anginal pain, or need for rehospitalization because of unstable angina. It should be noted that short and not long-acting nifedipine was used.

1. Acute Myocardial Infarction
g. Thrombolytic Misc

ASK

Australian Streptokinase Trial Study Group

Title	Streptokinase for acute ischemic stroke with relationship to time of administration.
Author	Donnan GA, Davis SM, Chamber BR et al.
Reference	JAMA 1996; 276:961-966.
Disease	Stroke
Purpose	To determine whether intravenous streptokinase given within 4 h of onset of acute ischemic stroke reduces morbidity and mortality at 3 months. To assess whether administration of drug within 3 h of onset results in better outcome than when given after 3 h of onset of stroke.
Design	Randomized, double blind, placebo-controlled trial, multicenter.
Patients	340 patients, ages 18-85 years with moderate to severe stroke.
Follow-up	3 months.
Treatment regimen	1.5 million U of intravenous streptokinase or placebo in 100 mL of normal saline administered over 1 h.

ASK

Australian Streptokinase Trial Study Group

(continued)

Results	Main endpoint was combined death and disability score. There was a nonsignificant trend toward unfavorable outcomes for streptokinase vs placebo (RR = 1.08; 95% CI = 0.74-1.56) and excess of hematomas with therapy (13.2% vs 3 %, p<0.01). The poor outcomes were observed in patients who received streptokinase therapy more than 3 h after stroke. Among 70 patients who received therapy within 3 h of onset of stroke there was a trend toward improved outcomes for those receiving streptokinase (RR =0.66; 95% CI = 0.28-1.58) and this improvement was better than in patients who received therapy after 3 h (p=0.04). Outcome of death was greater in patients treated with streptokinase after 3 h; but not in those treated within 3 h. Hypotension occurred in 33% of treated vs 6% of the placebo group.
Conclusions	Thrombolytic therapy with streptokinase therapy within 4 h increased morbidity and mortality at 3 months. Treatment was safer when instituted within 3 h than when instituted later; however even early treatment was not significantly better than placebo.

2. Unstable Angina/ Non Q Wave Infarction

RISC

Risk of Myocardial Infarction and Death During Treatment with Low Dose Aspirin and Intravenous Heparin in Men with Unstable Coronary Artery Disease

Title	Risk of myocardial infarction and death during treatment with low dose aspirin and intravenous heparin in men with unstable coronary artery disease.
Authors	The RISC Group.
Reference	Lancet 1990;336:827-830.
Disease	Unstable angina pectoris, non Q wave myocardial infarction.
Purpose	To evaluate the efficacy and safety of low dose aspirin and IV heparin therapy for patients with unstable angina or non Q wave infarction.
Design	Randomized, double blind, placebo-controlled, 2X2 factorial, multicenter.
Patients	796 men, <70 years old, with unstable angina or non Q wave infarction. Patients with left ventricular dysfunction from previous infarction or valvular disease, previous coronary bypass grafting surgery, permanent pacemaker, left bundle branch block, or inability to complete exercise test were excluded.
Follow-up	>3 months.
Treatment regimen	Randomization within 72 h after admission to oral aspirin 75 mg/d or placebo for 1 year, and to IV placebo or heparin 10,000 U X4/d as a bolus for the first day and 7,500 U X4/d for 4 more days.

RISC

Risk of Myocardial Infarction and Death During Treatment with Low Dose Aspirin and Intravenous Heparin in Men with Unstable Coronary Artery Disease

(continued)

Additional therapy	No drug containing aspirin, NSAID, or anticoagulant was permitted. If not contraindicated, metoprolol 100-200 mg/d. Nitrates and calcium channel blockers were permitted.
Results	Myocardial infarction or death occurred in 5.8% vs 2.5% of the oral placebo and aspirin groups respectively after 5 days (RR 0.43, 95% CI 0.21-0.91, p=0.033). After 30 days the incidence was 13.4% vs 4.3% (RR 0.31, 95% CI 0.18-0.53, p<0.0001), while after 90 days it was 17.1% vs 6.5% (RR 0.36, 95% CI 0.23-0.57, p<0.0001), respectively. Treatment with intermittent bolus injections of heparin did not alter the rates of myocardial infarction or death, although the group treated with aspirin and heparin had the lowest number of events during the initial 5 days. Treatment was associated with few side effects and was well tolerated.
Conclusions	Low dose aspirin, but not intermittent bolus injections of heparin, reduced mortality and myocardial infarction rates in patients with unstable angina or non Q wave infarction.

UNASEM

Unstable Angina Study using Eminase

Title	Thrombolysis in patients with unstable angina improves the angiographic but not the clinical outcome. Results of UNASEM, a multicenter, randomized, placebo-controlled, clinical trial with anistreplase.
Authors	Bär FW, Verheugt FW, Col J, et al.
Reference	Circulation 1992;86:131-137.
Disease	Unstable angina.
Purpose	To evaluate the role of thrombolytic therapy in unstable angina.
Design	Randomized, double blind, placebo controlled, multicenter.
Patients	126 patients, age 30-70 years, with unstable angina with electrocardiographic evidence of ischemia. Patients with previous infarction, angioplasty, cardiac surgery, cardiac pacemaker, intraventricular conduction abnormalities, valvular heart disease, hypertension, cardiomyopathy, heart failure, renal failure, anticoagulant therapy, or contraindication to thrombolysis were excluded. Patients with left main stenosis ≥70% or <50% stenosis of the coronary arteries were excluded.
Follow-up	Coronary angiography before randomization and after 12-28 h.
Treatment regimen	IV injection of 30 U anistreplase (APSAC) or placebo over 5 min after the first cardiac catheterization.

UNASEM

Unstable Angina Study using Eminase

(continued)

Additional therapy	IV nitroglycerin started before angiography. IV heparin 5,000 U bolus followed by infusion at a rate of 1,000 U/h. ß blockers or calcium blockers were given routinely. Aspirin was given after the second angiogram. Angioplasty was recommended only for recurrent angina in spite of medical therapy.
Results	Anistreplase compared to placebo was associated with decrease in diameter stenosis between the baseline to follow-up angiography (11% change (70% to 59%) vs 3% change (66% to 63%), p=0.008). However, clinical outcome was not different. Bleeding complications were higher in the anistreplase group (32% vs 11%, p=0.001).
Conclusions	Anistreplase infusion was associated with angiographic, but not clinical improvement. Moreover, it was associated with excess of bleeding.

TIMI IIIA

Thrombolysis in Myocardial Ischemia Trial IIIA

Title	Early effects of tissue-type plasminogen activator added to conventional therapy on the culprit coronary lesion in patients presenting with ischemic cardiac pain at rest. Results of the Thrombolysis in Myocardial Ischemia (TIMI IIIA) Trial.
Authors	The TIMI IIIA Investigators.
Reference	Circulation 1993;87:38-52.
Disease	Unstable angina, non Q wave myocardial infarction.
Purpose	To assess the early effects of t-PA on the culprit coronary lesion in patients with unstable angina or non Q wave myocardial infarction.
Design	Randomized, placebo-controlled, multicenter.
Patients	306 patients age 22-75 years with ≥5 min but ≤6 h of chest pain occurring at rest accompanied by ECG changes or documented coronary artery disease.
Follow-up	Coronary angiography at baseline and after 18-48 h.
Treatment regimen	Tissue plasminogen activator (t-PA) at a total dose of 0.8 mg/kg (maximum total dose 80 mg) or placebo infusion over 90 min (1/3 of the total dose was given as a bolus).
Additional therapy	Bed rest, oxygen, nitrates, calcium antagonists and/or ß blockers, heparin 5000 U bolus, and infusion for 18-48 h.

Results	Reduction of stenosis by ≥20% or improvement of TIMI flow by 2 grades was seen in 15% and 5% of the culprit lesions in the t-PA and placebo-treated patients (p=0.003). Substantial improvement was seen more often with t-PA (36%) than placebo (15%) among lesions containing thrombus (p<0.01), and among patients with non Q wave infarction (33% vs 8%, respectively, p<0.005). By multi-variate analysis, the adjusted p value for substantial improvement of the culprit lesion by t-PA was 0.01.
Conclusions	Angiographic improvement of the severity of the culprit lesion after conventional therapy with and without additional t-PA was only modest. However, substantial improvement of the culprit lesions was seen more frequently with t-PA than placebo, especially in 2 subgroups: those with apparent thrombus and those with non Q wave infarction.

TIMI IIIB

Thrombolysis in Myocardial Ischemia Trial IIIB

Title	Effects of tissue plasminogen activator and a comparison of early invasive and conservative strategies in unstable angina and non Q wave myocardial infarction. Results of the TIMI IIIB Trial.
Authors	The TIMI IIIB Investigators.
Reference	Circulation 1994;89:1545-1556.
Disease	Unstable angina, non Q wave myocardial infarction.
Purpose	To assess the early effects of t-PA and of an early invasive strategy on clinical outcome of patients with unstable angina or non Q wave myocardial infarction.
Design	Randomized, placebo-controlled, multicenter.
Patients	1473 patients age 22-79 years with ≥ 5 min but ≤ 6 h of chest pain occurring at rest accompanied by ECG changes or documented coronary artery disease.
Follow-up	24 h Holter monitoring that began 60-120 h after randomization. Predischarge thallium scintigraphy. Clinical evaluation and exercise tolerance test at 6 weeks.
Treatment regimen	Tissue plasminogen activator (t-PA) at a total dose of 0.8 mg/kg (maximum total dose 80 mg) or placebo infusion over 90 min (1/3 of the total dose was given as a bolus). Patients were also randomized to early invasive and early conservative strategies. In the early invasive group patients underwent coronary angiography 18-48 h after randomization and followed by revascularization if suitable. In the conservative arm patients were referred to coronary angiography only after failure of initial therapy.

TIMI IIIB

Thrombolysis in Myocardial Ischemia Trial IIIB

(continued)

Additional therapy	Bed rest, oxygen, a long acting nitrate, ß blockers, calcium antagonists, and heparin 5000 U bolus and infusion for 18-48 h. Aspirin 325 mg/d was began on the second day and continued for 1 year.
Results	The primary end point of death, myocardial infarction, or failure of initial therapy at 6 weeks occurred in 54.2% and 55.5% of the t-PA and placebo treated groups. Acute myocardial infarction was more prevalent in the t-PA (7.4%) than placebo treated patients (4.9%, p=0.04). Intracranial hemorrhage occurred in 0.55% and 0 of the t-PA and placebo groups (p=0.06). The primary end point for comparison between the early invasive and conservative group (death, myocardial infarction, or an unsatisfactory symptom-limited exercise test at 6 weeks) occurred in 18.1% and 16.2% of the early conservative and early invasive strategies, respectively (p=NS). However, the initial hospitalization was shorter and the incidence of rehospitalization was lower in the early invasive treated patients.
Conclusions	The addition of t-PA was not beneficial and may even be harmful. There was no difference in the primary end points between the early invasive and conservative strategies, although the former resulted in a shorter hospitalization and lower rate of readmission.

TAUSA

Thrombolysis and Angioplasty in Unstable Angina

Title	a. Adjunctive thrombolytic therapy during angioplasty for ischemic rest angina: results of the TAUSA Trial. b. Angioplasty of complex lesions in ischemic rest angina: results of the Thrombolysis and Angioplasty in Unstable Angina (TAUSA) Trial.
Authors	a. Ambrose JA, Almeida OD, Sharma S, et al. b. Mehran R, Ambrose JA, Bongu RM, et al.
Reference	a. Circulation 1994;90:69-77. b. J Am Coll Cardiol 1995;26:961-966.
Disease	Coronary artery disease, unstable angina.
Purpose	To assess the role of prophylactic intracoronary thrombolytic therapy during coronary angioplasty in unstable angina.
Design	Randomized, double blind, placebo controlled, multicenter.
Patients	469 patients with unstable angina with ischemic rest pain or non Q wave infarction <7 d before angioplasty, or recurrent rest pain within 7 days <30 d after myocardial infarction. All patients had ≥70 % stenosis of a native artery or vein graft that was suitable for angioplasty. Patients >80 years old, with severe hypertension, prior stroke or contraindications to thrombolytic therapy were excluded.
Follow-up	Angiography 15 min after angioplasty. In-hospital clinical follow-up.

Thrombolysis and Angioplasty in Unstable Angina

(continued)

Treatment regimen	Urokinase 150,000 U or placebo over 3 min (Phase I) or 250,000 U or placebo over 10-15 min (Phase II), before wire placement. Additional 100,000 U (Phase I) or 250,000 U (Phase II) or placebo 1 min post angioplasty.
Additional therapy	Aspirin 80-325 mg and IV heparin 10,000 U before procedure. 75 µg intracoronary nitroglycerin before wire placement. IV heparin infusion overnight.
Results	a. 257 and 212 patients were included in phase I and II, respectively. Angioplasty was successful in 97% and 94% of the placebo and urokinase groups (p=NS). Definite filling defects were present at 15 min in 18.0% vs 13.8% of the placebo and urokinase patients (p=NS). Acute closure was more common with urokinase (10.2%) than placebo (4.3%, p<0.02). These differences were more pronounced in phase II (8.7% vs 1.9%, p=0.031) than in phase I. There was no difference in detection of coronary dissection between the groups. Emergency bypass surgery (5.2% vs 2.1%, p=0.09) and post procedure ischemia (9.9% vs 3.4%, p=0.005) were more common in the urokinase group, however, there was no difference in the occurrence of myocardial infarction. Bleeding complications were reported in 12.9% and 8.9% of the urokinase and placebo groups (p=NS). b. Complex lesions were associated with higher abrupt closure than simple lesions (10.6% vs 3.3%, p<0.003), and higher recurrent angina. Abrupt closure of the complex lesions was more common in the urokinase group (15.0% vs 5.9%, p<0.03).
Conclusions	Prophylactic urokinase intracoronary administration was associated with adverse angiographic and clinical outcome in patients with unstable angina undergoing coronary angioplasty.

ATACS

Antithrombotic Therapy in Acute Coronary Syndromes

Title	Combination antithrombotic therapy in unstable rest angina and non Q wave infarction in nonprior aspirin users. Primary end points analysis from the ATACS trial.
Authors	Cohen M, Adams PC, Parry G, et al.
Reference	Circulation 1994;89:81-88.
Disease	Unstable angina, non Q wave myocardial infarction.
Purpose	To compare the efficacy of combination of aspirin + anticoagulation vs aspirin alone in patients with rest unstable angina or non Q wave infarction.
Design	Randomized, open label, multicenter.
Patients	214 patients, >21 years of age, with unstable rest angina or non Q wave infarction. Patients that received ≥150 mg aspirin within 3 days of randomization were excluded.
Follow-up	12 weeks.
Treatment regimen	Aspirin 162.5 mg/d or aspirin 162.5 mg/d + heparin 100 U/kg IV bolus and then continuous infusion of heparin for 3-4 days. Warfarin was started on the second and third day, if coronary angiography did not appear imminent. Heparin was discontinued after INR reached 2.0-3.0.
Additional therapy	Antianginal therapy: low risk patients received metoprolol and oral isosorbide dinitrate; high risk patients received additional nifedipine. If ß blockers were contraindicated, diltiazem was given instead of metoprolol. Patients already on ß blockers, received maximal dose of ß blockers + nifedipine.

Results	Trial therapy was begun by 9.5 ± 8.8 h of qualifying pain. By intention to treat analysis, after 14 days 27% of the aspirin vs 10% of the aspirin+anticoagulation experienced death, recurrent angina, or infarction (adjusted p=0.004). After 12 weeks 28% of the aspirin vs 19% of the aspirin+anticoagulation experienced death, recurrent angina, or infarction (adjusted p=0.09). Major bleeding complications occurred in 0 and 2.9%, respectively, while minor bleeding or medication intolerance was found in 2.8% and 6.7%, respectively. Withdrawal from the study or occurrence of a secondary end point (major bleeding or coronary revascularization) occurred in 31% and 45%, respectively.
Conclusions	Combination of anticoagulation therapy and aspirin, compared with aspirin alone, significantly reduced recurrent ischemic events in the early phase of unstable angina or non Q wave infarction.

Title	Recombinant hirudin for unstable angina pectoris. A multicenter, randomized angiographic trial.
Authors	Topol EJ, Fuster V, Harrington RA, et al.
Reference	Circulation 1994;89:1557-1566.
Disease	Unstable angina pectoris.
Purpose	To compare the efficacy of hirudin and heparin in preventing accumulation of coronary artery thrombus in patients with unstable angina.
Design	Randomized, open label, comparing 2 regimens of heparin and 4 regimens of hirudin in multifactorial fashion, multicenter.
Patients	166 patients, ≤75 years of age, with ≥5 min of rest ischemic pain within 48 h, and ≥60% stenosis of a major epicardial coronary artery or vein graft interpreted as having an intraluminal thrombus. Patients with renal failure, hemodynamic instability, previous stroke, or history of significant bleeding were excluded.
Follow-up	Coronary angiography at baseline and after 72-120 h. Clinical follow-up for 30 days.
Treatment regimen	1. Hirudin 0.15 mg/kg bolus, 0.05 mg/kg/h infusion. 2. Hirudin 0.30 mg/kg bolus, 0.1 mg/kg/h infusion. 3. Hirudin 0.60 mg/kg bolus, 0.2 mg/kg/h infusion. 4. Hirudin 0.90 mg/kg bolus, 0.3 mg/kg/h infusion. 5. Hirudin 0.60 mg/kg bolus, 0.3 mg/kg/h infusion. 6. Hirudin 0.60 mg/kg bolus, 0.3 mg/kg/h infusion. In all regimens: heparin 5000 U bolus, 1000 U/h infusion. PTT was adjusted to 65-90 s in regimens 1-5, and to 90-110 s in regimen 6. Infusion was continued for 3-5 days.

Additional therapy	Aspirin 160-325 mg/d. ß blockers, calcium channel blockers, and long acting nitrate. Coronary revascularization was discouraged until completion of the second angiogram.
Results	Hirudin led to a dose-dependent prolongation of the PTT that appeared to plateau at the 0.2 mg/kg/h infusion rate. 16% of the heparin and 71% of the hirudin treated patients had their aPTT within the therapeutic range (p<0.001). The hirudin treated patients showed better improvement in minimal cross sectional area of the culprit lesion (0.29 vs 0.10 mm2 , p=0.028), minimal luminal diameter (0.18 vs 0.03 mm, p=0.029), and % diameter stenosis (-5.19% vs -2.11%, p=0.071). There was no difference in any of the clinical events at 30 days between heparin and hirudin. There was no major adverse effects associated with hirudin.
Conclusions	Recombinant hirudin in patients with unstable angina improved the angiographic results, but not the clinical outcome.

TIMI-7

Thrombin Inhibition in Myocardial Ischemia 7

Title	Hirulog in the treatment of unstable angina. Results of the thrombin inhibition in myocardial ischemia (TIMI) 7 trial.
Authors	Fuchs J, Cannon CP, and the TIMI 7 Investigators.
Reference	Circulation 1995;92:727-733.
Disease	Unstable angina.
Purpose	To assess whether a dose response existed in the efficacy of hirulog used in conjunction with aspirin in unstable angina.
Design	Randomized, double blind, multicenter.
Patients	401 patients, age 21-75 years, with unstable angina (ischemic rest pain of 5-60 min) within 24 h of randomization, >24 h after myocardial infarction (if present).
Follow-up	6 weeks.
Treatment regimen	One of 4 doses of hirulog infusion for 72 h: 0.02, 0.25, 0.50, and 1.0 mg/kg/h.
Additional therapy	Aspirin 325 mg/d. No restriction on conventional therapy, excluding heparin during hirulog infusion.

TIMI-7

Thrombin Inhibition in Myocardial Ischemia 7

(continued)

Results   There was no difference among the groups in the primary end point (death, myocardial infarction, rapid clinical
deterioration, or recurrent ischemia with ECG changes) at
72 h (primary end point occurred in 8.1%, 6.2%, 11.4%,
and 6.2% of the patients in the 4 groups, respectively,
p=0.56). Primary end points occurred in 15.0%, 7.4%,
14.8%, and 12.3% of the patients respectively at discharge
(p=0.38). However, death or recurrent infarction at discharge occurred in 10% of the 0.02 mg/kg/h group vs 3.2%
of the patients assigned to the 3 other groups (p=0.008).
After 6 weeks end point occurred in 12.5% of the lower
dose vs 5.2% of the upper 3 doses (p=0.009). Only 0.5%
(2 patients) experienced a major bleeding attributed to
hirulog.

Conclusions   Hirulog in conjunction with aspirin is a safe and promis-
ing therapy for unstable angina.

A Comparison of Hirudin with Heparin in the Prevention of Restenosis after Coronary Angioplasty

Title	A comparison of hirudin with heparin in the prevention of restenosis after coronary angioplasty.
Authors	Serruys PW, Herrman JP, Simon R, et al.
Reference	N Engl J Med 1995;333:757-763.
Disease	Coronary artery disease, unstable angina.
Purpose	To compare the efficacy of 2 regimens of recombinant hirudin with heparin in preventing restenosis following coronary angioplasty.
Design	Randomized, double blind, multicenter.
Patients	1141 patients with unstable angina with ≥1 lesion suitable for coronary angioplasty.
Follow-up	30 week clinical follow-up, coronary angiography after 26 weeks.
Treatment regimen	1. Recombinant hirudin IV 40 mg bolus followed by infusion of 0.2 mg/kg/h for 24 h, and then placebo X2/d SC for 3 days. 2. Recombinant hirudin IV 40 mg bolus followed by infusion of 0.2 mg/kg/h for 24 h, and then 40 mg X2/d SC for 3 days. 3. Heparin 10,000 U bolus followed by infusion of 15 U/kg/h for 24 h, and then placebo X2/d SC for 3 days.
Additional therapy	Aspirin 100-500 mg/d for ≥14 days.

Results   At 30 weeks, event-free survival was 67.3%, 63.5%, and 68.0% for the heparin, hirudin IV, and hirudin IV+SC (p=0.61). However, early cardiac events (within 96 h) were reduced by hirudin (occurrence in 11.0%, 7.9%, and 5.6%, respectively, combined relative risk with hirudin vs heparin 0.61, 95% CI 0.41-0.90, p=0.023). In patients with severe unstable angina (Braunwald class III) the 96 h event rates were 21.6%, 5.3%, and 12.3% (combined relative risk 0.41, 95% CI 0.21-0.78, p=0.006). The minimal luminal diameter on the follow-up angiography was 1.54, 1.47, and 1.56 mm, respectively (p=0.08).

Conclusions   Although hirudin reduced the occurrence of early complications, long-term results were the same as with heparin.

FRISC

Fragmin During Instability in Coronary Artery Disease Study

Title	Low molecular weight heparin during instability in coronary artery disease.
Authors	Fragmin during Instability in Coronary Artery Disease (FRISC) Study Group.
Reference	Lancet 1996;347:561-568.
Disease	Unstable angina, non Q wave infarction.
Purpose	To assess the efficacy of subcutaneous low molecular weight heparin, in combination with aspirin and antianginal medications, to prevent new cardiac events in patients with unstable angina.
Design	Randomized, double blind, placebo controlled, multicenter.
Patients	1506 patients, >40 years old, with unstable angina (<72 h from the last episode of chest pain). Premenopausal women, patients with an increased risk of bleeding, current treatment with anticoagulants, or coronary revascularization within 3 months were excluded.
Follow-up	150 days clinical follow-up. Predischarge and 40-50 day exercise test.
Treatment regimen	Placebo or dalteparin sodium 120 U/kg (maximum 10,000 U)X2/d SC for 6 days, and then 7,500 U X1/d for the next 35-45 days.
Additional therapy	Aspirin 75 mg/d (initial dose 300 mg), ß blockers, nitrates, and calcium channel blockers.

Results	6 day mortality or development of new myocardial infarction was 4.8% in the placebo and 1.8% in the dalteparin group (RR 0.37, 95% CI 0.20-0.68, p=0.001). 1.2% vs 0.4%, respectively needed revascularization (RR 0.33, 95% CI 0.10-1.10, p=0.07), while 7.7% vs 3.8% needed intravenous heparin (RR 0.49, 95% CI 0.32-0.75, p=0.001). After 40 days the rate of death, myocardial infarction, revascularization, or the need for IV heparin was 25.7% in the placebo vs 20.5% in the dalteparin group (RR 0.79, 95% CI 0.66-0.95, p=0.011). There was an increased event rate during the first few days after the change of the dose in the dalteparin group, especially in smokers. There was no difference in the rates of end points after 150 days. The regimen was relatively safe with rare side effects and compliance was good.
Conclusions	Long-term dalteparin and aspirin therapy is safe and effective in patients with unstable angina.

Title	Platelet membrane receptor glycoprotein IIb/IIIa antagonism in unstable angina. The Canadian Lamifiban study.
Authors	Thèroux P, Kouz S, Roy L, et al.
Reference	Circulation 1996;94:899-905.
Disease	Coronary artery disease, unstable angina.
Purpose	To assess the clinical benefit of GP IIb/IIIa inhibition by Lamifiban in patients with unstable angina.
Design	Randomized, double blind, placebo-controlled, dose ranging multicenter.
Patients	365 patients, <75 years old, with unstable angina or myocardial infarction without ST segment elevation. Patients with identifiable precipitating secondary factors, or <6 months after PTCA or <2 months after coronary artery bypass surgery were excluded. Additional exclusion criteria were previous stroke, high risk for bleeding, uncontrolled hypertension, congestive heart failure or shock, thrombocytopenia, use of oral anticoagulants, concomitant life threatening disease, and left bundle branch block.
Follow-up	1 month.
Treatment regimen	Patients were randomized to 1 of 5 parallel arms: placebo and 4 doses of lamifiban. All arms included an IV bolus followed by an infusion for 72-120 hours. The bolus plus infusion doses were 1. 150 µg + 1µg/min; 2. 300 µg + 2 µg/kg; 3. 600 µg + 4 µg/min; and 4. 750 µg + 5 µg/min. 3 patients were randomized to lamifiban 600 µg bolus + 4 µg/min or to placebo for 1 patient in each of the other 3 groups.

(continued)

Additional therapy	Aspirin 325 mg/d. Heparin was permitted. The use of nitrates, ß blockers, and/or calcium channel blockers was recommended.

Results

During the infusion period the lamifiban-treated patients (all doses) had lower rate of primary end-point (death, myocardial infarction, or the need for an urgent revascularization) from 8.1% in the placebo group to 3.3% (odds ratio 0.39; 95% CI 0.15 to 0.99; p=0.04). The rates were 2.5%, 4.9%, 3.3%, and 2.4%, respectively for the 4 lamifiban dosage groups. The highest dose (5 µg/min) had an additional benefit on recurrent ischemia over the 3 other lower doses (odds ratio compared with placebo 0.32; 95% CI 0.12 to 0.89; p=0.02). At 1 month, mortality was 4.1% in the placebo vs 1.2% in the lamifiban-treated patients. Death or myocardial infarction occurred in 8.1% of the placebo, 6.2% of the 2 lower lamifiban doses, and 2.5% of the patients treated with the higher doses of lamifiban. The odds ratio with the 2 high doses compared with placebo was 0.29 (95% CI 0.09 to 0.94; p=0.03). Lamifiban inhibited platelet aggregation in a dose dependent fashion. Bleeding was more frequent with lamifiban than placebo (11.1% vs 1.6% of minor bleeding (p=0.002), and 2.9% vs 0.8% of minor bleeding (p=NS)). Concomitant heparin therapy increased significantly the bleeding risk.

Conclusions

3 to 5 days lamifiban therapy reduced the rate of mortality, myocardial infarction, or the need for revascularization during the infusion period and at 1 month in patients with unstable angina.

CAPTURE

C7E3 Fab AntiPlatelet Therapy in Unstable REfractory Angina.

Title	Randomized placebo-controlled trial of abciximab before and during coronary intervention in refractory unstable angina: the CAPTURE study.
Authors	The CAPTURE investigators.
Reference	Lancet 1997;349:1429-1435.
Disease	Unstable angina.
Purpose	To evaluate the efficacy of abciximab, a platelet glycoprotein IIb/IIIa receptor blocker, started 18-24 h before procedure and continued until 1 h after procedure, in improving outcome among patients with refractory unstable angina who are undergoing coronary balloon angioplasty.
Design	Randomized, placebo-controlled, multicenter.
Patients	1265 patients with refractory unstable angina, that continued to be active despite therapy with intravenous heparin and nitrates. Therapy should have been started within 48 h of last episode of pain. All patients should have an angiographically proven culprit coronary artery lesion suitable for angioplasty. Patients with recent myocardial infarction, persistent ischemia that mandated immediate intervention, >50% stenosis of the left main coronary artery, a culprit lesion in a bypass graft, bleeding diathesis, cerebrovascular accident within 2 years, planned administration of anticoagulants, intravenous dextran, or a thrombolytic agent before or during angioplasty, thrombocytopenia, or serious other medical conditions were excluded.
Follow-up	6 months.
Treatment regimen	Randomization to abciximab (0.25 mg/kg bolus followed by continuous infusion of 10 µg/min) or placebo. Treatment was given for 18-24 h before angioplasty and continued for 1 h after completion of angioplasty.

CAPTURE

C7E3 Fab AntiPlatelet Therapy in Unstable REfractory Angina.
(continued)

Additional therapy	Aspirin ≥50 mg/d. Intravenous heparin from before randomization until >1 h after angioplasty. Intravenous glyceryl trinitrate. The use of stents was avoided when feasible.
Results	The study was terminated prematurely by the Clinical Endpoint Committee. Angioplasty was attempted in 1241 patients (98%), and was successful in 88.8% of the placebo group vs 94.0% of the abciximab group (p=0.001). Death, myocardial infarction, or urgent intervention within the first 30 days of study occurred in 15.9% of the placebo vs 11.3% of the abciximab group (p=0.012). There was no difference in mortality (1.3% vs 1.0% in the placebo and abciximab groups, respectively; p>0.1). However, myocardial infarction occurred less frequently in the abciximab group than in the placebo group, both before intervention (0.6% vs 2.1%; p=0.029), and within the first 24 h of angioplasty (2.6% vs 5.5%; p=0.009), but not after the procedure (day 2-30)(1.0% vs 0.9%; p>0.1). The abciximab treated patients needed less urgent interventions (7.8%) than the placebo treated patients (10.9%)(p=0.054). Major bleeding episodes were more common in the abciximab group (3.8%) than in the placebo group (1.9%)(p=0.043), and more patients in the abciximab group needed transfusions (7.1% vs 3.4%, respectively; p=0.005). There were no excess strokes in the abciximab group. At 6 months, death or myocardial infarction occurred in 9.0% of the abciximab group vs 10.9% of the placebo group (p=0.19). 5.4% of the abciximab vs 7.1% of the placebo group needed coronary artery bypass surgery (p=0.20), and angioplasty in 21.4% vs 20.7%, respectively. Less events (death, myocardial infarction, or repeated intervention) per patients occurred in the abciximab treated patients during the 6 months follow-up (274 events were recorded in 193 placebo-treated patients compared with 242 events in 193 abciximab treated patients; p=0.067).
Conclusions	Abciximab infusion, started 18-24 h before and continued for 1 h after coronary angioplasty, reduced the rates of peri-procedure myocardial infarction and the need for reintervention among patients with unstable angina undergoing coronary balloon angioplasty. However abciximab did not alter the rate of myocardial infarction after the first few days after angioplasty or the need for subsequent reintervention.

Effects of Integrelin, a platelet glycoprotein IIb/IIIa receptor antagonist, in unstable angina. A randomized multicenter trial.

Title	Effects of Integrelin, a platelet glycoprotein IIb/IIIa receptor antagonist, in unstable angina. A randomized multicenter trial.
Author	Schulman SP, Goldschmidt-Clermont PJ, Topol EJ, et al.
Reference	Circulation 1996; 94:2083-2089.
Disease	Coronary artery disease, unstable angina.
Purpose	To determine the effect of the GPIIb/IIIa antagonist, Integrelin on the frequency and duration of Holter monitored ischemic events in patients with unstable angina.
Design	Randomized, double blind, placebo controlled.
Patients	227 patients with unstable angina.
Follow-up	In-hospital.
Treatment regimen	Patients were randomized to oral aspirin and placebo Integrelin, placebo aspirin and low dose Integrelin (45 µg/kg bolus plus 0.5 µg/kg/min infusion); or placebo aspirin and high dose Integrelin (90 µg/kg bolus followed by 1.0 µg/kg/min constant infusion). Drug was continued for 29-72 h. Patients received aspirin.

Effects of Integrelin, a platelet glycoprotein IIb/IIIa receptor antagonist, in unstable angina. A randomized multicenter trial.

(continued)

Results

Patients randomized to high dose Integrelin experienced fewer ischemic episodes (0.24 ± 0.11) compared to aspirin (1.0 ± 0.33, $p < .05$) and shorter ischemic episodes (8.41 ± 5.29 min.) compared to aspirin (26.2 ± 9.8 min, $p = 0.01$). Platelet aggregation was rapidly inhibited by Integrelin in a dose-dependent fashion. There were no differences in bleeding among the 3 arms.

Conclusions

Intravenous integrelin reduces the number and duration of ischemic events on Holter monitoring in patients with unstable angina.

FRIC

Fragmin in Unstable Coronary Artery Disease Study (FRIC)

Title	Comparison of low molecular weight heparin with unfractionated heparin acutely and with placebo for 6 weeks in the management of unstable coronary artery disease. Fragmin in unstable coronary artery disease study (FRIC).
Author	Klein W, Buchwald A, Hillis SE.
Reference	Circulation 1997; 96:61-68.
Disease	Coronary artery disease, unstable angina, non Q wave myocardial infarction.
Purpose	To compare the efficacy and safety of dalteparin with unfractionated heparin in the acute treatment of unstable angina or non Q wave myocardial infarction.
Design	Prospective, randomized, multicenter with 2 phases. During days 1-6 patients received either dalteparin given subcutaneously and weight adjusted or dose adjusted unfractionated heparin. Days 6-45 days was double blind prolonged treatment phase in which patients received either dalteparin or placebo.
Patients	1482 patients with unstable angina or non Q wave myocardial infarction.
Follow-up	45 days.

FRIC

Fragmin in Unstable Coronary Artery Disease Study (FRIC)

(continued)

Treatment regimen	In the acute phase dalteparin 120 IU/kg x2/d, subcutaneously. In the prolonged treatment phase dalteparin 7500 IU x1/d, subcutaneously. Those randomized to heparin received a bolus of 5000 IU followed within 2 h by a continuous infusion of 1000 IU/h, adjusted to maintain the aPTT at 1.5 times control values. Aspirin was given to all patients.
Results	There were no differences in mortality, myocardial infarction, and recurrent angina between the unfractionated heparin and dalteparin treated patients during the first 6 days. Between days 6 and 45 the rate of death, infarction, or recurrence of angina was 12.3% for placebo and dalteparin groups. Revascularization procedures were performed in 14% of patients in both of these groups.
Conclusions	Low molecular weight heparin dalteparin given twice daily may be an alternative to unfractionated heparin for patients with unstable angina or non Q wave myocardial infarction. Prolonged therapy with dalteparin at a lower once-a -day dose did not confer benefit over aspirin plus heparin.

HASI

Hirulog Angioplasty Study Investigators

Title	a. Treatment with bivalirudin (hirulog) as compared with heparin during coronary angioplasty for unstable or postinfarction angina. b. Bivalirudin compared with heparin during coronary angioplasty for thrombus-containing lesions.
Authors	a. Bittl JA, Strony J, Brinker JA, et al. b. Shah PB, Ahmed WH, Ganz P, Bittl JA.
Reference	a. N Engl J Med 1995;333:764-769. b. J Am Coll Cardiol 1997;30:1264-1269.
Disease	Unstable angina
Purpose	To compare the efficacy of hirulog and heparin as an adjunctive therapy after angioplasty for unstable or postinfarction angina.
Design	Randomized, double blind, multicenter.
Patients	4098 patients, >21 years old, with unstable or postinfarction angina <2 week after infarction.
Follow-up	In-hospital, 3 and 6 months clinical course
Treatment regimen	1. Hirulog: 1.0 mg/kg bolus before angioplasty, followed by 4 h infusion at a rate of 2.5 mg/kg/h, and a 14-20 h infusion at a rate of 0.2 mg/kg/h. 2. Heparin: IV bolus 175 U/kg followed by infusion at a rate of 15 U/kg/h for 18-24 h.
Additional therapy	Aspirin 300-325 mg/d

HASI

Hirulog Angioplasty Study Investigators

(continued)

Results   a. In the total population the occurrence of the primary end point (death, myocardial infarction, abrupt closure, or rapid clinical deterioration requiring coronary bypass surgery, intra-aortic balloon counterpulsation, or repeated angioplasty) were similar between hirulog (11.4%) and heparin (12.2%). However, hirulog resulted in lower incidence of major bleeding (3.8% vs 9.8%, p<0.001). In the subpopulation of postinfarction angina, hirulog resulted in a lower incidence of the in-hospital primary end points (9.1% vs 14.2%, p=0.04), lower incidence of myocardial infarction (2.0% vs 5.1%, p=0.04), and a lower incidence of bleeding (3.0% vs 11.1%, p<0.001). However, the cumulative rate of death, myocardial infarction, and repeated revascularization in the postinfarction angina patients during the 6 months follow-up were similar (20.5% vs 25.1%, p=0.17).

b. In patients with thrombus-containing lesions on angiography (n=567) myocardial infarction (5.1% vs 3.2%; p=0.03) and abrupt vessel closure (13.6% vs 8.3%; p<0.001) occurred more frequently than in patients without angiographic evidence of a thrombus. However, the incidence of primary end points was not reduced by hirulog compared with heparin in patients with thrombus-containing lesions. The cumulative incidence of ischemic events at 6 months was comparable between the hirulog group (26.9%) and the heparin group (27.1%)(p=0.95).

Conclusions   Hirulog (bivalirudin) was as effective as high dose heparin in preventing the ischemic complications following angioplasty for unstable angina. It was better than heparin in reducing the immediate complications in patients with postinfarction angina, however, heparin and hirulog had comparable efficacy in thrombus containing lesions. Hirulog was associated with a lower incidence of bleeding.

OASIS

Organization to Assess Strategies for Ischemic Syndromes

Title	Comparison of the effects of 2 doses of recombinant hirudin compared with heparin in patients with acute myocardial ischemia without ST elevation. A pilot study.
Author	Organization to Assess Strategies for Ischemic Syndromes (OASIS) investigators.
Reference	Circulation 1997; 96:769-777.
Disease	Coronary artery disease, unstable angina, suspected acute myocardial infarction.
Purpose	To compare the effects of 2 different doses of hirudin with heparin on composite primary endpoint of cardiovascular death, development of new myocardial infarction, or refractory angina, and on the above primary endpoint plus severe angina (secondary outcome).
Design	Randomized, multicenter.
Patients	909 patients with unstable angina or suspected acute myocardial infarction without ST segment elevation on the electrocardiogram.
Follow-up	7-180 days.

OASIS

Organization to Assess Strategies for Ischemic Syndromes

(continued)

Treatment regimen	Patients randomized to receive 72 h infusion of heparin or hirudin at varying doses: 1. heparin: bolus of 5000 U followed by an infusion of 1200 U/h, or 1000 U/h for patients with body weight < 60 kg; 2. low dose hirudin: bolus of 0.2/mg/kg followed by infusion of 0.10 mg/kg/h; or 3. medium dose hirudin: initial bolus 0.4mg/kg followed by infusion of 0.15 mg/kg/h. Infusions lasted 72 h. APPT monitored every 6-8 h; heparin and hirudin adjusted to maintain a PTT between 60-100 seconds.
Results	At 7 days, 6.5%, 4.4%, and 3.0% of patients developed primary outcome (cardiovascular death, recurrent myocardial infarction, or refractory angina) in heparin, low dose hirudin and medium dose hirudin groups, respectively (p=.047 heparin vs medium dose hirudin). The percentage of patients developing secondary outcome (primary plus severe angina) were 15.6%, 12.5%, and 9.4%, (p=0.02 for heparin vs medium dose hirudin). New myocardial infarctions developed in fewer patients on medium hirudin dose (1.9%) than heparin (4.9%; p=.046). Fewer patients required CABG in the 2 hirudin groups (3.7% low dose, 1.1% medium dose) vs heparin (4.0%; p=.028 for heparin vs medium dose hirudin). While there was an increase in ischemic events after study drugs were stopped, the difference between heparin and hirudin persisted for 180 days.
Conclusions	Hirudin, especially at medium dose was better than heparin in reducing ischemic outcomes in patients with unstable angina or acute myocardial infarction without ST segment elevation.

PRISM

The Platelet Receptor Inhibition in Ischemic Syndrome Management (PRISM) Study Investigators

Title	A comparison of aspirin plus tirofiban with aspirin plus heparin for unstable angina.
Author	The PRISM Investigators.
Reference	N Engl J Med 1998; 378:1498-1505.
Disease	Coronary artery disease, unstable angina.
Purpose	To determine whether the glycoprotein IIb/IIIa receptor antagonist tirofiban would improve clinical outcome in patients with unstable angina.
Design	Randomized, double blind, multicenter.
Patients	3232 patients with unstable angina already receiving aspirin.
Follow-up	30 days.
Treatment regimen	All patients received aspirin. Patients randomized to tirofiban (loading dose of 0.6 μg per kilogram per minute for 30 minutes followed by 0.15 μg per kilogram per minute for 47.5 hours). Patients randomized to heparin group received 5000 units IV bolus followed by an infusion of 1000 Units per h for 48 h.

PRISM

The Platelet Receptor Inhibition in Ischemic Syndrome Management (PRISM) Study Investigators

(continued)

Results

The incidence of attaining the composite endpoint (death, myocardial infarction, or refractory ischemia at 48 h) was 3.8% with tirofiban vs 5.6% with heparin (risk ration, 0.67; 95% CI = 0.48 -0.92, p= 0.01). At 30 days there was a trend toward a reduction in death or myocardial infarction with tirofiban (5.8% vs 7.1%, p = 0.11). At 30 days, mortality was 2.3% in the tirofiban group vs 3.6% in the heparin group (p =0.02). The incidence of refractory ischemia and myocardial infarction was not reduced by tirofiban at 30 days. Major bleeding was present in 0.4% of both groups.

Conclusions

Platelet inhibition with tirofiban plus aspirin may play a role in the treatment of unstable angina.

PRISM - PLUS

The Platelet Receptor Inhibition in Ischemic Syndrome Management in Patients Limited by Unstable Signs and Symptoms (PRISM-PLUS)

Title	Inhibition of the platelet glycoprotein IIb/IIIa receptor with tirofiban in unstable angina and non Q wave myocardial infarction.
Author	PRISM-PLUS Investigators.
Reference	N Engl J Med. 1998; 338:1488-1497.
Disease	Coronary artery disease, unstable angina, non Q wave myocardial infarction.
Purpose	To evaluate the effectiveness of tirofiban in treating unstable angina and non Q wave infarctions.
Design	Randomized, double blind, multicenter.
Patients	1915 patients with unstable angina or non Q wave infarcts.
Follow-up	6 months.
Treatment regimen	All patients received aspirin. They were randomized to tirofiban, heparin, or tirofiban plus heparin. Study drugs were infused for a mean of 71 h. Coronary angiography and angioplasty performed when indicated after 48 h.

PRISM - PLUS

The Platelet Receptor Inhibition in Ischemic Syndrome Management in Patients Limited by Unstable Signs and Symptoms (PRISM-PLUS)

(continued)

Results	Tirofiban alone was associated with an excess of mortality at 7 days (4.6%) compared with patients on heparin alone (1.1%). The incidence of the composite endpoint (death, myocardial infarction, or refractory ischemia) was lower among patients on tirofiban plus heparin (12.9%) compared to patients on heparin alone (17.9%, risk ratio, 0.68, 95% CI = 0.53 - 0.88, p=0.004). This benefit persisted at 30 days (18.5% vs 22.3%, p = 0.03) and 6 months (27.7% vs 32.1%, p = 0.02) Tirofiban plus heparin was also associated with a lower rate of death or myocardial infarction at 7, 30, and 60 days. Major bleeding was present in 3% of heparin group and 4% in combination group.
Conclusions	Tirofiban alone (without heparin) caused excess mortality early. However, when administered with heparin it was associated with a better clinical outcome than patients who received heparin.

ROXIS PILOT STUDY

Title	Randomized trial of roxithromycin in non Q wave coronary syndromes: ROXIS pilot study.
Author	Gurfinkel E, Bozovich A, Daroca A, et al.
Reference	Lancet 1997;August 9; 350:404-407.
Disease	Coronary artery disease, unstable angina or non-Q wave myocardial infarction.
Purpose	To determine the effectiveness of the antibiotic roxithromycin for reducing severe recurrent angina, acute myocardial infarction, and death in patients with unstable angina or non Q wave infarction.
Design	Randomized, double blind, placebo-controlled study.
Patients	202 patients with unstable angina or non Q wave infarction.
Follow-up	31 days.
Treatment regimen	Oral roxithromycin, 150 mg x2/d for 30 days vs placebo. All patients received, aspirin, IV nitroglycerin, heparin.
Results	No difference between groups for individual outcomes of angina, myocardial infarction, or death. There was a trend (p =.06) for reduced triple end-point of angina plus infarction plus death.
Conclusions	Nonsignificant trend toward improvement with antibiotic when examined in an intention-to-treat analysis.

TIMI 11A

Enoxaparin for Unstable Angina

Title	Dose ranging trial of enoxaparin for unstable angina: results of TIMI 11A.
Authors	The Thrombolysis In Myocardial Infarction (TIMI) 11A Trial Investigators.
Reference	J Am Coll Cardiol 1997;29:1474-1482.
Disease	Unstable angina, non Q wave myocardial infarction.
Purpose	To assess the tolerability and safety of 2 weight-adjusted doses of subcutaneous injections of enoxaparin, a low molecular weight heparin, in unstable angina and non Q wave myocardial infarction.
Design	Open label, dose ranging trial, multicenter.
Patients	630 patients with unstable angina or non Q wave myocardial infarction. Patients with evolving Q wave myocardial infarction, patients who had received thrombolytic therapy within 24 h of enrollment, renal failure, CABG within 2 months, history of heparin induced thrombocytopenia, contraindications to anticoagulation or aspirin, on continuous unfractionated heparin infusion, or a need for continuous anticoagulation were excluded.
Follow-up	14 days.
Treatment regimen	Intravenous bolus 30 mg followed by subcutaneous injection of either 1.25 mg/kg body weight or 1.0 mg/kg BID during in-hospital phase, and a fixed dose of either 60 mg (body weight ≥65 kg) or 40 mg (body weight <65 kg) subcutaneously BID after discharge.

Enoxaparin for Unstable Angina

(continued)

Results	In the initial cohort of patients a dose of 1.25 mg/kg BID was used during hospitalization. This regimen was terminated prematurely after enrollment of 321 patients due to high major bleeding rate (6.5%), mainly at instrumented sites. Additional 309 patients received a regimen of 1.0 mg/kg BID during hospitalization. The duration of the in-hospital phase was a median of 3 days. In this cohort 6% of the patients stopped treatment because of bleeding, 7% due to coronary artery bypass surgery, and 3% at their request. The duration of the outpatient phase was a median of 10 days. Enoxaparin was stopped by 17% of the patients in this phase. Major bleeding occurred in 6 patients (1.9%; 95% CI 0.8% - 4.4%) of the 1.0 mg/kg BID regimen, in 5 of them (1.6%) bleeding was at a puncture site and occurred a median of 34.5 h after a procedure. In only 1 patient, a major bleeding occurred spontaneously. Thrombocytopenia was noted in 2 patients (0.7%). The incidence of death was 2.2% in the first regimen and 0.6% in the second regimen. Myocardial infarction occurred in 2.2% and 2.9%, respectively, and recurrent ischemia requiring intervention in 1.2% and 1.6%, respectively (p=NS for all comparisons).
Conclusions	Enoxaparin therapy at a dose of 1.0 mg/kg was associated with an acceptable rate of major bleeding during the in-hospital phase, whereas a dose of 1.25 mg/kg was associated with excess of major bleeding. Efficacy should be tested in phase III trial.

TIMI 12

Title	Randomized trial of an oral platelet glycoprotein IIb/IIIa antagonist, sibrafiban, in patients after an acute coronary syndrome. Results of the TIMI 12 Trial.
Author	Cannon CP, McCabe CH, Borzak S, et al.
Reference	Circulation 1998; 97:340-349.
Disease	Coronary artery disease, acute coronary syndromes.
Purpose	To evaluate pharmacokinetics, pharmacodynamics, safety and tolerability of sibrafiban.
Design	Double blind, dose ranging trial.
Patients	106 patients - pharmacokinetics, pharmacodynamics, 223 safety cohort. Patients had acute coronary syndromes - unstable angina, non Q wave myocardial infarction, or Q wave myocardial infarction.
Follow-up	28 days.
Treatment regimen	In the pharmacokinetic/pharmacodynamic cohort, 106 patients received 1 of 7 doses of sibrafiban ranging from 5mg daily to 10 mg x2/d for 28 days. In the safety cohort patients were randomized to 1 of 4 dose regimens (5 mg twice daily to 15 mg once daily) or aspirin.

TIMI 12

Results   Sibrafibran successfully inhibited platelets from 47-97%
           inhibition of ADP-induced platelet aggregation across
           doses.There was a correlation between concentration of
           drug and degree of ADP-induced placebo inhibition.
           Twice daily dosing obtained more sustained inhibition,as
           with once daily dosing inhibition returned to baseline val-
           ues by 24 h. Major hemorrhage occurred in 1.5% of
           patients receiving sibrafiban and in 1.9% of those receiv-
           ing aspirin. Minor bleeding (usually mucocutaneous)
           occurred in 0-32% of patients on various doses of
           sibrafiban and none of aspirin.Minor bleeding correlated
           with total daily dose, twice daily dosing, renal function,
           and presence of unstable angina.

Conclusions Sibrafiban, an oral glycoprotein IIb/IIIa antagonist is an
           effective long-term platelet antagonist with a dose
           response.There was a relatively high incidence of minor
           bleeding.Further studies are warranted to assess outcome
           in acute coronary syndromes.

TRIM

Thrombin Inhibition in Myocardial Ischaemia

Title	A low molecular weight, selective thrombin inhibitor, inogatran, vs heparin, in unstable coronary artery disease in 1209 patients.
Authors	Thrombin Inhibition in Myocardial Ischaemia (TRIM) study group.
Reference	Eur Heart J 1997;18:1416-1425.
Disease	Unstable angina and non Q wave myocardial infarction.
Purpose	To assess the effects of Inogatran, a novel low molecular weight selective thrombin inhibitor in unstable angina and in non Q wave myocardial infarction.
Design	Randomized, double blind, multicenter.
Patients	1209 patients with unstable angina or non Q wave myocardial infarction. Patients with increased risk of bleeding, uncontrolled hypertension, history of stroke, active peptic ulcer, recent anticoagulant or fibrinolytic therapy, recent CABG, and uncompensated congestive heart failure or arrhythmia were excluded.
Follow-up	Clinical follow-up for 30-40 days.
Treatment regimen	Randomization to: 1. low-dose inogatran (1.1 mg bolus, 2 mg/h infusion); 2. medium-dose inogatran (2.75 mg bolus, 5 mg/h infusion); 3. high-dose inogatran (5.5 mg bolus, 5.5 mg/h infusion); and 4. heparin (5000 u bolus, 1,200 u/h infusion). All treatment regimens were given for 72h, within 24h of the end of the qualifying episode of pain. If the activated partial thromboplastin time (aPTT) was >3 times normal, infusion rate was reduced.

TRIM

Thrombin Inhibition in Myocardial Ischaemia

(continued)

Additional therapy	Aspirin was recommended. Ticlopidine and oral antico-agulants were prohibited.
Results	aPTTs were higher in the heparin-treated group than in the 3 inogatran groups after 6h. However, after 24h and 48h aPTTs were comparable. 41.3% of the heparin-treated patients vs only 1.3%-4.4% of the inogatran-treated patients needed infusion rate reduction due to prolonged aPTT. At the end of the 72h infusion, death or myocardial (re)infarction occurred in 3.6%, 2.0%, and 4.0% of the low medium, and high dose inogatran groups vs only 0.7% in the heparin group (odds ratio 5.02; 95% CI 1.19-21.17). The composite end-point (death, myocardial (re)infarction, refractory angina or recurrence of angina after 7 days) at the end of treatment occurred in 39.4%, 37.6%, and 36.1% of the inogatran groups, respectively vs only 29.5% in the heparin group (odds ratio 1.48; 95% CI 1.12-1.96). However, the composite end-point at 7 days was not significantly different among groups (45.7%, 45.9%, 45.5% in the inogatran groups, respectively and 41.0% in the heparin group; odds ratio 1.23; 95% CI 0.95-1.61). The composite event rates at 30 days were also comparable (51.7%, 52.2%, 53.2%, and 47.9%; odds ratio 1.21; 95% CI 0.93-1.57). Major bleeding within 7 days occurred in 1.1% of the patients, with similar rates among the groups. No intracerebral hemorrhages were noted.
Conclusions	During the 3 days of therapy, event rates were lower with heparin than with inogatran. However, after cessation of infusion there was an increase in event rates in all treatment arms. Since the high inogatran dose was not associated with increased bleeding, a higher dose may be more effective.

VANQWISH

Veterans Affairs Non Q Wave Infarction Strategies In-Hospital

Title	Outcome in patients with acute non Q wave myocardial infarction rendomly assigned to an invasive as compared with a conservative management.
Author	Boden WE, O'Rourke RA, Crawford MH, et al.
Reference	a. J Am Coll Cardiol 1998;31:312-320. b. J Am Coll Cardiol 1997;30:1-7. c. N Engl J Med 1998;338:1785-1792
Disease	Non Q wave myocardial infarction.
Purpose	To compare outcomes in patients with non Q wave myocardial infarctions randomized to early invasive strategy vs conservative management.
Design	Randomized, multicenter.
Patients	920 patients, ≥18 years old, with suspected non Q wave myocardial infarction. Patients with unstable angina or refractory angina after the non Q wave infarction, persistent left bundle branch block, congestive heart failure, pericarditis, ventricular tachyarrhythmias, revascularization within 3 months prior randomization, or concomitant severe illness were excluded.
Follow-up	12-44 months (mean 23 months).

VANQWISH

Veterans Affairs Non Q Wave Infarction Strategies In-Hospital

(continued)

Treatment regimen	Randomization within 1-7 days of infarction to early (3-7 days) coronary angiography (invasive strategy) or to conservative strategy (radionuclide left ventriculography and symptom-limited treadmill exercise test with thallium scintigraphy). In the invasive strategy, angioplasty was performed in patients with single vessel disease, whereas coronary bypass surgery was considered for patients with multivessel disease. Patients assigned to the conservative strategy were referred to angiography only if they had post infarction angina, ≥2 mm ST deviation during exercise test, or if the thallium scan showed ≥2 redistribution defects or one redistribution defect or increased lung uptake of thallium.
Additional thearpy	All patients received aspirin 325 mg/d and diltiazem 180-300 mg/d. Nitrates, angiotensin-converting-enzyme inhibitors, β-blockers, heparin and thrombolytic thearpy were permitted.
Results	Overall 96% of the invasive-strategy vs only 48% of the conservative-strategy arm underwent coronary angiography. 44% vs 33% respectively underwent revascularization procedures. During an average of 23 months there were 152 cardiac events (80 deaths and 72 nonfatal infarctions) in 138 patients among the invasive-strategy arm whereas in the conservative arm there were 139 events (59 deaths and 80 nonfatal infarctions) in 123 patients (p=0.35; hazard ratio for the conservative-strategy vs the invasive-strategy 0.87; 95% CI 0.68–1.10). However, during the first 12 monthe death or nonfatal myocardial infarction were more common in the invasive-strategy arm (111 vs 85 events; p=0.05). Mortality rate among the invasive and conservative arms were 21 vs 6 before hospital discharge (p=0.007); 23 vs 9 at 1 month (p=0.21); and 58 vs 36 at 1 year (p=0.025), respectively. During long-term follow-up, cumulative all-cause mortality was comparable between the conservative and invasive-strategy arms (hazard ratio 0.72; 95% CI 0.51–1.01).

VANQWISH

Veterans Affairs Non Q Wave Infarction Strategies In-Hospital

(continued)

Conclusions   This study shows that the strategy of routine, early invasive management of patients with non Q wave myocardial infarction, consisting of coronary angiography and revascularization, is not better than the strategy of conservative, ischemia-guided approach.

ESSENCE

Efficacy and Safety of Subcutaneous Enoxaparin in Non Q Wave Coronary Events

Title	A comparison of low molecular weight heparin with unfractionated heparin for unstable coronary artery disease.
Author	Cohen M, Demers C, Gurfinkel EP, et al.
Reference	N Engl J Med 1997; 337:447-452.
Disease	Coronary artery disease.
Purpose	To determine the safety and efficacy of the low molecular weight heparin, enoxaparin vs intravenous unfractionated heparin in patients with unstable angina and non Q wave myocardial infarction.
Design	Double blind, placebo-controlled, randomized, multicenter.
Patients	3171 patients with angina at rest or non Q wave infarction. Average ages 63 - 64; 66% - 67% males.
Follow-up	30 days.
Treatment regimen	1 mg/kg enoxaparin given subcutaneously x2/d vs continuous IV unfractionated heparin. Therapy continued from 48 h - 8 days. Aspirin was given to all patients.

ESSENCE

Efficacy and Safety of Subcutaneous Enoxaparin in Non Q Wave Coronary Events

(continued)

Results
: The composite end point of death, myocardial infarction, or recurrent angina was significantly lower in the enoxaparin group compared to unfractionated heparin group at 14 days (16.6% vs 19.8%, p=0.019), and at 30 days (19.8% vs 23.3%, p=0.016). Mortality was 0.4% in the unfractionated heparin group vs 0.5% in the enoxaprin group (p=0.18) at 48 h, 2.3% vs 2.2% respectively at 14 days (p=0.92), and 3.6% vs 2.9%, respectively (p=0.25) at 30 days. Need for revascularization was lower in patients on enoxaparin vs unfractionated heparin (27.0% vs 32.2%, p = 0.001). The incidence of major bleeding was similar in the 2 groups (6.5% vs 7.0%), but overall incidence of bleeding was higher in enoxaparin group (18.4%) compared to unfractionated heparin (14.2% = 0.001) mainly related to ecchymoses at sites of injection.

Conclusions
: Enoxaparin plus aspirin was more effective than unfractionated heparin plus aspirin in reducing the incidence of death, myocardial infarction, or recurrent angina. Enoxaparin increased minor but not the incidence of major bleeding.

3. Stable Angina Pectoris and Silent Ischemia-Medical Therapy

ASIST

Atenolol Silent Ischemia Study

Title	Effects of treatment on outcome in mildly symptomatic patients with ischemia during daily life: the Atenolol Silent Ischemia Study (ASIST).
Authors	Pepine CJ, Cohn PF, Deedwania PC, et al.
Reference	Circulation 1994;90:762-768.
Disease	Coronary artery disease, silent myocardial ischemia.
Purpose	To assess whether atenolol therapy will decrease adverse outcome events in mildly symptomatic patients with coronary artery disease.
Design	Randomized, double blind, placebo-controlled, multicenter.
Patients	306 patients with >50% stenosis of a major coronary artery, or previous myocardial infarction and transient ischemia documented by exercise ECG. Only patients with Canadian Cardiovascular Society class I or II, and without an abnormal ECG that could interfere with ambulatory ECG ST segment monitoring were included. Patients with unstable angina, myocardial infarction, or coronary revascularization within 3 months were excluded. Patients with contraindications to ß-blockers or with a need for antianginal medications other than nitrates, and patients with heart failure were excluded. The atenolol group included 152 patients and the placebo 154 patients.
Follow-up	1 year.
Treatment regimen	Atenolol (100 mg/d, in cases where adverse effects occurred, the dose was lowered to 50 mg/d) or placebo.

ASIST

Atenolol Silent Ischemia Study

(continued)

Results
: After 4 weeks of therapy, the number (3.6±4.2 vs 1.7±4.6 episodes, p<0.001) and mean duration (30.0±3.3 vs 16.4±6.7 min, p<0.001) of ischemic episodes detected by 48 h of ambulatory ECG monitoring were reduced in the atenolol treated patients, compared to baseline recording, but not in the placebo group. After 1 year less patients in the atenolol group experienced death, VT/VF, myocardial infarction, hospitalization, aggravation of angina, or revascularization (11% vs 25%; relative risk 44%; 95% CI 26-75%; p=0.001). The atenolol treated patients had a longer time to first event (120 vs 79 days; p<0.001). The most significant predictor of event-free survival in univariate and multivariate analysis was absence of ischemia on ambulatory ECG monitoring at 4 weeks. Side effects were comparable in both groups.

Conclusions
: Treatment of asymptomatic or mildly symptomatic patients with coronary artery disease with atenolol reduced number and duration of ischemic episodes at 4 weeks and the risk for adverse events at 1 year.

CAPE

Circadian Anti-Ischemia Program in Europe

Title	Amlodipine reduces transient myocardial ischemia in patients with coronary artery disease: double blind circadian anti-ischemia program in Europe (CAPE Trial).
Authors	Deanfield JE, Detry J-M RG, Lichtlen PR, et al.
Reference	J Am Coll Cardiol 1994;24:1460-1467.
Disease	Coronary artery disease, angina pectoris.
Purpose	To evaluate the effect of once-daily amlodipine on the circadian pattern of myocardial ischemia in patients with stable angina pectoris.
Design	Randomized, double blind, placebo-controlled, multicenter.
Patients	315 males, age 35-80 years, with stable angina with ≥3 attacks/week. Patients with heart failure, uncontrolled arrhythmias, bradycardia, hypertension or hypotension, chronic therapy with calcium channel blockers, and ECG features that interfere with interpretation of ST segment changes were excluded. All patients had ≥4 ischemic episodes or ≥20 min of ST depression over 48 h ambulatory ECG monitoring.
Follow-up	Clinical follow-up and 48 h ambulatory monitoring at 8 weeks of phase II.
Treatment regimen	Phase I: 2 weeks of single blind placebo run-in period. Phase II: randomization to amlodipine (started at 5 mg/d and increased to 10 mg/d) or placebo treatment for 8 weeks.

CAPE

Circadian Anti-Ischemia Program in Europe

(continued)

Additional therapy	Patients were instructed to maintain on stable doses of all concomitant cardiovascular medications. Nitroglycerin tablets were provided.
Results	Only 250 patients were fully evaluated for ambulatory ECG analysis. Amlodipine therapy resulted in greater reduction of the frequency of ST depression episodes (median reduction 60.0% vs 43.8%, p=0.025), ST segment integral (mm-min of ST depression)(median reduction 61.6% vs 49.5%, p=0.042), and total duration of ST depression (56% vs 49.5%, p=0.066) than placebo. The intrinsic circadian pattern of ischemia was maintained in both groups. Patients' diaries showed a significant reduction of anginal pain (70% vs 44%, p=0.0001) and in nitroglycerin consumption (67% vs 22%, p=0.0006) with amlodipine vs placebo. Adverse effects occurred in 17.3% of the amlodipine vs 13.3% of the placebo (p=0.422), discontinuation due to adverse events were 2.0% vs 4.4%, respectively (p=0.291).
Conclusions	Once-daily amlodipine, in addition to regular anti-anginal therapy, reduced both symptomatic and asymptomatic ischemic episodes in patients with chronic stable angina.

ACIP

Asymptomatic Cardiac Ischemia Pilot Study

Title	a. The asymptomatic cardiac ischemia pilot (ACIP) study: design of a randomized clinical trial, baseline data, and implications for a long-term outcome trial.
	b. Effects of treatment strategies to suppress ischemia in patients with coronary artery disease: 12 week results of the asymptomatic cardiac ischemia pilot (ACIP) study.
	c. Asymptomatic cardiac ischemia pilot (ACIP) study: impact of anti-ischemia therapy on 12 week rest electrocardiogram and exercise test outcomes.
	d. Asymptomatic cardiac ischemia pilot (ACIP) study. Improvement of cardiac ischemia at 1 year after PTCA and CABG.
	e. Prognostic significance of myocardial ischemia detected by ambulatory electrocardiography, exercise treadmill testing, and electrocardiogram at rest to predict cardiac events by one year (The Asymptomatic Cardiac Ischemia Pilot [ACIP] Study).
	f. Asymptomatic cardiac ischemia pilot (ACIP) study two-year follow-up. Outcomes of patients randomized to initial strategies of medical therapy vs revascularization.
Authors	a. Pepine CJ, Geller NL, Knatterud GL, et al.
	b. Knatterud GL, Bourassa MG, Pepine CJ, et al.
	c. Chaitman BR, Stone PH, Knatterud GL, et al.
	d. Bourassa MG, Knatterud GL, Pepine CJ, et al.
	e. Stone PH, Chaitman BR, Forman S, et al.
	f. Davies RF, Goldberg D, Forman S, et al.
Reference	a. J Am Coll Cardiol 1994;24:1-10.
	b. J Am Coll Cardiol 1994;24:11-20.
	c. J Am Coll Cardiol 1995;26:585-593.
	d. Circulation 1995;92:II-1–II-7.
	e. Am J Cardiol 1997; 80:1395-1401.
	f. Circulation 1997; 95:2037-2043.
Disease	Coronary artery disease.

ACIP

Asymptomatic Cardiac Ischemia Pilot Study

(continued)

Purpose	To compare 3 strategies of therapy (angina-guided medical therapy, ischemia-guided medical therapy, and coronary revascularization) in reduction of myocardial ischemia at exercise testing after 12 weeks of therapy. f. As above. Purpose of this study was to describe 2 year clinical outcome of angina-guided drug therapy, angina plus ischemia-guided drug therapy, or revascularization by angioplasty or coronary artery bypass surgery.
Design	Randomized, open label, multicenter.
Patients	a+b. 618 patients, c+d. 558 patients with obstructive coronary artery disease suitable for revascularization, ≥1 episode of ischemia on 48 h ambulatory ECG monitoring, or evidence of ischemia on exercise test. Follow-up 12 week repeated exercise test. 1 year clinical follow-up. f. 558 patients with coronary anatomy suitable to revascularization, randomized to: angina-guided drug therapy (n=183), angina plus ischemia-guided drug therapy (n=183) or revascularization (n=192).
Follow-up	12 week repeated exercise test. 1 year clinical follow-up. f. 2 years.
Treatment regimen	1. Angina guided medical therapy. 2. Angina + ambulatory ECG monitoring-guided medical therapy. 3. Coronary revascularization. The medical therapy included randomization to either atenolol or diltiazem as the first drug, and addition of nifedipine to atenolol and isosorbide dinitrate to diltiazem.
Results	a + b. Ambulatory ECG ischemia was no longer present at 12 weeks in 39%, 41%, and 55% of the angina-guided, ischemia-guided, and revascularization strategies. All strategies reduced the median number of episode and total duration of ST depression. Revascularization was the most effective strategy ($p<0.001$, and $p=0.01$ for the number of episodes and total duration, respectively). More

patients were ischemia free in the atenolol + nifedipine (47%) than diltiazem + nitrates (32%, p=0.03).

c. Peak exercise time was increased by 0.5, 0.7, and 1.6 min in the angina-guided, ischemia-guided, and revascularization strategies from baseline to 12 weeks (p<0.001). The sum of exercise induced ST depression was similar at baseline. However, at 12 weeks ST depression during exercise was 7.4±5.7, 6.8±5.3, and 5.6±5.6 mm, (p=0.02).

d. At 12 weeks, ischemia on the ambulatory ECG monitoring was suppressed in 70% of the 78 CABG patients and in 46% of the 92 PTCA patients (p=0.002). Myocardial infarction or repeated revascularization occurred in 1 vs 7 of the CABG and PTCA patients (p<0.001).

e. In the two groups treated medically, there was an association between number of ischemic episodes on ambulatory monitoring and combined cardiac events at 1 year (p=0.003). In the ambulatory ECG monitored group there was a trend toward an association between reduction in number of ambulatory ECG ischemic episodes and reduction in combined cardiac events (p=0.06). This association was absent in the revascularization group. In the medically-treated groups, the exercise duration on baseline exercise treadmill test was inversely associated with poor prognosis. Medical therapy only slightly improved exercise time. Exercise duration remained a significant prognosticator of outcome in the medically treated but not revascularization-treated patients.

f. After 2 years, total mortality was 6.6% with angina-guided therapy; 4.4% with ischemia guided therapy; and 1.1% with revascularization (p<.02). Rates of death or myocardial infarction were 12.1%, 8.8%, and 4.7%, respectively (p<.04). Rates of death, myocardial infarction or recurrent hospitalization for cardiac disease were 41.8%, 38.5%, and 23.1%, respectively (p<.001). P values were significant for comparisons between revascularization and angina guided strategies.

Conclusions	Coronary revascularization significantly reduced the duration of silent ischemia on ambulatory ECG monitoring and the extent and frequency of exercise induced ischemia compared to the medical strategies.
	f. Initial revascularization improved prognosis in these coronary artery disease patients at 2 years, compared to angina-guided medical therapy.

TIBBS

Total Ischemic Burden Bisoprolol Study

Title	Medical treatment to reduce total ischemic burden: total ischemic burden bisoprolol study (TIBBS), a multicenter trial comparing bisoprolol and nifedipine.
Authors	von Arnim T, for the TIBBS Investigators.
Reference	J Am Coll Cardiol 1995;25:231-238.
Disease	Coronary artery disease, stable angina pectoris.
Purpose	To compare the effects of bisoprolol and nifedipine on transient myocardial ischemia in patients with stable angina.
Design	Randomized, double blind, multicenter.
Patients	330 patients with stable angina pectoris, positive exercise test with ST depression, and ≥ 2 episodes of transient myocardial ischemia on 48 h ambulatory ECG monitoring. Patients with unstable angina, myocardial infarction within 3 months, bradycardia <50 bpm, AV block, or hypotension were excluded.
Follow-up	Exercise test and ambulatory ECG monitoring during the placebo phase, after 4 weeks of the first dose period and after 8 weeks (double dose period).
Treatment regimen	10 day placebo phase, and then randomization to either bisoprolol 10 mg/d or nifedipine slow release 20 mg X2/d for 4 weeks, and then the doses were doubled for an additional 4 weeks.

TIBBS

Total Ischemic Burden Bisoprolol Study

(continued)

Additional therapy	Long acting nitrates, ß blockers, calcium channel blockers, vasodilators, tricyclic antidepressants, digoxin, antiarrhythmic agents, and ß mimetic agents were not permitted during the study.
Results	4 weeks of bisoprolol 10 mg/d reduced the mean number of transient ischemic episodes from 8.1±0.6 to 3.2±0.4 episodes/48 h (mean change -4.9, 95% CI -5.8 to -4.0). Nifedipine 20 mg X2/d reduced the number of ischemic episodes from 8.3±0.5 to 5.9±0.4 episodes/48 h (mean change -2.5, 95% CI -4.3 to -1.5). The effect of bisoprolol was almost twice that of nifedipine (bisoprolol vs nifedipine p=0.0001). Total duration of ischemic episodes were reduced from 99.3±10.1 to 31.9±5.5 min/48 h by bisoprolol (mean change -67.4, 95% CI -84.0 to -50.7), and from 101.0±9.1 to 72.6±8.1 min/48 h by nifedipine (mean change -28.4, 95% CI -45.9 to -10.9)(bisoprolol vs nifedipine p=0.0001). Doubling the dose of the medications resulted in only small additional effects that were significant only for bisoprolol. Bisoprolol reduced the heart rate at onset of ischemia by 13.7±1.4 bpm (p<0.001). Heart rate was not changed by nifedipine. 73.7% of the bisoprolol 10 mg/d vs 42.4% of the nifedipine 20 mg X2/d showed ≥50% reduction in the number of ischemic episodes (p<0.0001). The corresponding rates for the higher dose were 80.5% vs 49.2% (p<0.0001). Only bisoprolol showed a marked circadian effect by reducing the morning peak of ischemia.
Conclusions	Both agents reduced the number and duration of ischemic episodes in patients with stable angina. Bisoprolol was more effective than nifedipine.

IMAGE

International Multicenter Angina Exercise Study

Title	Combination therapy with metoprolol and nifedipine vs monotherapy in patients with stable angina pectoris. Results of the International Multicenter Angina Exercise (IMAGE) Study.
Authors	Savonitto S, Ardissino D, Egstrup K, et al.
Reference	J Am Coll Cardiol 1996;27:311-316.
Disease	Angina pectoris.
Purpose	To compare the efficacy of combination therapy with metoprolol and nifedipine vs either drug alone in patients with stable angina pectoris.
Design	Randomized, double blind, placebo-controlled (second stage), multicenter.
Patients	280 patients, age ≤75 years, with stable angina for ≥6 months and a positive exercise test. Patients with myocardial infarction within 6 months, heart failure, inability to perform ≥3 min exercise test, or those with severe angina that preclude temporary cessation of medications, were excluded.
Follow-up	Exercise test at baseline, after the 6 weeks of monotherapy and after 10 weeks.
Treatment regimen	After 2 week placebo run-in period, patients were randomized to metoprolol 200 mg/d or nifedipine retard 20 mg X2/d for 6 weeks. Then, patients were randomized to addition of the second drug or placebo for 4 more weeks.

International Multicenter Angina Exercise Study
(continued)

Results	249 patients completed the study. By the end of 6 weeks the nifedipine treated group increased the mean duration of exercise time until 1 mm ST depression by 43 sec compared with baseline (95% CI 16-69 sec, $p<0.01$), and the metoprolol group by 70 sec (95% CI 47-92 sec, $p<0.01$). The improvement was greater with metoprolol ($p<0.05$). At week 10, the exercise time did not increase further in the patients who received placebo in addition to the metoprolol or nifedipine. However, addition of nifedipine to metoprolol resulted in further increase of the time 108 sec more than in the baseline test (95% CI 71-145 sec), and addition of metoprolol to nifedipine in 107 sec (95% CI 64-151 sec) more than in the baseline test ($p<0.05$ vs placebo). Analysis of the results in individual patients revealed that the additive effect was seen mainly in those who respond poorly to monotherapy.
Conclusions	Both drugs were effective as monotherapy in prolongation the exercise time (metoprolol more than nifedipine). The prolongation of exercise time, observed in the combination therapy, is not the result of an additive effect, but probably due to the effect of the second class of drug in patients not responding to the first one.

TREND

Trial on Reversing ENdothelial Dysfunction

Title	Angiotensin-converting enzyme inhibition with quinapril improves endothelial vasomotor dysfunction in patients with coronary artery disease. The TREND (trial on reversing endothelial dusfunction) study.
Authors	Mancini GBJ, Henry GC, Macaya C, et al.
Reference	Circulation 1996;94:258-265.
Disease	Coronary artery disease.
Purpose	To evaluate whether quinapril, an ACE inhibitor, improves endothelial dysfunction in normotensive patients with coronary artery disease and no heart failure, cardiomyopathy, or major lipid abnormalities.
Design	Randomized, double blind, placebo-controlled, multicenter.
Patients	129 patients, ≤75 years old, with documented coronary artery disease: single or double vessel disease (>50% diameter stenosis) that required a nonsurgical revascularization, and one adjacent coronary artery with <40% stenosis that had never been revascularized. This artery had to show endothelial dysfunction defined as either constriction or no response to acetylcholine. Patients with LDL cholesterol >165 mg/dL, hypertension (>160 mmHg systolic or >90 mmHg diastolic blood pressure), previous CABG, history of coronary spasm, coronary revascularization within 3 months, myocardial infarction within 7 days, left ventricular ejection fraction <0.40, type I diabetes mellitus, valvular heart disease, hepatic or renal dysfunction, 2nd or 3rd degree AV block, or lipid lowering therapy within 6 months were excluded.

TREND

Trial on Reversing ENdothelial Dysfunction
(continued)

Follow-up	Cardiac catheterization with assessment of the response to intracoronary injection of acetylcholine 10-6 and 10-4 mol/L over 2 min before revascularization and after 6 months of therapy.
Treatment regimen	Quinapril 40 mg/d or placebo for 6 months.
Additional therapy	All vasoactive medications, except for ß-blockers and sublingual nitrates, were discontinued 12 h before angiography.
Results	105 patients underwent repeated angiography at 6 months. At baseline, before initiation of study medications, the constrictive response to acetylcholine was comparable between the placebo and quinapril groups (4.4% vs 6.1% after infusion of 10-6 mol/L and 9.4% vs 14.3% after infusion of 10-4 mol/L (p=0.125), respectively). After 6 months of therapy there was no change in the response to acetylcholine in the placebo group (4.5% and 10.5% after acetylcholine 10-6 mol/L and 10-4 mol/L, respectively), whereas the quinapril-treated patients showed less constrictor response (1.6% and 2.3%, respectively) compared with the baseline study (p<0.014). Responses, expressed as net change from baseline, improved by 4.5±3.0% and 12.1±3.0% at each acetylcholine dose in the quinapril group, whereas the placebo group responses did not change (-0.1±2.8% and -0.8±2.9%, respectively, p<0.002). The analysis of the response to a nitroglycerin bolus (100-700 µg) revealed no difference between the groups at baseline (p=0.349) and after 6 months (p=0.336).
Conclusions	Angiotensin-converting enzyme inhibition with quinapril improved endothelial function in normotensive patients without severe hyperlipidemia or heart failure.

Efficacy of mibefradil compared with amlodipine in suppressing exercise-induced and daily silent ischemia. Results of a multicenter, placebo-controlled trial.

Title	Efficacy of mibefradil compared with amlodipine in suppressing exercise-induced and daily silent ischemia. Results of a multicenter, placebo-controlled trial.
Author	Tzivoni D, Kadr H, Braat S. et al.
Reference	Circulation 1997; 96: 2557-2564.
Disease	Coronary artery disease, stable angina pectoris.
Purpose	To determine the effects of mibefradil (a new calcium channel blocker which blocks the T-type channel) on exercise-induced and daily silent ischemia in patients with stable angina pectoris and compare its efficacy to amlodipine.
Design	Prospective, randomized, double blind, placebo-controlled, parallel-design trial, multicenter. 1 to 2 week washout period of long-acting antianginals. 1 week placebo run-in phase with exercise tests and 48 h ECG ambulatory monitoring. 2 week treatment phase with repeat exercise test and ambulatory monitoring.
Patients	309 patients with coronary artery disease, stable angina, and positive exercise tests.
Follow-up	3 weeks.
Treatment regimen	For initial treatment period patients were randomized to 1 of 5 groups: placebo; 25, 50, or 100 mg of mibefradil; amlodipine 5 mg. At one week mibefradil doses were increased to 50, 100, or 150 mg, and amlodipine to 10 mg.

Efficacy of mibefradil compared with amlodipine in suppressing exercise-induced and daily silent ischemia. Results of a multicenter, placebo-controlled trial.

(continued)

Results	At 100 mg and 150 mg (but not 50 mg) mibefradil increased exercise duration by 55.5 and 51.0 sec, respectively vs placebo, $p < .001$. At 100 and 150 mg mibefradil increased time to onset of angina (by 98.3 and 82.7 sec, respectively; $p < .001$) and increased time to 1-mm ST depression (by 81.7 and 94.3 sec, respectively, $p < .001$). Amlodipine at 10 mg/day increased time to onset of angina (by 38.5 seconds; $p = .036$). Mibefradil 100 mg and 150 mg decreased the number of episodes of silent ischemia on ambulatory monitoring as did 10 mg of amlodipine. There was a nonsignificant trend toward a greater reduction in number of silent ischemic episodes at higher doses of mibefradil than amlodipine. As expected, mibefradil but not amlodipine reduced heart rate.
Conclusions	Mibefradil 100 or 150 mg once-daily was effective in improving exercise tolerance and reducing ischemic episodes during ambulatory electrocardiographic monitoring. Amlodipine 10 mg improved time to onset of angina during exercise and had somewhat less of an effect of reducing silent ischemic episodes. (Note-mibefradil was taken off the U.S. market in 1998, in part due to interactions with other drugs).

THE ESBY STUDY

Electrical Stimulation Bypass Surgery

Title	Electrical stimulation vs coronary artery bypass surgery in severe angina pectoris. The ESBY study.
Author	Mannheimer C, Eliasson T, Augustinsson L-E.
Reference	Circulation 1998; 97:1157-1163.
Disease	Coronary artery disease; angina pectoris.
Purpose	To determine whether spinal cord stimulation (SCS) can be used as an alternative to coronary artery bypass grafting (CABG) in selected patients with coronary artery disease.
Design	Randomized, prospective, open comparison between SCS and CABG.
Patients	104 patients with symptomatic coronary artery disease who were considered to have only symptomatic (not prognostic) benefit from CABG, to be at increased risk of surgery, and to be ineligible for percutaneous transluminal coronary angioplasty.
Follow-up	6 months.
Treatment regimen	53 patients were randomized to SCS and 51 to CABG.

THE ESBY STUDY

Electrical Stimulation Bypass Surgery

(continued)

Results	Both treatments reduced angina to a similar extent. CABG resulted in an increase in exercise capacity, less ST segment depression on exercise compared to SCS; rate-pressure product on maximum and comparable workloads were higher for the CABG patients. 7 patients died in the CAGB group and 1 died in the SCS group. By intention-to-treat mortality was lower in the SCS group (p=0.02). There also was less cerebrovascular morbidity in the SCS group.
Conclusions	SCS may be a therapeutic alternative for this group of patients with coronary artery disease.

FEMINA

Felodipine ER and Metoprolol CR in Angina

Title	Addition of felodipine to metoprolol vs replacement of metoprolol by felodipine in patients with angina pectoris despite adequate beta-blockade. Results of the felodipine ER and metoprolol CR in angina (FEMINA) study.
Authors	Dunselman P, Liem AH, Verdel G, et al.
Reference	Eur Heart J 1997;18:1755-1764.
Disease	Angina pectoris-stable.
Purpose	To compare the effect of metoprolol alone, adding felodipine to metoprolol or replacement of metoprolol by felodipine in patients with angina pectoris despite metoprolol therapy.
Design	Randomized, double blind, parallel, multicenter.
Patients	356 patients, aged 18-75 years, with angina pectoris, who had been receiving metoprolol controlled release 100-200 mg/d before enrollment and who had positive exercise tests despite therapy.
Follow-up	Clinical follow-up and repeated exercise tests at baseline, 2 and 5 weeks.
Treatment regimen	Randomization to continuation of metoprolol, replacement of metoprolol by felodipine ER 5-10 mg/d or a combination of metoprolol and felodipine ER.

FEMINA

Felodipine ER and Metoprolol CR in Angina

(continued)

Results	A total of 324 patients completed the study. After 5 weeks of therapy there was no difference among groups in time until end of exercise and time until onset of pain. The felodipine/metoprolol treated patients had 43 sec increase in the time until 1 mm ST depression (95% CI 20-65 sec; p<0.05). Both ST depression at highest comparable workload (0.46 mm, 95% CI 0.19-0.72; p<0.05) and maximal ST depression (difference from baseline) decreased in the combination group (0.49 mm; 95% CI 0.23-0.74; p<0.05). Exercise results in the felodipine alone treated patients were comparable to that of patients who received metoprolol alone. However, felodipine resulted in an increase in heart rate and in rate-pressure product. Adverse effects occurred in 19 of the metoprolol alone treated patients, 28 in the metoprolol/felodipine treated patients (p=0.15 vs metoprolol alone), and 50 in the felodipine treated patients (p<0.01 vs metoprolol alone).
Conclusions	Adding felodipine to metoprolol is preferred to replacement of metoprolol with felodipine in patients with angina pectoris despite beta-blocker therapy.

SAPAT

The Swedish Angina Pectoris Aspirin Trial

Title	Double blind trial of aspirin in primary prevention of myocardial infarction in patients with stable chronic angina pectoris.
Authors	Juul-Moller S, Edvardsson N, Jahmatz B, et al.
Reference	Lancet 1992;340:1421-1425.
Disease	Angina pectoris.
Purpose	To assess the efficacy of aspirin in stable angina.
Design	Randomized, double blind, placebo-controlled, multicenter.
Patients	2035 patients, 30-80 years old with stable angina pectoris. Patients already on aspirin, anticoagulants, nonsteroidal anti-inflammatory drugs, class I antiarrhythmic drugs or verapamil, patients with resting heart rate <55/min, history of myocardial infarction, chronic obstructive lung disease, active peptic ulcer, type I or uncontrolled diabetes mellitus, or hypersensitivity to aspirin were excluded.
Follow-up	A median of 50 (range 23-76) months.
Treatment regimen	Randomization to aspirin 75 mg/d (n=1009) or placebo (n=1026).
Additional therapy	Sotalol in increasing dose until symptoms were controlled.

SAPAT

The Swedish Angina Pectoris Aspirin Trial

(continued)

Results
At the end of the follow-up period there were 81 prima-ry events (myocardial infarction or sudden death) in the aspirin group vs 124 in the placebo group (34% reduc-tion; p=0.003). Aspirin therapy decreased the occurrence of sudden death by 38% (p=0.097), and nonfatal myocar-dial infarction by 39% (p=0.006). However, the incidence of fatal myocardial infarction was not changed. Vascular events were reduced by 32% with aspirin (p<0.001), stroke by 25% (p=0.246), and all cause mortality by 22% (p=0.103). There was no difference in the number of coro-nary artery bypass procedures between the aspirin and placebo groups. Treatment withdrawal due to adverse effects occurred in 109 patients of the aspirin group vs 100 patients of the placebo group (p=NS), bleedings in 27 patients vs 16 patients (p=NS), and major bleeding in 20 patients and 13 patients (p=NS), respectively. In a mul-tivariate regression model the only variables found to be independently associated with primary events were aspirin therapy, gender, diabetes mellitus type II, and serum cholesterol levels. The relative risk of aspirin ther-apy vs placebo was 0.68 (95% CI 0.49-0.93).

Conclusions
Low dose aspirin, added to sotalol therapy reduced the occurrence of cardiovascular events, especially nonfatal myocardial infarction and vascular events in patients with stable angina pectoris without prior myocardial infarc-tion. However, the effect on total mortality, fatal myocar-dial infarction, sudden death, and stroke were not statistically significant.

TIBET

The Total Ischaemic Burden European Trial

Title	a. The total ischaemic burden European trial (TIBET). Effects of atenolol, nifedipine SR and their combination on the exercise test and total ischaemic burden in 608 patients with stable angina. b. The total ischaemic burden European trial (TIBET). Effects of atenolol, nifedipine SR, and their combination on outcome in patients with chronic stable angina.
Authors	a. Fox KM, Mulcahy D, Findlay I et al. b. Dargie HJ, Ford I, Fox KM, on behalf of the TIBET study group.
Reference	a. Eur Heart J 1996;17:96-103. b. Eur Heart J 1996;17:104-112.
Disease	Angina pectoris.
Purpose	To compare the effects of atenolol, nifedipine and their combination on exercise parameters, ambulatory ischemic activity, and prognosis in patients with mild stable angina pectoris and to evaluate the relationship between presence of ischemic events on ambulatory 48 h Holter ECG monitoring and outcome.
Design	Randomized, double blind, parallel group, multicenter.
Patients	(a. 608, b. 682) patients (86% men), 40-79 years old, with stable angina pectoris over the preceding 3 months who were not being considered for revascularization and who had positive exercise test after a 2 week washout phase. Patients with recent (<3 months) coronary revascularization or myocardial infarction, conduction disturbances, contraindications to either nifedipine or atenolol, or medications that might affect the interpretation of the ST segment shift during exercise test were excluded.

TIBET

The Total Ischaemic Burden European Trial

(continued)

Follow-up	a. 1 year. Exercise test (treadmill Bruce protocol or bicycle protocol) at baseline, 2 and 6 weeks after randomization. 48 h Holter ambulatory ECG monitoring at baseline and 6 weeks. b. An average of 2 years or until death had occurred (range 1 to 3 years).
Treatment regimen	a.+ b. After 2 single blind run-in phases of 2 weeks active combination therapy (to confirm tolerance) followed by 2 weeks placebo treatment, patients were randomized to atenolol 50 mg BID (n=205), nifedipine slow release 20 mg BID (n=202), or their combination (n=201). b. At the 6 week visit, the nifedipine dose could be increased to 40 mg BID.
Results	a. Atenolol alone and in combination caused a significant fall in resting heart rate (sitting heart rate decreased by 15.4 and 13.5 BPM in the atenolol alone and atenolol+nifedipine group, respectively), whereas nifedipine alone caused a 2.9 BPM increase in sitting heart rate. All three regimens caused a significant fall in blood pressure ($p<0.01$), which was more pronounced in the combination group. All three treatment regimens caused significant improvements in total exercise time, time to pain, time to 1 mm ST depression and maximum ST depression during exercise. Changes from baseline were significant for all these variables in all groups, but there was no significant difference among the three groups. All three groups had a significant reduction in the incidence of ischemic episodes during therapy, without a significant difference between the groups. b. There was no evidence of a relationship between the presence, frequency or total duration of ischemic ECG changes during continuous ambulatory Holter monitoring, either at baseline or during therapy, and cardiac mortality, the occurrence of myocardial infarction, unstable angina, revascularization, and treatment failure. Cardiac mortality, myocardial infarction, or unstable angina occurred in 12.8% of the atenolol group, 11.2% of the nifedipine group, and 8.5% of the combination group (p=NS). Comparison of the time to these events among

the 3 groups, using the logrank test, was insignificant (p=0.32). However, there was a non-significant trend towards less events in the combination group. During follow-up 27% of the atenolol group, 40% of the nifedipine, and 29% of the combination group withdrew from the study (p=0.001).

| Conclusions | a. Combination of nifedipine and atenolol provided no additional benefit over either drug alone in patients with mild chronic angina pectoris. |

a. Combination of nifedipine and atenolol provided no additional benefit over either drug alone in patients with mild chronic angina pectoris.

b. Ischemic ECG changes on ambulatory Holter monitoring failed to predict prognosis in patients with mild chronic stable angina. Compliance was poorest with the nifedipine alone group, but there was no significant difference in prognosis among the three treatment groups.

4. Interventional Cardiology

a. PTCA or CABG Vs Medical Therapy

CASS

Coronary Artery Surgery Study

Title	a. Coronary artery surgery study (CASS): a randomized trial of coronary artery bypass surgery. Survival data. b. Myocardial infarction and mortality in the coronary artery surgery study (CASS) randomized trial. c. 10 year follow-up of survival and myocardial infarction in the randomized coronary artery surgery study. d. 10 year follow-up of quality of life in patients randomized to receive medical therapy or coronary artery bypass graft surgery. The coronary artery surgery study (CASS).
Authors	a.+b. CASS Principal Investigators and Their Associates. c. Alderman EL, Bourassa MG, Cohen LS, et al. d. Rogers WJ, Coggin CJ, Gersh BJ, et al.
Reference	a. Circulation 1983;68:939-950. b. N Engl J Med 1984;310:750-758. c. Circulation 1990;82:1629-1646. d. Circulation 1990;82:1647-1658.
Disease	Coronary artery disease, angina pectoris.
Purpose	To compare the effects of coronary artery bypass grafting surgery and medical therapy on mortality and morbidity in patients with mild angina or aymptomatic patients after myocardial infarction with coronary artery disease.
Design	Randomized, open label, multicenter.
Patients	780 patients, ≤65 years of age, with angina pectoris Canadian Cardiovascular Society Class I or II, or myocardial infarction >3 weeks before randomization. Patients with prior coronary bypass surgery, unstable angina, heart failure (NYHA class III or IV) were excluded.
Follow-up	10 years.

CASS

Coronary Artery Surgery Study

(continued)

Treatment regimen	Coronary artery bypass surgery or medical therapy.
Additional therapy	Common medical care including medications.
Results	The average annual mortality rate was 1.1% in the surgical group vs 1.6% in the medical group (p=NS). Annual mortality rates in patients with single, double, and 3 vessel disease were 0.7% vs 1.4%, 1.0% vs 1.2%, and 1.5% vs 2.1%, in the surgical and medical groups respectively. The differences were not significant. The annual mortality rate for patients with ejection fraction <0.50 was 1.7% vs 3.3% in the surgical and medical groups. In these patients the probability of survival after 5 years was 83±4% in the medical vs 93±3% in the surgical groups (p=0.11). The annual rate of bypass surgery in the medical group was 4.7%. 6% had surgery within 6 months and 40% within 10 years. Nonfatal Q wave myocardial infarction occurred in 14% vs 11% in the surgical and medical group after 5 years (p=NS). The 5 year probability of remaining alive and free from infarction was 83% vs 82% (p=NS). There was no significant difference in survival or myocardial infarction curves between subgroups of patients assigned to medical vs surgical therapy. At 10 years 82% of the surgical vs 79% of the medical groups were alive (p=NS), and 66% vs 69%, respectively were free of death and myocardial infarction (p=NS). However, 79% vs 61% of the surgical and medical patients with initial ejection fraction <0.50 were alive after 10 years (p=0.01), while more patients with ejection fraction ≥0.50 on the medical therapy were free of death and infarction after 10 years (75% vs 68%, p=0.04). 66% vs 30%, 63% vs 38%, and 47% vs 42% of the surgical and medical groups were free from angina after 1, 5, and 10 years. By 5 years indexes of quality of life appeared superior in the surgery group. However, after 10 years the differences were less apparent.
Conclusions	Coronary bypass surgery did not prolong life or prevent myocardial infarction as compared with medical therapy in patients with mild angina or patients who are asymptomatic after myocardial infarction. However, long-term survival was improved by surgical therapy in patients with initial ejection fraction <0.50.

ACME

Angioplasty Compared to Medicine

Title	A comparison of angioplasty with medical therapy in the treatment of single vessel coronary artery disease.
Authors	Parisi AF, Folland ED, Hartigan P, et al.
Reference	N Engl J Med 1992;326:10-16.
Disease	Coronary artery disease, stable angina pectoris.
Purpose	To compare the results after 6 months of angioplasty vs medical therapy in patients with stable angina pectoris and single vessel coronary artery disease.
Design	Randomized, multicenter.
Patients	212 patients with stable angina pectoris, positive exercise test, or myocardial infarction within the past 3 months, and 70-99% stenosis of the proximal 2/3 of a coronary artery.
Follow-up	Clinical evaluation every month. Exercise test and angiography after 6 months.
Treatment regimen	1. Medical therapy: a stepped-care approach including nitrates, ß-blockers, and calcium blockers. 2. Coronary angioplasty + calcium blocker for 1 month, and nitroglycerin during and for 12 h after the angioplasty.
Additional therapy	Oral aspirin 325 mg/d.

ACME

Angioplasty Compared to Medicine

(continued)

Results   Angioplasty was successful in 80 of the 100 patients who actually underwent the procedure. 2 patients in the angioplasty group required emergency coronary artery bypass surgery. After 6 months, 16 of the angioplasty group had repeated angioplasty. Of the 107 patients assigned to medical therapy, 11 underwent angioplasty. Myocardial infarction occurred in 5 and 3 of the patients assigned to angioplasty and medical therapy. After 6 months, 64% and 46% of the angioplasty and medical groups were free of angina ($p<0.01$). The angioplasty group were able to increase their total duration of exercise by 2.1 min, while the medical group by only 0.5 min ($p<0.0001$). The maximal heart rate blood pressure product decreased by 2800 units in the medical group, while it increased by 1800 units in the angioplasty group ($p<0.0001$). The overall psychological-well-being score improved by 8.6 and 2.4 in the angioplasty and medical therapy groups ($p=0.03$).

Conclusions   Angioplasty offers earlier and better relief of angina than medical therapy and is associated with better performance on the exercise test in patients with single vessel disease. However, the initial costs and the complication rates are higher with angioplasty.

RITA-2

Coronary Angioplasty vs Medical Therapy for Angina.

Title	Coronary angioplasty vs medical therapy for angina: the second randomized intervention treatment of angina (RITA-2).
Authors	RITA-2 trial participants.
Reference	Lancet 1997;350:461-468.
Disease	Coronary artery disease.
Purpose	To compare 2 initial strategies for patients with coronary artery disease: initial coronary angioplasty vs conservative medical therapy.
Design	Randomized, multicenter.
Patients	1018 patients, >18 years old, with angiographically proven coronary artery disease considered to be suitable for both medical therapy and coronary angioplasty. Patients in whom myocardial revascularization was mandatory, patients with previous myocardial revascularization, left main coronary artery disease, significant valvular disease, or concomitant life-threatening non cardiac disease were excluded.
Follow-up	5 years (the present study summarized interim results after a minimum of 6 months and a median of 2.7 years)
Treatment regimen	Randomization to conservative medical therapy or balloon angioplasty (PTCA). Patients assigned to PTCA underwent the procedure within 3 months of randomization.
Additional therapy	Stents and atherectomy were permitted if the initial standard PTCA results were unsatisfactory. All patients received aspirin unless contraindicated. Lipid lowering medications were prescribed at the discretion of the treating physician.

RITA-2

Coronary Angioplasty vs Medical Therapy for Angina.
(continued)

Results

Of the 504 patients randomized to initial PTCA strategy, 471 (93%) underwent the intended procedure within a median time of 5 weeks from randomization. PTCA was successful in 93% of the 642 attempted coronary lesions. 7 patients (1.5%) randomized to PTCA underwent emergency CABG. During follow-up 2.2% of the PTCA vs 1.4% of the conservative therapy group died (p=0.32). Cardiac mortality was 0.99% vs 0.60%, respectively. Nonfatal myocardial infarction occurred in 4.2% of the PTCA group vs only 1.9% in the medical group. The difference was due to 7 randomized-procedure-related myocardial infarctions in the PTCA group. Death or definite myocardial infarction occurred in 6.3% of the PTCA group vs 3.3% of the medical group (relative risk 1.92; 95% CI 1.08-3.41; p=0.02). The absolute treatment difference was 3.0% (95% CI 0.4%-5.7%). During follow-up 7.9% of the PTCA group and 5.8% of the medical group underwent CABG. Additional nonrandomized PTCA was performed in 12.3% of the PTCA group vs 19.6% of the medical group. In this group, the risk of requiring CABG or PTCA within 1 year of randomization was 15.4%. Improvement in reported angina was greater in the PTCA group, with a 16.5% excess of grade 2+ angina in the medical group after 3 months of therapy (p<0.001). However, after 2 years of follow-up, the medical group had only 7.6% excess of grade 2+ angina (p=0.02). Bruce treadmill exercise test was performed by about 90% of the patients at each follow-up. After 3 months the PTCA group exercised longer than the medical group (mean difference 35 seconds; 95% CI 20-51 seconds; p<0.001). However, the difference was attenuated at 1 year to 25 sec (95% CI 7-42 sec; p= nonsignificant). The beneficial effects of PTCA over medical therapy were more pronounced in patients with more severe angina at baseline.

Conclusions

In patients with stable coronary artery disease suitable for either medical therapy or PTCA, initial strategy of PTCA was associated with greater symptomatic improvement, especially in patients with more severe baseline symptoms. However, the differences between the PTCA and medical therapy tended to decrease over time and the initial PTCA strategy was associated with a significant excess of mortality and nonfatal myocardial infarction.

4. Interventional Cardiology
b. PTCA Vs CABG

RITA

Randomized Intervention Treatment of Angina (RITA) Trial

Title	a. The randomized intervention treatment of angina (RITA) trial protocol: a long-term study of coronary angioplasty and coronary artery bypass surgery in patients with angina b. Coronary angioplasty vs coronary artery bypass surgery: the Randomized Intervention Treatment of Angina (RITA) trial. c. Health service costs of coronary angioplasty and coronary artery bypass surgery: the Randomized intervention Treatment of Angina (RITA) trial.
Authors	a. Henderson RA, for the RITA Trial. b. RITA Trial Participants. c. Sculpher MJ, Henderson RA, Buxton MJ, et al.
Reference	a. Br Heart J 1989;62:411-414. b. Lancet 1993;341:573-580. c. Lancet 1994;344:927-930.
Disease	Coronary artery disease.
Purpose	To compare the long-term effects of percutaneous transluminal coronary angioplasty (PTCA) vs coronary artery bypass surgery (CABG) in patients with 1, 2, and 3 vessel disease.
Design	Randomized, multicenter.
Patients	1011 patients with coronary artery disease with a need for revascularization. Patients with left main coronary artery disease, previous PTCA or CABG, or significant valvular disease were excluded.
Follow-up	> 6 months, median 2.5 years.
Treatment regimen	CABG vs PTCA.

RITA

Randomized Intervention Treatment of Angina (RITA) Trial
(continued)

Results   Angioplasty was successful in 87% of the lesions. Emergency CABG was required in 4.5% of the PTCA group. Additional 1.4% underwent CABG before hospital discharge due to unsuccessful PTCA. Among the CABG patients 0.6% had pulmonary embolism and 4.9% wound-related complications. Median hospital stay was 12 and 4 days for CABG and PTCA, respectively. Mortality was 3.6% in the CABG and 3.1% in the PTCA group. Definite myocardial infarction occurred in 4.0% vs 6.5% of the CABG and PTCA patients. However, there was no difference in the rate of the primary end point (myocardial infarction or mortality) between the groups (RR CABG vs PTCA 0.88, 95% CI 0.59-1.29, p=0.47). Within 2 years an estimated 38% of the PTCA vs 11% of the CABG patients had experienced either further CABG, PTCA, myocardial infarction, or death (p<0.001). The prevalence of angina during follow-up was 32% in the PTCA vs 11% in the CABG group after 6 months (RR 0.35, 95% CI 0.26-0.47, p<0.001) and 31% vs 22% after 2 years (p=0.007).

Conclusions   While there was no difference in mortality, CABG was associated with less recurrent angina and need for revascularization.

ERACI

Argentine Randomized Trial of Percutaneous Transluminal Coronary Angioplasty vs Coronary Artery Bypass Surgery in Multivessel Disease.

Title	Argentine randomized trial of percutaneous transluminal coronary angioplasty vs coronary artery bypass surgery in multivessel disease (ERACI): in-hospital results and 1 year follow-up.
Authors	Rodriguez A, Boullon F, Perez-Baliño N, et al.
Reference	J Am Coll Cardiol 1993;22:1060-1067.
Disease	Coronary artery disease.
Purpose	To compare outcome following coronary artery bypass surgery (CABG) vs percutaneous transluminal coronary angioplasty (PTCA) in patients with multivessel coronary artery disease.
Design	Randomized, 1 center.
Patients	127 patients, age 33-76 years, with stable angina and multivessel disease which was suitable to either PTCA or CABG.
Follow-up	1 year clinical follow-up.
Treatment regimen	CABG vs PTCA.

ERACI
Argentine Randomized Trial of Percutaneous Transluminal Coronary Angioplasty vs Coronary Artery Bypass Surgery in Multivessel Disease.

(continued)

Results   The overall primary success rate of angioplasty was 91.7% per lesion. There was no significant difference with in-hospital mortality (4.6% vs 1.5%), myocardial infarction (6.2% vs 6.3%), stroke (3.1% vs 1.5%), or need for repeated emergency procedure (1.5% vs 1.5%) between the CABG and the PTCA groups. Complete revascularization was achieved in 88% vs 51% of the CABG and PTCA groups (p<0.001). Mortality after 1 year was 3.2% in the PTCA vs 0% in the CABG patients (p=NS). New Q wave infarction occurred in 3.2% of the PTCA and 1.8% of the CABG (p=NS). 32% of the PTCA group needed revascularization vs 3.2% of the CABG patients (p<0.001). However, freedom from angina (including patients with repeated procedure) after 1 year was similar.

Conclusions No significant differences were found in major in-hospital complications and 1 year outcome between the groups. However, after 1 year more patients treated with PTCA needed repeated revascularization.

GABI

The German Angioplasty Bypass Surgery Investigation

Title	A randomized study of coronary angioplasty compared with bypass surgery in patients with symptomatic multi vessel coronary disease.
Authors	Hamm CW, Reimers J, Ischinger T, et al.
Reference	N Engl J Med 1994;331:1037-1043.
Disease	Coronary artery disease.
Purpose	To compare the outcomes of coronary revascularization with coronary artery bypass grafting (CABG) and percutaneous transluminal coronary angioplasty (PTCA) in patients with multivessel disease.
Design	Randomized, multicenter.
Patients	337 patients, <75 years old, with symptomatic multivessel disease (Canadian Cardiovascular Society class ≥II, and ≥70% stenosis) and a need for revascularization of ≥2 major coronary arteries. Patients with 100% occlusion or >30% stenosis of the left main coronary artery were excluded. Patients who underwent prior CABG or PTCA and patients with myocardial infarction within 4 weeks were excluded.
Follow-up	1 year.
Treatment regimen	CABG vs PTCA.

GABI

The German Angioplasty Bypass Surgery Investigation

(continued)

Results   Among the CABG patients an average of 2.2±0.6 vessels
                   were grafted and among the PTCA patients 1.9±0.5 ves-
                   sels were dilated. Complete revascularization was
                   achieved in 86% of the PTCA patients. Hospitalization was
                   longer after CABG (median days 19 vs 5) and Q wave
                   infarction related to the procedure was more common
                   (8.1% vs 2.3%, p=0.022). However, there was no signifi-
                   cant difference in mortality (2.5% vs 1.1%, p=0.43). At dis-
                   charge 93% vs 82% of the CABG and PTCA patients were
                   angina-free (p=0.005). During the following year 6% of the
                   CABG patients vs 44% of the PTCA patients underwent
                   repeated interventions (p<0.001). The cumulative risk of
                   death or myocardial infarction was 13.6% in the CABG
                   and 6.0% in the PTCA patients (p=0.017). 1 year after the
                   procedure 74% vs 71%, respectively were angina-free
                   (p=NS). Exercise capacity was similar. However, 22% of
                   the CABG vs only 12% of the PTCA patients did not
                   require antianginal medication (p=0.041). 219 patients
                   underwent coronary angiography after 6 months. The clin-
                   ical course of these patients did not differ from that of
                   those who refused to undergo repeated catheterization.
                   13% of the vein grafts were occluded and 7% of the inter-
                   nal thoracic artery anastomoses did not function, where-
                   as 16% of the vessels dilated by angioplasty were ≥70%
                   stenotic.

Conclusions   In selected patients with multivessel disease PTCA and
                   CABG resulted in similar improvement after 1 year.
                   However, the PTCA treated patients needed more addi-
                   tional interventions and antianginal medication, whereas
                   CABG was more associated with procedure related
                   myocardial infarction.

EAST

The Emory Angioplasty Vs Surgery Trial

Title	a. A randomized trial comparing coronary angioplasty with coronary bypass surgery. b. A comparison of the costs of and quality of life after coronary angioplasty or coronary surgery for multivessel coronary artery disease: results from the Emory Angioplasty vs Surgery Trial (EAST).
Authors	a. King SB III, Lembo NJ, Weintraub WS, et al. b. Weintraub WS, Mauldin PD, Becker E, et al.
Reference	a. N Engl J Med 1994;331:1044-1050. b. Circulation 1995;92:2831-2840.
Disease	Coronary artery disease.
Purpose	To compare the outcome following coronary artery bypass surgery (CABG) vs percutaneous transluminal coronary angioplasty (PTCA) in patients with multivessel coronary artery disease.
Design	Randomized, single center.
Patients	392 patients of any age with 2- to 3-vessel disease and had not previously undergone PTCA or CABG. Patients with old 100% occlusion of vessels serving viable myocardium, ≥ 2 total occlusions, >30% left main artery stenosis, ejection fraction $\leq 25\%$, or myocardial infarction <5 d, were excluded.
Follow-up	3 year clinical follow-up. Repeated angiography and thallium scan after 1 and 3 years.
Treatment regimen	PTCA vs CABG.

EAST

The Emory Angioplasty Vs Surgery Trial

(continued)

Results

In hospital mortality was 1.0% in each group. Q wave infarction occurred in 10.3% of the CABG and 3.0% of the PTCA patients (p=0.004). Stroke occurred in 1.5% vs 0.5%, respectively (p=0.37). 0% and 10.1% of the patients, respectively underwent emergency CABG during hospitalization. 3 year mortality was 6.2% in the CABG and 7.1% in the PTCA groups (p=0.72). Q wave infarction within 3 years occurred in 19.6% vs 14.6%, respectively (p=0.21). Large ischemic defect on thallium scan were found in 5.7% vs 9.6%, respectively (p=0.17). There was no difference in the occurrence of the composite end point (death, Q wave infarction, or a large ischemic defect on thallium scan)(27.3% vs 28.8%, p=0.81). After 3 years 1% of the CABG vs 22% of the PTCA group underwent CABG (p<0.001), while PTCA was performed in 13% vs 41%, respectively (p<0.001). Initially, 99.1% vs 75.1% of the index segments per patients were revascularized in the CABG and PTCA, respectively. 1 year later, 88.1% vs 58.8% of the index segment per patients were revascularized (p<0.001). However, by 3 years the differences were narrowed (86.7% vs 69.9%, respectively, p<0.001). There was no difference in ejection fraction between the groups. However, angina was present in 12% and 20% of the patients after 3 years, respectively.

Conclusions

PTCA and CABG did not differ significantly with respect to the occurrence of the composite end points. However, PTCA was associated with more repeated procedures and residual angina.

CABRI

Coronary Angioplasty Vs Bypass Revascularization Investigation

Title	First year results of CABRI (Coronary Angioplasty vs Bypass Revascularization Investigation).
Authors	CABRI Trial Participants.
Reference	Lancet 1995;346:1179-1184.
Disease	Coronary artery disease.
Purpose	To compare the effects of percutaneous transluminal coronary angioplasty (PTCA) vs coronary artery bypass surgery (CABG) in patients with multivessel disease.
Design	Randomized, multicenter.
Patients	1054 patients, <76 years old, with >1 vessel disease with left ventricular ejection fraction >0.35. Patients with left main or severe triple vessel disease, overt cardiac failure, myocardial infarction within 10 days, a previous coronary revascularization, or a recent cerebrovascular event were excluded. At least 1 lesion had to be suitable for PTCA.
Follow-up	1 year.
Treatment regimen	CABG or PTCA (stents and atherectomy were permitted).
Additional therapy	Aspirin. The use of fish oil and lipid-lowering agents were allowed.

CABRI

Coronary Angioplasty Vs Bypass Revascularization Investigation
(continued)

Results

After 1 year 2.7% of the CABG and 3.9% of the PTCA allocated patients had died (RR 1.42, 95% CI 0.73-2.76, p=0.3). Kaplan-Meier survival curves did not demonstrate a difference in survival at 28 months. The PTCA allocated group required more repeated interventions. 20.8% vs 2.7% needed angioplasty, while 15.7% vs 0.8% needed CABG. 66.4% of the PTCA vs 93.5% of the CABG group had only a single procedure in the first year. The rate of reintervention was 5 times higher in the PTCA group (RR 5.23, 95% CI 3.90-7.03, p<0.001). The PTCA group needed more antianginal medications (RR 1.30, 95% CI 1.18-1.43, p<0.001). After 1 year 67 % of the PTCA vs 75% of the CABG were angina-free. The presence of angina at 1 year was greater in the PTCA than in the CABG group (RR 1.54, 95% CI 1.09-2.16, p=0.012).

Conclusions

CABG as the initial revascularization strategy for multivessel disease was associated with decreased need for repeated procedure. However, 1 year survival was similar.

BARI

The Bypass Angioplasty Revascularization Investigation

Title	a. Comparison of coronary bypass surgery with angioplasty in patients with multivessel disease. b. 5 year clinical and functional outcome comparing bypass surgery and angioplasty in patients with multivessel coronary disease. A multicenter randomized trial. c. 5 year clinical and functional outcome comparing bypass surgery and angioplasty in patients with multivessel coronary disease. A multicenter randomized trial. d. Influence of diabetes on 5 year mortality and morbidity in a randomized trial comparing CABG and PTCA in patients with multivessel disease. The bypass angioplasty revascularization investigation (BARI). e. Medical care costs and quality of life after randomization to coronary angioplasty or coronary bypass surgery.
Authors	a. + b. The Bypass Angioplasty Revascularization Investigation (BARI) Investigators. c. The writing group for the bypass angioplasty revascularization investigation (BARI) investigators. d. The BARI Investigators. e. Hlatky MA, Rogers WJ, Johnstone I, et al.
Reference	a. N Engl J Med 1996;335:217-225. b. JAMA 1997;277:715-721. c. JAMA 1997;277:715-721. d. Circulation 1997; 96:1761-1679. e. N Engl J Med. 1997; 336:92-99.
Disease	Coronary artery disease. d. Coronary artery disease, diabetes mellitus.
Purpose	a. + b. To compare the long-term effects of percutaneous transluminal coronary balloon angioplasty (PTCA) and coronary artery bypass grafting surgery (CABG) in patients with multivessel coronary artery disease. c. To assess the clinical and functional status of patients with similar 5 year survival following coronary artery bypass grafting (CABG) vs percutaneous transluminal coronary angioplasty (PTCA).

BARI

The Bypass Angioplasty Revascularization Investigation

(continued)

	d. More details on original trial in regards to diabetes. Examination of course-specific mortality, CABG efficacy by using internal mammary artery (IMA) grafts vs saphenous vein grafts (SVGs) only. e. To compare quality of life, employment, and costs of medical care in patients treated with PTCA vs CABG in the BARI study.
Design	Randomized, multicenter. c. Randomized trial. Symptoms, use of medications, quality of life questionnaire and exercise test, results obtained at 4-14 weeks, 1, 3, and 5 years after randomization. Multicenter. e. As per BARI study. Data on quality of life collected annually; economic data collected quarterly.
Patients	1829 patients with angiographically documented multivessel coronary artery disease, clinically severe angina, or evidence of ischemia requiring revascularization, and were suitable for both PTCA and CABG. c. 1829 patients with multivessel coronary artery disease with clinically severe angina or objective evidence for ischemia requiring either CABG or PTCA as suitable therapies. Average age 61.5 years; 73% male. d. 353 treated diabetic patients and 1476 patients classified as not having treated diabetes. e. 934 of the 1829 patients enrolled in the BARI study.
Follow-up	Mean follow-up 5.4 years (range 3.8–6.8 years). c. 5.4 years. d. Average 5.4 years. e. 3 - 5 years.

BARI

The Bypass Angioplasty Revascularization Investigation

(continued)

Treatment regimen	PTCA vs CABG. New interventional devices, such as stents and atherectomy devices were not used during the initial revascularization procedure. c. CABG or PTCA within 2 weeks of randomization. d. CABG vs PTCA e. Coronary angioplasty vs coronary artery bypass surgery.
Results	Of the 915 patients randomized to PTCA, 904 (99%) actually underwent the procedure, 9 underwent CABG, and 2 received medical therapy alone. Of the 914 patients randomized to CABG, 892 (98%) underwent the procedure, 15 underwent PTCA as the initial procedure, and 7 were treated medically. Among the 892 patients who underwent CABG as assigned, an average of 3.1 coronary arteries were bypassed with a mean of 2.8 grafts. In 91% of patients all intended vessels were revascularized. At least 1 internal-thoracic-artery was used in 82% of patients. Among the 904 patients who underwent PTCA as assigned, angioplasty was attempted on an average of 2.4 lesions. Multilesion angioplasty was attempted in 78% of patients and multivessel angioplasty in 70% of patients. Immediate angiographic success was achieved in 78% of the attempted angioplasties. Rates of in-hospital mortality were comparable between the CABG and PTCA groups (1.3% vs 1.1% in the CABG and PTCA group, respectively; p=NS). Q wave myocardial infarction during hospitalization occurred in 4.6% vs 2.1%, respectively (p<0.01). There was no statistically significant difference between the groups in the occurrence of stroke, congestive heart failure, cardiogenic shock, and nonfatal cardiac arrest. However, more of the CABG patients experienced respiratory failure (2.2% vs 1.0%, p<0.05), wound dehiscence or infection (4.1% vs 0.4%, p<0.001), and reoperation for bleeding (3.1% vs 0.4%, p<0.001). Emergency CABG (6.3% vs 0.1%; p<0.001) and PTCA (2.1% vs 0; p<0.001) following the initial procedure were performed more often in the PTCA group. Nonemergency CABG was also performed more often in the PTCA patients (3.9% vs 0; p<0.001). The median hospital stay was longer after CABG (7 days) than after PTCA (3 days). The cumulative survival rates at 5 years were 89.3% and 86.3% for the CABG and PTCA groups, respectively

(2.9% difference, 95% CI -0.2% to 6.0%; p=0.19). The cumulative rates of Q wave myocardial infarction at 5 years were 11.7% and 10.9%, respectively (p=0.45). At 5 years 80.4% and 78.7% of the CABG and PTCA patients were alive and free of Q wave myocardial infarction (1.6% difference, 95% confidence interval -2.2% to 5.4%, p=0.84). During the 5 year follow-up, 8% of the CABG patients underwent repeated revascularization procedures (1% underwent repeated CABG and 7% PTCA), while 54% of the PTCA group underwent at least 1 additional procedure (31% underwent CABG and 34% repeated PTCA, 11% underwent both CABG and PTCA). Multiple additional revascularization procedures were required for 19% of the PTCA patients vs 3% of the CABG patients. Patients undergoing PTCA had more frequent hospitalizations than the CABG patients (an average of age of 2.5 per patient vs 1.9, p<0.001). At 4 - 14 weeks 95% of the CABG vs 73% of the PTCA patients reported no angina (p<0.001). At the 5 year visit 86% of the CABG vs 78% of the PTCA patients were angina-free (p=0.003). At the 4 - 14 weeks visit, 20% of the CABG vs 31% of the PTCA group had abnormal exercise-induced ST segment changes (p<0.001), however, at 5 years there was no difference (28% vs 31%). At 5 years there was no difference in the proportion of patients experiencing exercise induced angina. During follow-up, patients in the PTCA were more likely to receive anti-ischemic medications than the CABG group (89% vs 44% at 4-14 weeks (p<0.001), 76% vs 57% by the fifth year (p<0.001). At follow-up of 1 year and later, quality of life, return to work, modification of smoking and exercise behaviors, and cholesterol levels were similar for the 2 groups. Subgroup analysis did not reveal a difference in survival between CABG and PTCA in patients with unstable angina or non Q wave infarction, stable angina, severe ischemia, normal or reduced left ventricular function, double or triple vessel disease, and presence of type C coronary lesions (complicated lesions). However, a significant survival benefit was observed in patients with treated diabetes mellitus assigned to CABG. The 5 year survival in diabetic patients was 80.6% in the CABG compared to 65.5% in the PTCA group (15.1% difference, 99.5% confidence interval 1.4% to 28.9%, p=0.003).

BARI

The Bypass Angioplasty Revascularization Investigation

(continued)

c. At each follow-up period CABG patients were more likely to be angina free compared to PTCA group. At 4 - 14 weeks 95% of CABG patients had no angina vs 73% of PTCA patients (p<.001). This difference narrowed by 5 years at which time 86% of CABG patients and 78% of PTCA patients were angina - free (p=.003). Among the asymptomatic CABG patients 94% did not require additional revascularization procedures. Among the asymptomatic PTCA patients 48% did not require additional revascularization procedures. Quality of life and return to work were similar at 1 year between groups. Antianginal medicines were more commonly used among PTCA patients. A larger percent of PTCA patients experienced angina pectoris on exercise and exercise induced ST segment changes than CABG patients except at 5 years when there was no difference between groups.

d. The improved 5.4 year survival with CABG over PTCA in the treated diabetics was due to a reduction in cardiac mortality (5.8% vs 20.6%, p=.0003) and confined to patients receiving at least one internal mammary artery graft.

e. During the first 3 years, functional status scores that measure the ability to perform common activities of daily living improved to a greater extent in patients that received CABG compared to PTCA (p = 0.05). Patients receiving PTCA returned to work 5 weeks sooner than patients in the surgery group (p <0.001). While the initial cost of PTCA was 65% of the surgical cost, after 5 years the total medical cost of angioplasty was 95% that of surgery. 5 year cost of PTCA was significantly lower than surgery in patients with 2 vessel disease (p < 0.05), but not among patients with 3 vessel disease. CABG was especially cost-effective in diabetes because of their better survival.

BARI

The Bypass Angioplasty Revascularization Investigation

(continued)

Conclusions
The 5 year survival of patients assigned to initial strategy of PTCA was comparable to that of patients assigned to CABG. However, subsequent repeated revascularization was required more often in the PTCA group. In patients with diabetes mellitus, 5 year survival was significantly worse with PTCA than with CABG.

c. There was a narrowing of treatment benefits of CABG over PTCA in these 5 year survivors. The narrowing of benefits in angina and exercise-induced ischemia are related to return of symptoms among patents assigned to CABG and an increase in surgical procedures among patients originally assigned to PTCA.

d. Patients with treated diabetes mellitus have a marked reduction in cardiac mortality when initially treated with CABG rather than PTCA which appears to be related to long term patency of the internal mammary artery.

e. CABG resulted in a better quality of life than PTCA in patients with multivessel disease, after the initial morbidity associated with the procedure. In patients with double (but not triple) disease PTCA had a lower 5 year cost.

4. Interventional Cardiology

c. PTCA Vs Stenting Vs Other Percutaneous Devices

CAVEAT-1

Coronary Angioplasty Vs Excisional Atherectomy Trial

Title	a. A comparison of directional atherectomy with coronary angioplasty in patients with coronary artery disease. b. 1 year follow-up in the coronary angioplasty vs excisional atherectomy trial (CAVEAT I).
Authors	a. Topol EJ, Leya F, Pinkerton CA, et al. b. Elliott JM, Berdan LG, Holmes DR, et al.
Reference	a. N Engl J Med 1993;329:221-227. b. Circulation 1995;91:2158-2166.
Disease	Coronary artery disease, angina pectoris.
Purpose	To compare outcome of percutaneous transluminal coronary angioplasty (PTCA) with that of directional coronary atherectomy (DCA).
Design	Randomized, controlled trial.
Patients	1012 patients (median age 59 years, 73% men) with symptomatic coronary artery disease. Only patients with angiography-proven native coronary artery lesions ≥60% stenosis, and <12 mm length, with no prior intracoronary interventions were included. Patients who had acute myocardial infarction within 5 days of procedure were excluded. 512 and 500 patients were assigned to DCA and PTCA, respectively.
Follow-up	1 year.
Treatment regimen	Percutaneous transluminal coronary angioplasty (PTCA) or directional coronary atherectomy (DCA).

CAVEAT-1

Coronary Angioplasty Vs Excisional Atherectomy Trial

(continued)

Additional therapy	Before procedure, all patients received ≥160 mg aspirin, ≥1 dose of calcium channel blocker, and heparin as a bolus of 10000 U with additional boluses to maintain clotting time >350 sec during the procedure.
Results	Reduction of stenosis to ≤50% was more successful with DCA (89%) than PTCA (80%), p<0.001. The success rates (≤50% residual stenosis and no major complications) were higher in the DCA group (82%) than the PTCA group (76%, p=0.016). The immediate gain in luminal diameter was greater in the DCA (1.05 mm) than PTCA (0.86 mm, p<0.001) patients. However, early complications were more frequent in the DCA than PTCA patients (11% vs 5%, p<0.001). At 6 months 50% and 57% of the DCA and PTCA patients had restenosis, respectively (p=0.06). 1 year mortality was 2.2% and 0.6% in the DCA and PTCA groups, respectively (p=0.035). Myocardial infarction within 1 year occurred in 8.9% of the DCA and 4.4% of the PTCA patients (p=0.005). By multivariate analysis, DCA was the only variable predictive of the combined end point of death or myocardial infarction. Rates of repeated interventions at the target site were similar.
Conclusions	DCA, as compared with PTCA, was associated with an increase rates of restenosis at 6 months, and 1 year mortality and occurrence of myocardial infarction.

Title	A comparison of directional atherectomy with balloon angioplasty for lesions of the left anterior descending coronary artery.
Authors	Adelman AG, Cohen EA, Kimball BP, et al.
Reference	N Engl J Med 1993;329:228-233.
Disease	Coronary artery disease, restenosis.
Purpose	To compare the rates of restenosis for directional atherectomy and balloon angioplasty in lesions of the proximal left anterior descending coronary artery.
Design	Randomized, open label, multicenter.
Patients	274 patients with de novo ≥60% stenosis of the proximal 1/3 of the left anterior descending coronary artery. Patients within 7 days of acute infarction or severe left ventricular dysfunction were excluded.
Follow-up	Clinical evaluation and repeated angiography at 4-7 months (median 5.9 months).
Treatment regimen	Directional atherectomy or balloon angioplasty.
Additional therapy	Aspirin, calcium channel blocker, and nitrates were started ≥12 h before procedure and continued for 24 h. Heparin was given during procedure. Antianginal medications were discontinued. The use of n-3 fatty acids was prohibited.

(continued)

Results	The procedural success rate was 94% in the atherectomy and 88% in the angioplasty patients (p=0.06). Major in-hospital complications occurred in 5% and 6%, respectively. Repeated angiography was performed in 257 patients. After 6 months, the restenosis rate was 46% and 43% (p=0.7). Despite a greater initial gain in minimal luminal diameter (1.45±0.47 vs 1.16±0.44 mm, p<0.001), there was a larger loss (0.79±0.61 vs 0.47±0.64 mm, p<0.001) in the atherectomy group, resulting in a similar minimal luminal diameter at follow-up (1.55±0.60 vs 1.61±0.68 mm, p=0.44). The clinical outcome was similar in the 2 groups.
Conclusions	Despite better initial success rate and gain in minimal luminal diameter, atherectomy did not result in better clinical outcome or late angiographic results with lesions of the proximal third of the left anterior descending coronary artery.

Title	a. A comparison of balloon-expandable stent implantation with balloon angioplasty in patients with coronary artery disease. b. Continued benefit of coronary stenting vs balloon angioplasty: 1 year clinical follow-up of Benestent Trial.
Authors	a. Serruys PW, de Jaegere P, Kiemenij F, et al. b. Macay a C, Serruys PW, Ruygrok P, et al.
Reference	a. N Engl J Med 1994;331:489-495. b. J Am Coll Cardiol 1996;27:255-261.
Disease	Coronary artery disease, restenosis.
Purpose	To compare elective balloon angioplasty with Palmaz-Schatz stent implantation in patients with stable angina and de novo coronary artery lesions.
Design	Randomized, multicenter.
Patients	516 patients, age 30-75 years, with stable angina and a single new lesion of the native coronary circulation <15 mm, located in vessels >3 mm and supplying normally functioning myocardium.
Follow-up	12 months (0.3-34 months). Exercise test and repeated angiography at 6 months.
Treatment regimen	Balloon angioplasty or Palmaz-Schatz stent implantation.
Additional therapy	Aspirin 250-500 mg/d and dipyridamole 75 mg X3/d, started ≥1 day before procedure and continued for >6 months. IV heparin 10,000 U bolus before procedure. Calcium channel blockers until discharge. Patients undergoing stent implantation received dextran infusion (1,000 ml over 6-8 h), heparin infusion (started after sheath removal and continued for ≥36 h), and warfarin for 3 months (target INR 2.5-3.5).

Results

The procedural success rate was 92.7% in the stent group and 91.1% in the angioplasty group, whereas the angiographic success was 96.9% vs 98.1%, respectively. There was no differences in the incidence of death, stroke, myocardial infarction, or the need for repeated procedures during the index hospitalization between the groups. There was no difference in the composite end point of all in-hospital clinical events (6.2% in the angioplasty vs 6.9% in the stent group (RR 1.12, 95% CI 0.58-2.14)). Subacute vessel closure occurred in 2.7% of the angioplasty and 3.5% of the stent group (p=NS). The incidence of bleeding and vascular complications was higher in the stent group 13.5% vs 3.1%, RR 4.34, 95% CI 2.05-9.18, p<0.001). Mean hospitalization was 8.5±6.8 days in the stent vs 3.1±3.3 days in the angioplasty group (p=0.001). After 7 months primary events occurred in 29.6% vs 20.1% of the angioplasty and stent groups (RR 0.68, 95% CI 0.50-0.92, p=0.02). The major difference was the need for repeated angioplasty in the angioplasty group (20.6% vs 10.0%, RR 0.49, 95% CI 0.31-0.75, p=0.001). The minimal luminal diameter after the procedure was 2.48±0.39 vs 2.05±0.33 mm (p<0.001), and at follow-up it was 1.82± 0.64 vs 1.73±0.55 mm (p=0.09), in the stent and angioplasty groups. The incidence of >50% restenosis was 22% vs 32%, respectively (p=0.02). After 1 year a primary end point occurred in 32% of the angioplasty vs 23% of the stent group (RR 0.74, 95% CI 0.55-0.98, p=0.04). However, the only significant difference was the rate of repeated interventions.

Conclusions

Implantation of stent is associated with better initial gain in luminal stenosis, a larger minimal diameter after 7 months and a significant reduction of the need for repeated interventions that was maintained to at least 1 year. However, stent implantation is associated with longer hospital stay and more bleeding and vascular complications.

Stent Restenosis Study

Title	a. A randomized comparison of coronary-stent placement and balloon angioplasty in the treatment of coronary artery disease. b. 1 year follow-up of the Stent Restenosis (STRESS -1) Study.
Authors	a. Fischman DL, Leon MB, Baim DS, et al. b. George CJ, Baim DS, Brinker JA, et al.
Reference	a. N Engl J Med 1994;331:496-501. b. Am J Cardiol. 1998; 81:860-865.
Disease	Coronary artery disease, restenosis.
Purpose	a. To compare the results of Palmaz-Schatz stent placement and conventional balloon angioplasty on restenosis and clinical outcome.
Design	Randomized, open label, multicenter.
Patients	a. 407 patients with new ≥70% stenotic lesions, ≤15 mm in length, in ≥3.0 mm of a native coronary artery. Patients with myocardial infarction within 7 days, ejection fraction <40%, diffuse coronary or left main artery disease, or angiographic evidence of thrombus were excluded.
Follow-up	a. Clinical follow-up for 6 months. Repeated angiography at 6 months.
Treatment regimen	Palmaz-Schatz stent placement or balloon angioplasty.

STRESS

Stent Restenosis Study

(continued)

Additional therapy	For the stent arm: aspirin 325 mg/d, dipyridamole 75 mg X3/d, and calcium channel blocker. IV low-molecular weight dextran started 2 h before procedure at a dose of 100 ml/h for 2 h, and during and after procedure 50 ml/h. IV heparin 10,000-15,000 U before procedure, and IV infusion 4-6 h after removal of the sheath. Warfarin sodium started on the day of procedure. Dipyridamole and warfarin were administered for 1 month, and aspirin indefinitely. For the angioplasty arm: aspirin 325 mg/d, without warfarin sodium or dipyridamole.
Results	a. Clinical success was achieved in 96.1% and 89.6% of the stent and angioplasty groups (p=0.011). The stent group had a larger immediate gain in minimal diameter of the lumen (1.72±0.46 vs 1.23±0.48 mm, p<0.001), and a larger luminal diameter after the procedure (2.49±0.43 vs 1.99±0.47 mm, p<0.001). There was no statistical significant difference in the rate of any of the early clinical events (days 0-14) between the groups. At 6 months, the stent group had a larger luminal diameter (1.74±0.60 vs 1.56±0.65 mm, p=0.007), and a lower rate of ≥50% restenosis (31.6% vs 42.1%, p=0.046). 80.5% and 76.2% of the stent and angioplasty groups were event-free after 6 months (p=0.16). Revascularization of the original lesion was performed in 10.2% and 15.4% of the stent and angioplasty patients (p=0.06). b. 1 year follow-up results: 75% of patients assigned to stent implantation were free of all clinical events (death, myocardial infarction, revascularization, procedures) compared to 70% of PTCA patients. 79% of stent patients were alive vs 74% of PTCA patients. These differences were not significantly different. There was no difference in freedom from angina at 1 year between groups (84%).
Conclusions	a. In selected patients, placement of Palmaz-Schatz stent was associated with better immediate results, lower rate of 6 months restenosis, and less revascularization procedures. b. Authors note that although there was no statistically significant improvement in outcome in stented group, the study had a relatively low statistical power.

CAVEAT-II

Coronary Angioplasty Vs Directional Atherectomy- II

Title	A multicenter, randomized trial of coronary angioplasty vs directional atherectomy for patients with saphenous vein bypass graft lesions.
Authors	Holmes DR, Topol EJ, Califf RM, et al.
Reference	Circulation 1995;91:1966-1974.
Disease	Coronary artery disease, saphenous vein grafts.
Purpose	To compare outcome after directional coronary atherectomy vs angioplasty in patients with de novo venous bypass graft stenosis.
Design	Randomized, open label, multicenter.
Patients	305 patients with de novo saphenous vein graft lesions, ≥60% and <100% stenosis, who required revascularization and were suitable for either angioplasty or atherectomy.
Follow-up	Clinical evaluation and repeated coronary angiography at 6 months.
Treatment regimen	Balloon angioplasty or directional atherectomy.
Additional therapy	Aspirin ≥160 mg and a calcium blocker <24 h before procedure. A bolus of 10,000 U heparin before procedure. Aspirin 325 mg/d and a calcium channel blocker for 1 month.

CAVEAT-II

Coronary Angioplasty Vs Directional Atherectomy- II

(continued)

Results
: Initial angiographic success was 89.2% with atherectomy vs 79.0% with angioplasty (p=0.019), as was initial luminal gain (1.45 vs 1.12 mm, p<0.001). Distal embolization occurred in 13.4% and 5.1% of the patients, respectively (p=0.012), and non Q wave infarction in 16.1% and 9.6%, respectively (p=0.09). The restenosis rates (>50% stenosis) were similar at 6 months (45.6% vs 50.5%, p=0.49). 13.2% of the atherectomy and 22.4% of the angioplasty patients required repeated interventions (p=0.41).

Conclusions
: Atherectomy of de novo vein graft lesion was associated with better initial angiographic success, but with increased distal embolization. There was no difference in restenosis rates, however, there was a trend towards less target vessel revascularization procedures.

AMRO

Amsterdam-Rotterdam trial

Title	Randomised trial of excimer laser angioplasty vs balloon angioplasty for treatment of obstructive coronary artery disease.
Authors	Appelman YEA, Piek JJ, Strikwerda S, et al.
Reference	Lancet 1996;347:79-84.
Disease	Coronary artery disease, restenosis.
Purpose	To compare the initial and 6 month clinical and angiographic outcome of excimer laser coronary angioplasty vs balloon angioplasty.
Design	Randomized, multicenter.
Patients	308 patients with stable angina pectoris, coronary lesions >10 mm, or total or functional occlusions (TIMI flow grade 0 or 1), either with single or multivessel disease, who were suitable for coronary angioplasty. Patients with unstable angina; myocardial infarction within 2 weeks; a life expectancy of <1 year; intended angioplasty of a venous graft; unprotected left main disease angulated, highly eccentric, ostial or bifurcation lesions; lesions with a thrombus or dissection; and total occlusions with low likelihood of passage with a guide wire were excluded.
Follow-up	Clinical follow up and repeated coronary angiography at 6 months.
Treatment regimen	Excimer laser angioplasty (wave-length 308 nm) or balloon angioplasty (PTCA).

AMRO

Amsterdam-Rotterdam trial

(continued)

Additional therapy	Nifedipine 20 mgX3/d during hospitalization. Aspirin 250-500 mg/d, started a day before the procedure and continued for 6 months. Intravenous heparin for ≥12 h after procedure.
Results	155 patients (162 lesions) were randomized to excimer laser and 158 patients (162 lesions) to PTCA. In 5 patients, the randomized segment was not treated. Excimer laser could not be done in 25 patients. Of the remaining 133 lesions, 98% (130 lesions) were treated with additional PTCA. Of the 167 lesions (157 patients) assigned to PTCA, PTCA was not done in 24 patients due to inability to cross the lesion. The angiographic success rate was 80% after laser and 79% after PTCA. There were no deaths. Myocardial infarction occurred in 4.6% vs 5.7% of the excimer laser and PTCA groups, respectively (p=0.67). There was no difference in the rates of coronary artery bypass surgery (10.6% vs 10.8%, respectively; p=0.95), repeated angioplasty (21.2% in the laser vs 18.5% in the PTCA group; p=0.55), or in the occurrence of primary end-point (death, myocardial infarction, or repeated revascularization; 33.1% vs 29.9%; p=0.55). The incidence of transient occlusions of the randomized segment was higher in the excimer laser (10 patients) than PTCA (1 patient) (relative risk 10.57; 95% CI 1.37 to 81.62; p=0.005). Arterial diameter stenosis was comparable between the groups before procedure, immediately after and at follow up. The restenosis (>50% diameter) rate was higher in the excimer laser group (51.6% vs 41.3%; difference 10.3%; 95% CI -2.0% to 22.6%; p=0.13). Minimal lumen diameter in the excimer laser and PTCA groups were 0.77±0.44 vs 0.77±0.47 mm before procedure, 1.69±0.41 vs 1.59±0.34 mm immediately after procedure (p=0.05), and 1.17±0.71 vs 1.25±0.68 mm at follow-up (p=0.34). Net gain in lumen minimal diameter (at follow-up minus before procedure) tended to be larger with PTCA (0.48±0.66 vs 0.40±0.69 mm; p=0.34). Late minimal lumen diameter loss (immediately after procedure minus at follow-up) was greater with excimer laser (0.52±0.70 vs 0.34±0.62 mm; 0.18 mm difference; 95% CI 0.15 to 0.35; p=0.04).
Conclusions	Excimer laser coronary angioplasty followed by PTCA was not better than conventional PTCA alone in the treatment of obstructive coronary lesions.

SICCO

Stenting In Chronic Coronary Occlusion

Title	Stenting in chronic coronary occlusion (SICCO): a randomized, controlled trial of adding stent implantation after successful angioplasty.
Authors	Sirnes PA, Golf S, Myreng Y, et al.
Reference	J Am Coll Cardiol 1996;28:1444-1451.
Disease	Coronary artery disease, restenosis.
Purpose	To investigate whether stent implantation improves long-term results after recanalization by angioplasty of chronic coronary artery occlusions.
Design	Randomized, multicenter.
Patients	117 patients, >18 years old, who underwent conventional balloon angioplasty (PTCA) of an occluded native coronary artery (TIMI flow grade 0 or I). Patients with occlusion of <2 weeks old, inability to tolerate anticoagulant therapy, reference artery diameter <2.5 mm, major dissection following angioplasty, elastic recoil >50% after angioplasty, lesions with complex anatomy, poor distal runoff, or angiographically visible thrombus were excluded.
Follow-up	Repeated coronary angiography after 6 months.
Treatment regimen	After conventional successful PTCA, patients were randomized to either a control group with no additional intervention, or to Palmaz-Schatz stent implantation.

SICCO

Stenting In Chronic Coronary Occlusion

(continued)

Addtional therapy	Aspirin 75 to 160 mg/d, started before angioplasty, heparin 10,000 to 15,000 IU before PTCA and then heparin infusion for 12 to 24 h in the control group and for 2 to 5 days in the stented group. The patients in the stent group received an infusion of dextran (1000 ml, 50 ml/h). The stented patients received dipyridamole 75 mgX3/d and warfarin (INR 3.5 to 4.0) for 3 months.
Results	There were no deaths throughout the follow-up period. Stent delivery was unsuccessful in one patient. One patient with stent implantation had a myocardial infarction. Stent implantation resulted in an increase in minimal luminal diameter from 2.21±0.50 to 2.78±0.49 mm (p<0.001). Vessel closure within 14 days occurred in 6.9% and 5.1% of the stent and control groups (p=NS). Inguinal hematoma was more common in the stent group (11 vs 0 patients; p=0.04). At follow-up, 57% vs 24% of the stent and control groups had no angina (p<0.001). There was no difference in late target revascularization during the 6 month follow-up (3 patients in each group), however, at 300 days after the procedure more patients in the control than stent group underwent repeated revascularization (42.4% vs 22.4%). Follow-up angiography was performed in 114 patients. ≥50% diameter stenosis developed in 32% vs 74% of the stent and control group, respectively (Odds ratio 0.165; 95% CI 0.07 to 0.37; p<0.001); reocclusion occurred in 12% vs 26%, respectively (p=0.058). Minimal luminal diameter at follow-up was larger in the stent group (1.92±0.95 vs 1.11±0.78 mm; p<0.001).
Conclusions	Stent implantation after successful balloon angioplasty of chronic coronary artery occlusions improved long-term angiographic results, and was associated with less recurrence of angina and less revascularization procedures.

A comparison of coronary-artery stenting with angioplasty for isolated stenosis of the proximal left anterior descending coronary artery.

Title	A comparison of coronary-artery stenting with angioplasty for isolated stenosis of the proximal left anterior descending coronary artery.
Author	Versaci F, Gaspardone A, Tomai F, et al.
Reference	N Engl J Med. 1997;336:817-822
Disease	Coronary artery disease.
Purpose	To compare treatment of isolated coronary artery stenosis with percutaneous transluminal coronary angioplasty vs coronary-artery stent deployment.
Design	Randomized, prospective.
Patients	120 patients with isolated stenosis of the proximal left anterior descending coronary artery.
Follow-up	12 months.
Treatment regimen	Stent implantation vs PTCA.
Results	The rates of procedural success (residual stenosis of less than 50%; absence of death, myocardial infarction, and need for coronary artery bypass surgery during hospital stay) were similar between the 2 groups (95% with stenting; 93% with angioplasty, p=NS). The 12 month rates of event-free survival (freedom from death, myocardial infarction, and the recurrence of angina) were 87% for stenting and 70% for angioplasty (p=0.04). Rates of restenosis were 19% after stenting and 40% after PTCA (p=0.02).

A comparison of coronary-artery stenting with angioplasty for isolated stenosis of the proximal left anterior descending coronary artery.

(continued)

Conclusions   Stenting resulted in a lower rate of restenosis and better long-term clinical outcome compared to PTCA in patients with asymptomatic isolated coronary artery stenosis.

BOAT

Balloon vs Optimal Atherectomy Trial (BOAT)

Title	Final results of the balloon vs optimal atherectomy trial (BOAT)
Author	Baim DS, Cutlip DE, Sharma SK et al.
Reference	Circulation 1998; 97:322-331
Disease	Coronary artery disease.
Purpose	To determine whether optimal directional coronary atherectomy provides short and long-term benefits compared to percutaneous transluminal coronary angioplasty.
Design	Randomized, multicenter.
Patients	1000 patients with single de novo atherosclerotic narrowing in a coronary artery.
Follow-up	1 year.
Treatment regimen	Optimal atherectomy included use of 7F cutters as the final device, removal of as much tissue as safe, postdilation with balloon, obtaining a final residual stenosis < 20%, and special training.

Balloon vs Optimal Atherectomy Trial (BOAT)

(continued)

Results   Optimal directional atherectomy resulted in a lesion suc-
           cess rate of 99%, vs PTCA at 97% (p=.02). Residual diam-
           eter stenosis was less with atherectomy at 15% vs 28% for
           PTCA (p<.0001). Atherectomy was associated with more
           patients exhibiting an increase in creatine kinase -MB >
           3x normal (16% vs 6%, p<.0001). Major clinical compli-
           cations (death, Q wave MI, or emergent CABG) were sim-
           ilar between groups. At 6.9 months angiographic restudy
           showed reduction of angiographic restenosis by atherec-
           tomy (31.4%) compared to angioplasty (39.8%, p=.016).
           Clinical follow-up showed nonsignificant trends toward
           lower mortality rate, target vessel revascularization, and
           target vessel failure (21.1% vs 24.8%, p=.17) with atherec-
           tomy compared to angioplasty.

Conclusions   Optimal directional coronary atherectomy improved
              short-term success compared to angioplasty, but did not
              significantly improve late clinical events.

ERBAC

Excimer Laser, Rotational Atherectomy, and Balloon Angioplasty Comparison (ERBAC) Study

Title	Randomized comparison of angioplasty of complex coronary lesions at a single center. Excimer laser, rotational atherectomy, and balloon angioplasty comparison (ERBAC) Study.
Author	Reifart N, Vandormael M, Krajcar M, et al.
Reference	Circulation 1997; 96:91-98.
Disease	Coronary artery disease.
Purpose	To test whether coronary revascularization with ablation of either excimer laser or rotational atherectomy improves initial angiographic and clinical outcomes vs percutaneous transluminal coronary angioplasty alone.
Design	Randomized, single center.
Patients	685 patients with symptomatic coronary artery disease warranting revascularization procedure.
Follow-up	6 months.
Treatment regimen	Patients randomized to balloon angioplasty, excimer laser angioplasty, or rotational atherectomy.

ERBAC

Excimer Laser, Rotational Atherectomy, and Balloon Angioplasty Comparison (ERBAC) Study

(continued)

Results

Procedural success was defined by diameter stenosis <50%, survival, no Q wave infarction, or coronary artery bypass surgery. Patients who received rotational atherectomy had higher rate of procedural success (89%) vs laser angioplasty (77%) or balloon angioplasty (80%; p = .0019). There were no differences in major in-hospital complications (3.1 - 4.3%). At 6 months, revascularization of target lesion was more frequently required in the rotational atherectomy group (42.4%) and the excimer laser group (46.0%) than the angioplasty group (31.9%, p=.013)

Conclusions

Although rotational atherectomy resulted in better early procedural success, it did not result in better late outcomes compared to laser atherectomy or balloon angioplasty.

SAVED

Saphenous Vein De Novo Trial

Title	Stent placement compared with balloon angioplasty for obstructed coronary bypass grafts.
Author	Savage MP, Douglas JS, Fischman DL, et al.
Reference	N Engl J Med 1997; 337:740-747.
Disease	Coronary artery disease, obstructed coronary bypass grafts.
Purpose	To compare the effects of stent placement with those of balloon angioplasty in patients with obstruction of saphenous vein grafts.
Design	Multicenter, randomized.
Patients	270 patients with new lesions in aortocoronary-venous bypass grafts.
Follow-up	6 months.
Treatment regimen	Randomized to Palmaz-Schatz stents vs standard balloon angioplasty.

SAVED

Saphenous Vein De Novo Trial

(continued)

Results   Patients receiving stents had a higher initial procedural
               success with reduction in stenosis to less than 50% of ves-
               sel diameter (92% vs 69% with angioplasty, p=0.001), but
               more hemorrhagic complications (17% vs 5%, P<0.01).
               The stent group had a greater mean increase in luminal
               diameter immediately after the procedure and a greater
               mean net gain in luminal diameter as well (0.85 ± 0.96
               with stents vs 0.54 ± 0.91 mm with angioplasty, p=0.002).
               At 6 months restenosis occurred in 37% of patients that
               received stents and 46% that received angioplasty
               (p=0.24). The stent group had a better clinical outcome
               at 6 months (freedom from death, myocardial infarction, repeat
               coronary artery bypass grafting, or repeat revasculariza-
               tion) compared to the angioplasty group at (58%, p
               =0.03).

Conclusions   Stenting of venous bypass graft stenoses resulted in a bet-
               ter initial outcome, larger gain in luminal diameter, but no
               significant long-term improvement in angiographic evi-
               dence of restenosis. Stents did reduce the frequency of
               major cardiac events.

4. Interventional Cardiology

d. Medical Therapy to Prevent Restenosis and/or Complications After Intracoronary Interventions or Occlusion After Coronary Artery Bypass Grafting

CARPORT

Coronary Artery Restenosis Prevention on Repeated Thromboxane-Antagonism Study

Title	Prevention of restenosis after percutaneous transluminal coronary angioplasty with thromboxane A2-receptor blockade. A randomized, double blind, placebo-controlled trial.
Authors	Serruys PW, Rutsch W, Heyndrick GR, et al.
Reference	Circulation 1991;84:1568-1580.
Disease	Coronary artery disease, restenosis.
Purpose	To evaluate the efficacy of GR32191B, a thromboxane A2-receptor antagonist, to prevent restenosis following coronary angioplasty.
Design	Randomized, double blind, placebo-controlled, multicenter.
Patients	697 patients, >21 years old, with coronary artery disease who were excluded for angioplasty for de novo lesions in native arteries. Patients with myocardial infarction within 2 weeks of procedure were excluded.
Follow-up	Clinical evaluation, exercise test, and repeated angiography at 6 months.
Treatment regimen	1. GR32191B 80 mg PO 1 h + saline infusion before procedure. 40 mg X2/d GR32191B thereafter. 2. Placebo PO + 250 mg aspirin IV before procedure. Placebo X2/d thereafter. Aspirin and NSAID were prohibited during the follow-up.
Additional therapy	Heparin IV 10,000 U bolus, 10 mg nifedipine every 2 h for 12 h, and then 20 mg of slow released nifedipine X3/d for 2 days.

CARPORT

Coronary Artery Restenosis Prevention on Repeated Thromboxane-Antagonism Study
(continued)

Results 522 compliant patients underwent repeated angiography. The mean minimal luminal diameter loss was 0.31±0.54 vs 0.31±0.55 mm in the control and treated group. A loss of ≥0.72 mm was found in 19% and 21% of the patients, respectively. 6 months after procedure 72% and 75% of the patients, respectively were symptom free. There was no difference in the rates of clinical events during the 6 months between the groups. There was no difference in exercise performance between the groups.

Conclusions Long term blockade of the thromboxane A2 receptor with GR32191B did not prevent restenosis or reduced clinical events after coronary angioplasty.

MERCATOR
Multicenter European Research Trial With Cilazapril After Angioplasty to Prevent Transluminal Coronary Obstruction and Restenosis

Title	Does the new angiotensin converting enzyme inhibitor cilazapril prevent restenosis after percutaneous transluminal coronary angioplasty? Results of the MERCATOR study: a multicenter, randomized, double blind, placebo-controlled trial.
Authors	The MERCATOR Study Group.
Reference	Circulation 1992;86:100-110.
Disease	Coronary artery disease, restenosis.
Purpose	To assess the effect of angiotensin-converting enzyme inhibition with cilazapril on restenosis after coronary angioplasty.
Design	Randomized, double blind, placebo-controlled, multicenter.
Patients	693 patients with successful angioplasty of a coronary artery.
Follow-up	Clinical evaluation, exercise test, and repeated angiography at 6 months
Treatment regimen	Medications were started in the evening following the angioplasty. Cilazapril 2.5 mg PO initially, and then 5 mg X2/d or placebo for 6 months.
Additional therapy	Aspirin 150-250 mg/d, started before angioplasty. IV heparin 10,000 U bolus before angioplasty, and infusion. calcium channel blockers for 48 h were permitted.

MERCATOR
Multicenter European Research Trial With Cilazapril After Angioplasty to Prevent Transluminal Coronary Obstruction and Restenosis
(continued)

Results
: The mean difference in minimal coronary luminal diameter between the baseline and follow-up angiography was −0.29±0.49 and -0.27±0.51 mm in the control and cilazapril treated patients, respectively. The occurrence of clinical events including death, myocardial infarction, coronary revascularization, or recurrent angina were similar in both groups. 63.6% and 62.2% of the control and cilazapril patients were event-free after 6 months. No difference in exercise test results were found between the groups.

Conclusions
: Long-term angiotensin converting enzyme inhibition with cilazapril did not prevent restenosis and did not reduce clinical events.

Title	Evaluation of ketanserin in the prevention of restenosis after percutaneous transluminal coronary angioplasty. A multicenter randomized, double blind placebo controlled trial.
Authors	Serruys PW, Klein W, Tijssen JPG, et al.
Reference	Circulation 1993;88:1588-1601.
Disease	Coronary artery disease, restenosis.
Purpose	To evaluate the role of ketanserin in prevention of restenosis after coronary angioplasty.
Design	Randomized, double blind, placebo controlled, multicenter.
Patients	658 patients, >30 years old, with angina due to a single or multivessel coronary artery disease who underwent coronary angioplasty.
Follow-up	Clinical evaluation and repeated angiography at 6 months.
Treatment regimen	Oral ketanserin 40 mg X2/d or placebo started 1 h before balloon insertion and continued for 6 months (the first 79 patients received IV infusion of ketanserin or placebo).
Additional therapy	Aspirin 250-500 mg/d, started before angioplasty. Heparin 10,000 U bolus before procedure.

Post-Angioplasty Restenosis Ketanserin

(continued)

Results
: Clinical follow-up of 525 patients was reported. There was no difference in the occurrence of any of the clinical end points (death, myocardial infarction, coronary bypass surgery, or repeated angioplasty) between the 2 groups. Any of the end points occurred in 28% and 32% of the ketanserin and placebo patients (RR 0.89, 95% CI 0.70-1.13). 592 patients underwent serial angiographic studies. The mean loss of minimal luminal diameter between the post-angioplasty and follow-up angiogram was 0.27 ± 0.49 and 0.24±0.52 mm in the ketanserin and placebo groups (difference 0.03 mm, 95% CI -0.05-0.11, p=0.5). Restenosis (>50%) occurred in 32% and 32% of the patients, respectively.

Conclusions
: Ketanserin at a dose of 80 mg/d failed to reduce restenosis rate and did not lower the incidence of adverse clinical events at 6 months.

Prevention of Coronary Artery Bypass Graft Occlusion by Aspirin, Dipyridamole, and Acenocoumarol/Phenoprocoumon Study

Title	a. Prevention of 1 year vein graft occlusion after aorto-coronary-bypass surgery: a comparison of low-dose aspirin, low dose aspirin plus dipyridamole, and oral anti-coagulants. b. Effects of low dose aspirin (50 mg/d), low dose aspirin plus dipyridamole, and oral anticoagulant agents after internal mammary artery bypass grafting: patency and clinical outcome at 1 year.
Authors	a. van der Meer J, Hillege HL, Kootstra GJ, et al. b. van der Meer J, de la Rivière AB, van Gilst WH, et al.
Reference	a. Lancet 1993;342:257-264. b. J Am Coll Cardiol 1994;24:1181-1188.
Disease	Coronary artery disease, coronary artery bypass grafting.
Purpose	To assess the benefits of low dose aspirin, aspirin+dipyridamole, and anticoagulation on 1 year patency rate of: a. vein grafts, b. internal thoracic artery bypass.
Design	Randomized, double blind (placebo-controlled for dipyridamole, open label for anticoagulation), multicenter.
Patients	a. 948 patients, ≤70 years old, who underwent elective aortocoronary bypass surgery with saphenous vein grafts. Patients with unstable angina or myocardial infarction within 7 days were excluded. b. 494 patients of the previous group, who received both internal thoracic artery and vein grafts.
Follow-up	Clinical follow-up and coronary angiography after 1 year.

*Prevention of Coronary Artery Bypass Graft Occlusion by Aspirin,
Dipyridamole, and Acenocoumarol/Phenoprocoumon Study*

(continued)

Treatment regimen	1. Aspirin 5θ mg/d started after surgery. 2. Aspirin 50 mg/d started after surgery + dipyridamole IV 5 mg/kg/d started before surgery and continued for 28 h, and then orally 200 mg X2/d. 3. Oral anticoagulation, started 1 d before surgery. Target INR 2.8-4.8.
Additional therapy	Coronary artery bypass grafting surgery. Paracetamol as an analgesic. Drugs that interfere with platelet aggregation were prohibited.
Results	a. After 1 year, occlusion rate of distal anastomosis was 11% in the aspirin+dipyridamole, 15% in the aspirin alone, and 13% in the oral anticoagulation (aspirin+dipyridamole vs aspirin RR 0.76, 95% CI 0.54-1.05, oral anticoagulants vs aspirin+dipyridamole RR 0.90, 95% CI 0.65-1.25). Clinical events (death, myocardial infarction, thrombosis, or major bleeding) occurred in 20.3%, 13.9% (RR 1.46, 95% CI 1.02-2.08), and 16.9% (RR 1.22, 95% CI 0.84-1.77), respectively. b. Occlusion rates were 4.6%, 5.3%, and 6.8% in the aspirin+dipyridamole, aspirin, and oral anticoagulants (p=NS). Overall clinical event rates were 23.3%, 13.3% (RR 1.75, 95% CI 1.09-2.81, p=0.025), and 17.1% (RR 1.29, 95% CI 0.77-2.15, p=0.42), respectively.
Conclusions	Addition of dipyridamole to low dose aspirin did not improve patency of either venous or internal thoracic artery grafts significantly. However, the overall clinical event rate was increased by adding dipyridamole.

EPIC

Evaluation of 7E3 for the Prevention of Ischemic Complications

Title	a. Randomized trial of coronary intervention with antibody against platelet IIb/IIIa integrin for reduction of clinical restenosis: results at 6 months. b. Use of monoclonal antibody directed against the platelet glycoprotein IIb/IIIa receptor in high-risk coronary angioplasty. c. Effects of platelet glycoprotein IIb/IIIa receptor blockade by a chimeric monoclonal antibody (Abciximab) on acute and 6 month outcomes after percutaneous transluminal coronary angioplasty for acute myocardial infarction. d. Increased risk of non Q wave myocardial infarction after directional atherectomy is platelet dependent: Evidence from the EPIC Trial. e. Long-term protection from myocardial ischemic events in a randomized trial of brief integrin (3 blockade with percutaneous coronary intervention. f. Role of platelet glycoprotein IIb/IIIa receptor inhibition on distal embolization during percutaneous revascularization of aortocoronary saphenous vein grafts.
Authors	a. Topol EJ, Califf RM, Weisman HF, et al. b. The EPIC Investigators. c. Lefkovits J, Ivanhoe RJ, Carliff RM, et al. d. Lefkovits J, Blankenship JC, Anderson KM, et al. e. Topol EJ, Ferguson JJ, Weisman HF, et al. f. Mak K-H, Challapalli R, Eisenberg MJ, et al.
Reference	a. Lancet 1994;343:881-886. b. N Engl J Med 1994;330:956-961. c. Am J Cardiol 1996; 77:1045-1051. d. J Am Coll Cardiol. 1996; 28:849-855. e. JAMA 1997, 278: 479-484. f. Am J Cardiol 1997; 80:985-988.
Disease	Coronary artery disease, restenosis.

EPIC

Evaluation of 7E3 for the Prevention of Ischemic Complications

(continued)

Purpose	To evaluate the effect of a monoclonal antibody Fab fragment (c7E3), directed against the IIb/IIIa integrin, to reduce restenosis following balloon angioplasty or directional atherectomy of coronary lesions in high risk coronary lesions. e. A previous study showed that abciximab improves outcomes for patients undergoing percutaneous transluminal coronary angioplasty (PTCA) at 30 days and 6 months. The purpose of this study was to determine if abciximab improves 3 year outcome following PTCA. f. 101 patients treated for narrowing of saphenous vein grafts in the EPIC study.
Design	Randomized, double blind, placebo controlled, multicenter. e. Double blind, placebo-controlled, randomized trial, multicenter. Primary outcome was composite of death, myocardial infarction, or coronary revascularization. Secondary endpoints were death, myocardial infarction, coronary revascularization, separately.
Patients	2099 patients, age <80 years, who needed coronary angioplasty or directional atherectomy and had an evolving or recent myocardial infarction, unstable angina, or high risk angiographic or clinical characteristics. e. 2099 high risk coronary artery disease patients undergoing PTCA.
Follow-up	6 month clinical follow-up. e. 2.5 years among 2001 patients; 3 years among 1559 patients.

EPIC

Evaluation of 7E3 for the Prevention of Ischemic Complications
(continued)

Treatment regimen	1. Placebo bolus and placebo infusion for 12 h; 2. c7E3 0.25 mg/kg bolus and placebo infusion for 12 h; and 3. c7E3 0.25 mg/kg bolus and 10 μg/min infusion for 12 h. The bolus was given at least 10 min before procedure. e. Abciximab bolus of 0.25mg/kg followed by infusion of 10μg/min for 12 h; abciximab bolus of 0.25mg/kg followed by placebo infusion; placebo bolus followed by placebo infusion.
Additional therapy	Aspirin 325 mg/d, with the first dose at least 2 h before procedure. IV heparin bolus 10,000-12,000 U before procedure and for ≥12 h after the procedure.
Results	Bleeding complications that mandated transfusion occurred in 7%, 14%, and 17% of the 3 groups, respectively (p<0.001). There was no difference in the events rates during the first 48 h. At 30 days, the composite end point of death, infarction, and repeated revascularization occurred in 12.8%, 11.5%, and 8.3%, respectively (c7E3 bolus+infusion vs placebo p=0.008). >48 h-6 months, the composite end point occurred in 25.4%, 24.3%, and 19.2%, respectively (p=0.007). Total events rates within 6 months were 35.1%, 32.6%, and 27.0%, respectively (p=0.001). The favorable long-term effect was mainly due to reduced need for repeated revascularization (22.3%, 21.0%, and 16.5%, respectively p=0.007). By regression analysis the c7E3 bolus+infusion was independently associated with fewer events during the 6 month follow-up (hazard ratio 0.75, p=0.025). c. 42 patients underwent direct PTCA for acute myocardial infarction and 22 patients had rescue PTCA after failed thrombolysis. Patients receiving abciximab (as bolus and as bolus plus infusion) had a reduced primary composite end-point (death, reinfarction, repeat intervention, or bypass surgery) with 26.1% in the placebo group reaching the endpoint, vs 4.5% in the treated group (p=0.06). Major bleeding was more common with abciximab (24% vs 13%, p = 0.28). At 6 months there was a significant reduction in ischemic events in patients that received abciximab (47.8% in placebo vs

4.5% in abciximab p = 0.002) including reinfarction (p=0.05) and repeat revascularization (p=0.002).

d. Directional atherectomy was performed in 197 patients in the EPIC trial. These patients had a lower baseline risk for acute complications but had a higher rate of myocardial infarction, including non Q wave myocardial infarction than PTCA patients. Bolus and infusion of C7E3 decreased non Q wave myocardial infarctions after atherectomy (15.4% for placebo; 4.5% for treated, p = 0.046). Bolus and infusion of C7E3 reduced incidence of development of Q waves infarctions in PTCA patients (2.6% with placebo vs 0.8% with C7E3, p = 0.017).

e. At 3 years primary endpoint occurred in 41.1% on abciximab bolus plus infusion; 47.4% on abciximab bolus only; and 47.2% on placebo only (p=.009 for abciximab bolus plus infusion vs placebo). There was no significant difference in death among these groups (6.8%, 8.0%, 8.6%). Myocardial infarction occurred in 10.7%, 12.2%, and 13.6% respectively (p=.08 for abciximab bolus plus infusion vs placebo). Revascularization occurred in 34.8%, 38.6%, and 40.1%, respectively (p=.02 for abciximab bolus plus infusion vs placebo). In the subgroup of patients with refractory angina or evolving myocardial infarction death occurred in 5.1%, 9.2% and 12.7%, respectively (p=.01 for abciximab bolus plus infusion vs placebo). There was a correlation between the increase in periprocedural creatine kinase levels and mortality.

f. Bolus and infusion therapy of abciximab resulted in a significant reduction in distal embolization (2%) vs placebo (18%; p = 0.017), and a trend towards reduction in early large non Q wave acute myocardial infarction (2% vs 12%). At 30 days and 6 months the occurrence of composite end point were not different among the groups, in these patients undergoing revascularization of aortocoronary saphenous vein grafts.

EPIC

Evaluation of 7E3 for the Prevention of Ischemic Complications
(continued)

Conclusions
c7E3 bolus and infusion reduced the revascularization procedure rate during 6 month follow-up of high risk angioplasty patients. However, bleeding complications were increased.

e. Abciximab bolus plus infusion administered at the time of PTCA improved outcomes for as long as 3 years.

f. Adjunctive therapy with abciximab reduced the occurrence of distal embolization and possibly non Q wave myocardial infarction in patients undergoing percutaneous therapy for narrowed saphenous vein bypass grafts.

ERA

Enoxaparin Restenosis Trial

Title	Low molecular weight heparin in prevention of restenosis after angioplasty. Results of enoxaparin restenosis (ERA) trial.
Authors	Faxon DP, Spiro TE, Minor S, et al.
Reference	Circulation 1994;90:908-914.
Disease	Coronary artery disease, restenosis.
Purpose	To evaluate whether enoxaparin given subcutaneously for 28 days will reduce the restenosis rates after coronary angioplasty.
Design	Randomized, double blind, placebo controlled, multicenter.
Patients	458 patients, >21 years old, with ≥50% stenosis of a coronary artery, reduced to <50% with ≥20% change in diameter by angioplasty. Patients with asthma, hypertension, acute myocardial infarction within 5 days, angioplasty of venous grafts, or restenosis after prior angioplasty were excluded.
Follow-up	Clinical evaluation, exercise test, and repeated angiography at 24 weeks.
Treatment regimen	Enoxaparin 40 mg/d SC or placebo, started <24 h after angioplasty and continued for 28 days.
Additional therapy	Aspirin 325 mg/d started 1 day before procedure. IV heparin was given during angioplasty. Calcium channel blockers were given before and after angioplasty.

(continued)

Results	Restenosis (loss of >50% of the initial gain in luminal diameter or death, reinfarction, need for bypass surgery, or worsening of angina in patients without follow-up angiography) occurred in 51% of the placebo and 52% of the enoxaparin patients (RR 1.07, p=0.63). Restenosis occurred in 49% and 50% of the patients with follow-up angiography, respectively. The late loss of minimal luminal diameter was 0.49 and 0.54 mm, in the control and enoxaparin, respectively (p=0.78). Adverse clinical events were infrequent and similar between the groups. Minor bleeding complications were more common with enoxaparin (48% vs 34%). In a subset of patients, there was no difference in performance in exercise test.
Conclusions	Enoxaparin 40 mg/d did not reduce the occurrence of restenosis or of adverse clinical events.

MARCATOR

***Multicenter American Research Trial With Cilazapril
After Angioplasty to Prevent Transluminal Coronary
Obstruction and Restenosis***

Title	Effect of high dose angiotensin-converting enzyme inhibition on restenosis: final results of the MARCATOR study, a multicenter, double blind, placebo-controlled trial of cilazapril.
Authors	Faxon DP, MARCATOR Study Group.
Reference	J Am Coll Cardiol 1995;25:362-369.
Disease	Coronary artery disease, restenosis.
Purpose	To assess the effect of high and low dose angiotensin-converting enzyme inhibition on restenosis after coronary angioplasty.
Design	Randomized, double blind, placebo-controlled, multicenter.
Patients	1436 patients, age 25-80 years, without recent myocardial infarction (<5 days), prior revascularization, or severe hypertension or valvular disease.
Follow-up	Clinical evaluation and repeated angiography at 24 weeks.
Treatment regimen	Study medication were started <6 h after successful angioplasty and continued for 6 months. 1. Cilazapril 1mg X2/d 2. Cilazapril 5 mg X2/d. 3. Cilazapril 10 mg X2/d. 4. Placebo.
Additional therapy	Aspirin 325 mg/d, started before angioplasty. IV heparin 10,000 U before procedure, and infusion thereafter. Calcium channel blockers were recommended.

MARCATOR
Multicenter American Research Trial With Cilazapril
After Angioplasty to Prevent Transluminal Coronary
Obstruction and Restenosis

(continued)

Results	The mean difference in minimal coronary lumen diameter between the baseline and follow-up angiography was -0.35±0.51, -0.37±0.52, -0.45±0.52, and -0.41±0.53 mm for the placebo, 2, 10, and 20 mg/d cilazapril, respectively (p=NS). Restenosis >50% at follow-up occurred in 33%, 40%, 36%, and 34%, respectively. Clinical events during follow-up did not differ among the 4 groups.
Conclusions	Long-term angiotensin-converting enzyme inhibition with cilazapril did not prevent restenosis and did not reduce clinical event rate after angioplasty.

SHARP

The Subcutaneous Heparin and Angioplasty Restenosis Prevention (SHARP) Trial

Title	The Subcutaneous Heparin and Angioplasty Restenosis Prevention (SHARP) Trial. Results of a multicenter randomized trial investigating the effects of high dose unfractionated heparin on angiographic restenosis and clinical outcome.
Authors	Brack MJ, Ray S, Chauhan A, et al.
Reference	J Am Coll Cardiol 1995;26:947-954.
Disease	Coronary artery disease.
Purpose	To investigate whether high dose subcutaneous heparin will improve outcome after coronary angioplasty.
Design	Randomized, open label with blinded analysis of data, 3 centers.
Patients	339 patients who had undergone successful coronary angioplasty. Patients with restenotic lesions, chronic total occlusions, or conduit lesions were not included.
Follow-up	4 month clinical evaluation and repeated angiography.
Treatment regimen	Subcutaneous heparin 12,500 U X2/d for 4 months, started 2 h after femoral sheath removal, or no therapy.
Additional therapy	Coronary angioplasty, aspirin 300 mg, and heparin IV bolus 10,000 U before the procedure. After angioplasty, heparin infusion 1,000 U/h for up to 24 h. Aspirin 75-300 mg/d. Other medications according to operator choice.

The Subcutaneous Heparin and Angioplasty Restenosis Prevention (SHARP) Trial
(continued)

Results	Repeated angiography was performed in 90% of the patients. The difference in minimal luminal diameter between the post-angioplasty and follow-up study was -0.55±0.58 mm for the control and -0.43±0.59 mm for the heparin group (p=NS). The occurrence of myocardial infarction, coronary artery bypass surgery, repeated angioplasty, and angina at 4 months was comparable. There was no difference between the groups in the number of patients with ischemia during follow-up exercise test.
Conclusions	Long-term treatment with high dose subcutaneous heparin for 4 months failed to improve outcome and to prevent restenosis.

REDUCE

Reviparin in Percutaneous Transluminal Coronary Angioplasty

Title	Low molecular weight heparin (Reviparin) in percutaneous transluminal coronary angioplasty. Results of a randomized, double blind, unfractionated heparin and placebo-controlled, multicenter trial (REDUCE trial).
Authors	Karsch KR, Preisack MB, Baildon R, et al.
Reference	J Am Coll Cardiol 1996;28:1437-1443.
Disease	Coronary artery disease.
Purpose	To evaluate the effect of low molecular weight heparin on the incidence of restenosis in patients with coronary artery disease undergoing percutaneous transluminal coronary angioplasty (PTCA).
Design	Randomized, double blind, multicenter.
Patients	612 patients with single lesion coronary artery obstruction scheduled to undergo coronary angioplasty. Patients with class 3C unstable angina or unstable angina requiring continuous heparin infusion, myocardial infarction within 14 days, bleeding disorders, active peptic ulcer, uncontrolled asthma or hypertension, left main coronary artery stenosis >50%, and angioplasty of saphenous vein graft or previous angioplasty at the same site were excluded.
Follow-up	Clinical follow-up for 30 weeks. Repeated coronary angiography at 26±2 weeks after angioplasty.

REDUCE

Reviparin in Percutaneous Transluminal Coronary Angioplasty

(continued)

Treatment regimen	At the time of arterial access, patients were randomized to either a bolus of unfractionated heparin (10,000 IU), followed by infusion of 24,000 IU heparin over 16±4h, or reviparin (7,000 IU anti-Xa U), followed by infusion of reviparin 10,500 IU anti-Xa U over 16±4h. Then, patients received either 3,500 IU anti-Xa U of reviparin or placebo subcutaneously X2/d for 28 days.
Additional therapy	Standard balloon angioplasty. Aspirin 100 mg/d was started 1 day before angioplasty.
Results	By intention to treat analysis, treatment failure (death, myocardial infarction, bypass surgery, or emergency or elective repeat angioplasty) occurred in 33.3% of the reviparin and 32.0% of the controls (p=0.71). Angiographic restenosis was present in 33.0% of patients of the reviparin vs 34.4% of the control group. 16.4% of the reviparin vs 19.9% of the control group developed significant angina. Acute events within 24 hours after the procedure occurred less often in the reviparin-treated group (3.9% vs 8.2%, respectively; relative risk (RR) 0.49; 95% CI 0.26-0.92; p=0.027). Only 6 patients in the reviparin-treated group vs 21 patients in the control group needed emergency stent implantation (RR 0.29; 95% CI 0.13-0.66; p=0.003). Analysis of primary end-points after 30 weeks revealed that the occurrence of clinical events was comparable between the groups (31.7% vs 30% in the reviparin and control, respectively). There was no difference in late loss of minimal lumen diameter between the 2 groups. Bleeding complications were comparable (2.3% in the reviparin vs 2.6% in the control group; p=0.8).
Conclusions	Reviparin use started immediately before coronary balloon angioplasty and continued for 28 days did not reduce the rate of major clinical events or the incidence of restenosis over 30 weeks follow-up.

ISAR

Intracoronary Stenting and Antithrombotic Regimen trial

Title	a. A randomized comparison of antiplatelets and anticoagulant therapy after the placement of coronary-artery stents. b. Major benefit from antiplatelet therapy for patients at high risk for adverse cardiac events after coronary Palmaz-Schatz stent replacement. c. Restenosis after coronary stent placement and randomization to a 4 week combined antiplatelet or anticoagulant therapy. 6 month angiographic follow-up of the intracoronary stenting and antithrombotic regimen (ISAR) trial.
Authors	a. Schömig A, Neumann F-J, Kastrati A, et al. b. Schuhlen H, Hadamitzky M, Walter H, et al. c. Kastrati A, Schuhlen H, Hausleiter J, et al.
Reference	a. N Engl J Med 1996; 334:1084-1089. b. Circulation 1997; 95:2015-2021. c. Circulation 1997; 96:462-467.
Disease	a. Coronary artery disease, restenosis. b. Coronary artery disease. c. Coronary artery disease.
Purpose	a. To compare the efficacy of 2 therapeutic regimens after placement of coronary artery stents: 1. combined antiplatelet therapy with ticlopidine plus aspirin, and 2. anticoagulation with intravenous heparin, phenprocoumon, and aspirin. b. Comparison of antiplatelet therapy to anticoagulant therapy after coronary artery stent deployment. This study was an analysis of prospective risk stratification. c. The ISAR Trial compared outcomes of patients randomized to either combined anti-platelet therapy-aspirin plus ticlopidine or phenprocoumon (anticoagulant) with initial aspirin and heparin after coronary stent deployment. Within the first 4 weeks of therapy, combined antiplatelet therapy resulted in fewer ischemic complications. The purpose of this study was to determine whether 4 weeks of antiplatelet therapy could reduce angiographic evidence of restenosis at 6 months.

ISAR

Intracoronary Stenting and Antithrombotic Regimen trial (continued)

Design	a. Randomized, 1 center. b + c. Prospective, randomized study.
Patients	a. 257 patients in whom intracoronary Palmaz-Schatz stents were successfully implanted after balloon angioplasty. The indications for stenting were extensive dissection after angioplasty, complete vessel closure, residual stenosis ≥30%, and lesions in venous bypass grafts. Patients with absolute indication for anticoagulation, or contraindications to 1 of the drugs, cardiogenic shock, or who had needed mechanical ventilation were excluded. b. 517 patients from original ISAR study [N Engl J Med 1996;334:1084-1089]. Risk stratification performed based on clinical, procedural, and angiographic variables. 165 patients with 2 or fewer criteria = low risk; 148 patients with 3 criteria = intermediate risk; 204 with 4 or more criteria = high risk. c. 432 patients with 6 month follow-up angiograms.
Follow-up	a. Hospitalization for 10 days. Clinical follow-up for 30 days. b. 30 days. c. 6 months.
Treatment regimen	In patients assigned to antiplatelet therapy, heparin infusion was started after arterial sheath removal for 12 h. Ticlopidine 250 mgX2/d was administered for 4 weeks. In patients assigned to anticoagulation therapy, heparin infusion, started after sheath removal, was continued for 5 to 10 days. Phenoprocoumon was given for 4 weeks (target INR 3.5 to 4.5). Aspirin 100 mg bid given to both groups.
Additional therapy	a. Heparin and aspirin intravenously before PTCA. All patients received aspirin 100 mgX2/d throughout the study.

Results

a. 30 days after randomization, mortality was comparable (0.4% vs 0.8% in the antiplatelet and anticoagulant group, respectively). Myocardial infarction occurred in 0.8% vs 4.2% of the patients, respectively (relative risk (RR) 0.18; 95% CI 0.02 to 0.83; p=0.02) and the need for revascularization was 1.2% vs 5.4% (RR 0.22; 95% CI 0.04 to 0.77; p=0.01). A primary cardiac event (cardiac death, myocardial infarction, or revascularization) occurred in 1.6% of the antiplatelet vs 6.2% of the anticoagulant patients (RR 0.25; 95% CI 0.06 to 0.77; p=0.01). Occlusion of the stented vessel occurred less often in the antiplatelet group (0.8% vs 5.4%; RR 0.14; 95% CI 0.02 to 0.62; p=0.004). A primary noncardiac endpoint (noncardiac death, cerebrovascular accident, or severe peripheral vascular or hemorrhagic event) was reached by 1.2% vs 12.3% of the antiplatelet and anticoagulant groups, respectively (RR 0.09; 95% CI 0.02 to 0.31; p<0.001). Bleeding complications occurred only in the anticoagulant group (6.5%; p<0.001). Peripheral vascular events occurred in 0.8% of the antiplatelet group vs 6.2% of the anticoagulant group (RR 0.13; 95% CI 0.01 to 0.53; p=0.001).

b. At 30 day follow-up there was a decrease in risk for noncardiac and cardiac complications, especially occlusion of the stented vessel, in patients treated with antiplatelet vs anticoagulation therapy. Cardiac event rate (death, myocardial infarction, repeat intervention) was 6.4%, 3.4%, and 0% for high, intermediate and low risk patients, respectively (p<.01). Occlusion of the stented vessel occurred in 5.9%, 2.7%, and 0% respectively (P<.01). In high risk patients the cardiac event rate was 12.6% with anticoagulation therapy vs. 2.0% for antiplatelet therapy (p=.007) and rate of stent vessel occlusion was 11.5% vs 0% (P<.001). There were no significant differences between anticoagulant and antiplatelet in low and intermediate risk groups.

c. At 6 months there were no differences in minimal diameter, late lumen loss, or restenosis rates (26.8% in antiplatelet group and 28.9% in anticoagulation group, respectively p = .20).

Conclusions   a. After successful placement of coronary artery stents, the combination of aspirin and ticlopidine was associated with lower rate of cardiac events, fewer vascular, and hemorrhagic complications.

b. Patients in the high risk group had the greatest benefit from anitplatelet therapy.

c. Aspirin plus ticlopidine for 4 weeks after stent placement did not reduce restenosis rates compared to phenprocoumon with initial overlapping heparin plus aspirin treatment.

ACCORD

Angioplasie Coronaire Corvasal Diltiazem

Title	Effect of the direct nitric oxide donors linsidomine and molsidomine on angiographic restenosis after coronary balloon angioplasty. The ACCORD study.
Authors	Lablanche J-M, Grollier G, Lusson J-R, et al.
Reference	Circulation 1997;95:83-89
Disease	Coronary artery disease, restenosis.
Purpose	To evaluate the effect of molsidomine and linsidomine, direct nitric oxide donors, on restenosis after coronary balloon angioplasty.
Design	Randomized, multicenter.
Patients	700 patients, ≤70 years old, with angina and/or evidence of myocardial ischemia who were referred for balloon angioplasty. Patients with myocardial infarction within 3 months, recent unstable angina, ejection fraction <0.35, systolic blood pressure <100 mmHg, contraindications to aspirin, restenotic graft or left main coronary artery lesions and totally occluded lesions were excluded.
Follow-up	Clinical follow-up with repeated coronary angiography at 6 months.
Treatment regimen	Randomization to active treatment group or controls. The active treatment consisted of continuous infusion of linsidomine (1 mg/h), started 3-18 h before the angioplasty, and continued for 24 h after the procedure, and then, molsidomine 4mgX3/d PO for 6 months. The control group received diltiazem 60 mgX3/d.

ACCORD

Angioplasie Coronaire Corvasal Diltiazem

(continued)

Additional therapy	Aspirin 250 mg/d. Heparin 10,000 IU at the start of angio plasty, additional doses of heparin 5000 IU after each h of procedure. Long-acting nitrates, calcium channel blockers, oral anticoagulants, and angiotensin-converting enzyme inhibitors were prohibited.
Results	3520 patients had 3 angiograms (at baseline, immediately after angioplasty, and at follow-up). Despite the intra-coronary administration of isosorbide dinitrate before angiography, the mean reference luminal diameter was greater in the NO donor group than in the diltiazem group before angioplasty (2.94 vs 2.83 mm; p=0.014). The mean minimal luminal diameter (MLD) before angioplasty was comparable. However, immediately after angioplasty, MLD was 1.94 vs 1.81 mm, in the NO donor and the diltiazem group, respectively (p=0.001). Mean MLD remained larger in the NO donor group at follow-up (1.54 vs 1.38 mm; p=0.007). Late loss, loss index, and the slope of the regression between late loss and acute gain were comparable. At 6 months, restenosis ($\geq$50%) occurred in 38.0% of the NO donor treated patients vs 46.5% of the diltiazem group (p=0.062). After adjustment for center and hypercholesterolemia the p value was 0.026. The combined rate of major clinical events (death, myocardial infarction, and coronary revascularization) were comparable (32.2% in the NO donor group vs 32.4% in the diltiazem group). The incidence of side effects and the number of dropouts due to adverse effects were similar (13 vs 10, respectively).
Conclusions	NO donor therapy was associated with larger MLD immediately after and at follow-up following coronary balloon angioplasty and lower rate of restenosis. However, late luminal loss did not differ between the groups and there was no difference in the occurrence of major clinical events.

EMPAR

Enoxaparin MaxEPA Prevention of Angioplasty Restenosis

Title	Fish oils and low molecular weight heparin for the reduction of restenosis after percutaneous transluminal coronary angioplasty. The EMPAR Study.
Author	Cairns JA, Gill J, Morton B, et al.
Reference	Circulation 1996; 94:1553-1560.
Disease	Coronary artery disease, restenosis post-angioplasty.
Purpose	To determine whether fish oils reduce the incidence of restenosis following percutaneous transluminal coronary angioplasty.
Design	Randomized, placebo-controlled, multicenter.
Patients	814 patients with coronary artery disease, undergoing PTCA.
Follow-up	16 - >28 weeks.
Treatment regimen	Starting 6 days before PTCA patients were randomized to fish oils (5.4 g n - 3 fatty acids) or placebo and continued on this for 18 weeks post-PTCA. At the time of sheath removal patients were randomized to low molecular weight heparin or control.
Results	Restenosis rates per patient were 46.5% in the fish oil group and 44.7% in the placebo group. Rates were 45.8% of patients receiving low molecular weight heparin and 45.4% in controls.
Conclusions	Fish oils did not reduce restenosis rates. Low molecular weight heparin did not reduce restenosis rates.

EPILOG

Evaluation in PTCA to Improve Long-Term Outcome with Abciximab GPIIb/IIIa Blockade

Title	Platelet glycoprotein IIb/IIIa receptor blockade and low dose heparin during percutaneous coronary revascularization.
Author	The EPILOG Investigators
Reference	N Engl J Med.1997; 336:1689-1696.
Disease	Coronary artery disease, urgent or elective percutaneous coronary revascularization.
Purpose	To determine whether the clinical benefits of abciximab (known to diminish ischemic complications in patients undergoing high risk angioplasty and atherectomy procedures) could be extended to all patients undergoing coronary intervention, regardless of risk. To determine whether adjusting the heparin dose could limit the hemorrhagic complications associated with abciximab use.
Design	Prospective, double blind, randomized, multicenter.
Patients	2792 patients undergoing urgent or elective percutaneous coronary revascularization.
Follow-up	30 days.

EPILOG

*Evaluation in PTCA to Improve Long-Term Outcome
with Abciximab GPIIb/IIIa Blockade*

(continued)

Treatment regimen	1. Abciximab (0.25 mg per kg 10-60 min before inflation, followed by an infusion of 0.125 µg/kg/min, maximum of 10 µg per min for 12 h) plus standard dose heparin (bolus of 100 U per kg (maximum 10,000 U) prior to intervention, with additional boluses to achieve an activated clotting time of at least 300 sec or 2. Abciximab plus low dose weight adjusted heparin (bolus of 70 U/kg, maximum 7,000 U) with additional boluses to maintain activated clotting time of at least 200 sec) or 3. Placebo with standard dose, weight adjusted heparin.
Results	At 30 days the composite event rate of death, myocardial infarction, or urgent revascularization within 30 days was 5.4% in group assigned to abciximab plus standard dose heparin (hazard ratio 0.45, 95% CI = 0.32 - 0.63, p<0.001); 5.2% in group assigned to abciximab with low dose heparin (hazard ratio 0.43; 95% CI 0.30-0.60, p< 0.001) and 11.7% in group assigned to placebo with standard dose heparin. Major bleeding did not differ among groups. Minor bleeding was more frequent in patients receiving abciximab plus standard dose heparin.
Conclusions	Abciximab plus low dose, weight adjusted heparin reduced ischemic complications in patients undergoing percutaneous revascularization procedures and did not increase risk of hemorrhage.

EPILOG Substudy

*Evaluation in PTCA to Improve Long-term Outcome
with Abciximab GP IIb/IIIa blockade*

Title	Abciximab therapy and unplanned coronary stent deployment. Favorable effects on stent use, clinical outcomes, and bleeding complications.
Author	Kereiakes DJ, Lincoff AM, Miller DP.
Reference	Circulation 1998; 97:857-864.
Disease	Coronary artery disease.
Purpose	To describe the effects of abciximab on clinical outcomes in patients in the EPILOG study who required unplanned coronary stent deployment.
Design	Randomized, double blind, placebo-controlled trial.
Patients	326 patients that required unplanned coronary stent deployment.
Follow-up	6 months.
Treatment regimen	As per EPILOG protocol.

EPILOG Substudy

*Evaluation in PTCA to Improve Long-term Outcome
with Abciximab GP IIb/IIIa blockade*

(continued)

Results
: Patients requiring stents had greater coronary lesion complexity, longer lesion length, more lesion eccentricity, irregularity, and involvement of bifurcations, compared to nonstented patients. Patients that were treated with abciximab and low dose, weight adjusted heparin required unplanned stents less frequently (9.0%) than patients on placebo and standard dose heparin (13.7%, p = .001). Patients with unplanned stents had a more complicated course-more death, myocardial infarction, or urgent intervention (14.4%) vs patients with no stents (6.3%, p = .001). At 6 months abciximab reduced the incidence of death, infarction, or urgent revascularization compared to placebo in patients who had unplanned stents. Abciximab's benefit was somewhat greater in patients requiring compared to not requiring a stent. It did not cause an increase in bleeding in the stented patients.

Conclusions
: Patients that required unplanned stenting had more complex coronary artery lesions and a more complicated clinical course. Abciximab reduced the need for unplanned stent deployment and improved clinical outcome in those patients requiring a stent.

THE FACT STUDY

Fraxiparine Angioplastie Coronaire Transluminale

Title	Effect of nadroparin (Fraxiparine), a low-molecular weight heparin, on clinical and angiographic restenosis after coronary balloon angioplasty. The FACT Study.
Author	Lablanche J-M, McFadden EP, Meneveau N et al.
Reference	Circulation 1997; 96:3396-3402.
Disease	Coronary artery disease.
Purpose	To determine whether nadroparin, a low molecular-weight heparin, begun 3 days prior to percutaneous transluminal coronary angioplasty (PTCA) improved clinical outcome following the procedure.
Design	Prospective, multicenter, double blind, randomized.
Patients	354 patients with angina or objective evidence of myocardial ischemia, > 50% stenosis of a coronary artery, and scheduled for PTCA.
Follow-up	6 months.
Treatment regimen	Subcutaneous nadroparin (0.6mL of 10 250 antiXa IU/mL) or placebo from 3 days prior to angioplasty until 3 months after the procedure.

THE FACT STUDY

Fraxiparine Angioplastie Coronaire Transluminale

(continued)

Results   The primary endpoint of angiographic restenosis, determined by quantitative coronary angiography at 3 months did not differ between treated and control groups. Combined major cardiac related events also did not differ between groups (30.3% in treated vs 29.6% in controls).

Conclusions   Pretreatment with the low molecular weight heparin nadroparin did not affect angiographic restenosis or clinical outcome.

IMPACT-II

Integrillin to Minimise Platelet Aggregation and Coronary Thrombosis-II

Title	Randomized, placebo-controlled trial of effect of eptifibatide on complications of percutaneous coronary intervention: IMPACT-II.
Authors	The IMPACT-II Investigators.
Reference	Lancet 1997;349:1422-1428.
Disease	Coronary artery disease.
Purpose	To assess whether eptifibatide (integrillin), a platelet glycoprotein IIb/IIIa inhibitor, would prevent ischemic complications following percutaneous coronary interventions.
Design	Randomized, double blind, placebo-controlled, multicenter.
Patients	4010 patients, scheduled for elective, urgent, or emergency transcutaneous coronary intervention (balloon angioplasty, directional atherectomy, rotational atherectomy, or excimer laser ablation). Patients with bleeding diathesis, severe hypertension, major surgery within 6 weeks, stroke, other major illness, or pregnancy were excluded.
Follow-up	6 months.
Treatment regimen	Randomization to: 1. eptifibatide 135µg/kg bolus followed by an infusion of 0.5 µg/kg for 20-24 h (the 135/0.5 group); 2. eptifibatide 135µg/kg bolus followed by an infusion of 0.75 µg/kg for 20-24 h (the 135/0.75 group); or 3. placebo bolus and placebo infusion. Therapy was started after vascular access had been established and heparin 100 U/kg was administered.

IMPACT-II

Integrillin to Minimise Platelet Aggregation and Coronary Thrombosis-II

(continued)

Additional therapy | Aspirin 325 mg before the procedure. No further heparin was given after the coronary intervention and arterial sheath was removed within 4-6 h.

Results | By 30 days, mortality was 1.1% in the placebo group, 0.5% in the 135/0.5 group and 0.8% in the 135/0.75 group. The composite end-point of death, myocardial infarction, urgent or emergency revascularization (PTCA or CABG), or index insertion of an intracoronary stent for abrupt closure in 30 days occurred in 11.4% of the placebo group, 9.2% in the 135/0.5 group (p=0.063 vs placebo; OR 0.79; 95% CI 0.61-1.01) and in 9.9% of the 135/0.75 group (p=0.22 vs placebo; OR 0.86; 95% CI 0.67-1.10). Death or myocardial infarction occurred in 8.4% of the placebo, compared with 6.9% in the 135/0.5 group (p=0.13; OR 0.80; 95% CI 0.60-1.07) and 7.3% in the 135/0.75 group (p=0.27; OR=0.85; 95% CI 0.64-1.13). Most events occurred within the first 6 h of procedure. By the end of infusion of eptifibatide/placebo, the composite event rate was 9.3% in the placebo vs 6.8% in the 135/0.5 group (p=0.017) and 7.0% in the 135/0.75 group (p=0.026). There was no clustering of events after the end of infusion, suggesting that there is no rebound phenomenon. During 6 months of follow-up, death or myocardial infarction occurred in 11.6% of the placebo group, 10.5% in the 135/0.5 group (p=0.33), and 10.1% in the 135/0.75 group (p=0.19). Revascularization rates were comparable among the groups. There was no differences in the rates of major bleeding among the groups (4.8%, 5.1%, and 5.2%, respectively), or the need for transfusion (5.2%, 5.6%, and 5.9%, respectively). The rates of stroke were comparable.

Conclusions | Eptifibatide infusion reduced early abrupt closure and reduced the rates of 30 day ischemic events, without increasing the risk of bleeding complications. However, the effect on 30 day mortality or occurrence of myocardial infarction, and on 6 month cumulative ischemic event rate were not statistically significant.

M-HEART II

Multi-Hospital Eastern Atlantic Restenosis Trialists

Title	Effect of thromboxane A2 blockade on clinical outcome and restenosis after successful coronary angioplasty. Multi-Hospital Eastern Atlantic Restenosis Trial (M-Heart II).
Author	Savage MP, Goldberg S, Bove AA, et al.
Reference	Circulation 1995; 92:3194-3200.
Disease	Coronary artery disease.
Purpose	To determine the effects of aspirin (a nonselective inhibitor of thromboxane A2 synthesis) and sulotroban (a selective blocker of the thromboxane A2 receptor) on late clinical events and restenosis after coronary angioplasty.
Design	Prospective, randomized, multicenter.
Patients	752 patients with coronary artery disease.
Follow-up	6 months.
Treatment regimen	Aspirin (325 mg daily), sulotroban (800 mg 4 times a day) or placebo within 6 h before PTCA and for 6 months.
Results	Neither of the agents differed from placebo in the rate of angiographic restenosis. Aspirin significantly improved clinical outcome compared to placebo. Myocardial infarction was reduced by aspirin (1.2%), sulotroban (1.8%) compared to placebo (5.7%; p = .03).
Conclusions	Thromboxane A2 blockade protects against late ischemic events after angioplasty but not angiographic restenosis. Overall clinical outcome was superior for aspirin compared with sulotroban.

MVP

Multivitamins and Probucol

Title	a. Probucol and multivitamins in the prevention of restenosis after coronary angioplasty. b. Prevention of restenosis after angioplasty in small coronary arteries with probucol.
Author	a. Tardif J-C, Cote G, Lesperance J, et. al. b. Rodes J, Cote G, Lesperance J, et. al.
Reference	a. N Engl J Med. 1997; 337: 365-372. b. Circulation 1998; 97:429-436.
Disease	Coronary artery disease, patients undergoing angioplasty.
Purpose	a. To determine whether antioxidant drugs could decrease the incidence and severity of restenosis after angioplasty. b. To determine whether probucol therapy was successful in reducing restenosis in smaller coronary arteries (<3.0 mm).
Design	Double blind, placebo-controlled trial with 4 study groups.
Patients	a. 317 patients undergoing angioplasty. b. Subset of 189 patients undergoing angioplasty with at least 1 coronary segment with a diameter of <3.0mm.
Follow-up	6 months.

MVP

Multivitamins and Probucol

(continued)

Treatment regimen	1 month before angioplasty patients were randomized to placebo; probucol (500 mg); multivitamins (30,000 IU of beta carotene, 500 mg of vitamin C, and 700 IU of vitamin E) or both probucol and multivitamins taken twice-a-day. Patients were treated for 4 weeks prior to and 6 months after angioplasty. They received an extra 1000 mg of probucol, 2000 IU Vitamin E, both probucol and Vitamin E, or placebo 12 h prior to the procedure. Angiograms at baseline and at 6 months were read by blinded observer.
Results	a. Mean reduction in luminal diameter at 6 months was 0.12 ± 0.41, 0.22 ± 0.46, 0.33 ± 0.51 and 0.38 ± 0.50 mm in the probucol, combined treatment, multivitamin and placebo groups respectively ($p=0.006$ for probucol vs no probucol; $p = 0.70$ for multivitamins vs no multivitamins). Restenosis rates per coronary segment were 20.7, 28.9, 40.3, and 38.9 in the probucol, combined treatment, multivitamin, and placebo groups, respectively ($p=0.003$ for probucol vs no probucol). Patients receiving probucol also had lower rates of need for repeated angioplasty. b. In small coronary arteries restenosis rates were 20%, 29%, 45%, and 37% for probucol, combined therapy, vitamins and placebo ($p=0.006$ for probucol). Probucol also reduced absolute lumen loss.
Conclusions	a. Probucol was effective in reducing restenosis rates following coronary angioplasty. b. Probucol was effective in reducing restenosis in small coronary arteries.

RESTORE

Randomized Efficacy Study of Tirofiban for Outcomes and Restenosis

Title	Effects of platelet glycoprotein IIb/IIIa blockade with tirofiban on adverse cardiac events in patients with unstable angina or acute myocardial infarction undergoing coronary angioplasty.
Author	The RESTORE Investigators
Reference	Circulation 1997; 96: 1445-1453.
Disease	Coronary artery disease, myocardial infarction, unstable angina.
Purpose	To determine effect of tirofiban, a platelet glycoprotein IIb/IIIa blocker, in patients undergoing balloon angioplasty or directional atherectomy within 72 h of presentation of unstable angina or acute myocardial infarction on the following end points: death, myocardial infarction, coronary bypass surgery secondary to angioplasty failure or recurrent ischemia, need for repeat angioplasty (PTCA), stent insertion due to actual or threatened closure, and the primary endpoint-a composite of the above.
Design	Randomized, double-blind, placebo-controlled trial, multicenter.
Patients	2139, mean age 60 years, > 70% males.
Follow-up	30 days.
Treatment regimen	Tirofiban bolus 10μg/kg over a 3 min period followed by a 36 h infusion of 0.15 μg/kg/min or placebo. Patients were already receiving aspirin and heparin.

RESTORE

Randomized Efficacy Study of Tirofiban for
Outcomes and Restenosis
(continued)

Results   The primary composite endpoint was 12.2% in the place-bo group and 10.3% in the tirofiban group (p=.16), at 30 days. At 2 days post angioplasty tirofiban had a 38% relative reduction in the composite endpoint (p ≤.005); at 7 days there was a 27% relative reduction (p=.022) mainly secondary to reduction in nonfatal myocardial infarction and need for repeat PTCA. If only urgent or emergent repeat angioplasty or coronary bypass surgery were included in the composite endpoint, the 30 day event rates were 10.5% for placebo and 8.0% for tirofiban (p=.052). Major bleeding occurred in 3.7% of the place-bo group and 5.3% in the tirofiban group (p=.096).

Conclusions   Tirofiban protected against early adverse cardiac events related to thrombotic closure in patients undergoing PTCA for acute coronary syndromes; however at 30 days this reduction in adverse cardiac events was no longer statistically significant.

Results of a consecutive series of patients receiving only antiplatelet therapy after optimized stent implantation. Comparison of aspirin alone vs combined ticlopidine and aspirin therapy.

Title	Results of a consecutive series of patients receiving only antiplatelet therapy after optimized stent implantation. Comparison of aspirin alone vs combined ticlopidine and aspirin therapy.
Author	Albiero R, Hall P, Itoh A, et al.
Reference	Circulation 1997; 95:1145-1156.
Disease	Coronary artery disease.
Purpose	To determine whether ticlopidine combined with aspirin is superior to aspirin alone in preventing stent thrombosis.
Design	Retrospective analysis of consecutive patients assigned to receive either aspirin alone or a combination of ticlopidine plus aspirin after a successful intracoronary stent insertion.
Patients	801 consecutive coronary artery disease patients, average age 57-58 years; 86-89% male.
Follow-up	1-4 months.
Treatment regimen	Aspirin before stent employment plus heparin. Then aspirin 325 mg x1/d or ticlopidine 250 mg x2/d for 1 month and long term aspirin.

Results of a consecutive series of patients receiving only antiplatelet therapy after optimized stent implantation. Comparison of aspirin alone vs combined ticlopidine and aspirin therapy.

(continued)

Results	At 1 month the rate of stent thrombosis was 1.9% in the aspirin group as well as the combined ticlopidine plus aspirin group. The rates of major adverse clinical events were 1.9% and 2.0% respectively.
Conclusions	There was no difference in rates of stent thrombosis or clinical outcomes at 1 month follow-up in patients receiving either aspirin alone or aspirin plus ticlopidine. There was no benefit to adding ticlopidine to aspirin in these coronary artery disease patients that received stents.

5. Hypertension

SHEP

Systolic Hypertension in the Elderly Program

Title	a. Prevention of stroke by antihypertensive drug treatment in older persons with isolated systolic hypertension. Final results of the systolic hypertension in the elderly program (SHEP). b. Prevention of heart failure by antihypertensive drug treatment in older persons with isolated systolic hypertension. c. Effect of treatment of isolated systolic hypertension on left ventricular mass. d. Effect of diuretic-based antihypertensive treatment on cardiovascular disease risk in older diabetic patients with isolated systolic hypertension. e. Influence of long-term, low dose, diuretic-based antihypertensive therapy on glucose, lipid, uric acid, and potassium levels in older men and women with isolated systolic hypertension.
Authors	a. SHEP Cooperative Research Group. b. Kostis JB, Davis BR, Cutler J, et al. c. Ofili EO, Cohen JD, St. Vrain J, et al. d. Curb JD, Pressel SL, Cutler JA, et al. e. Savage PL, Precsel SL, Curb JD, et al.
Reference	a. JAMA 1991;265:3255-3264. b. JAMA 1997; 278:212-216. c. JAMA 1998; 279: 778-780. d. JAMA 1996; 276:1886-1892 e. Arch Intern Med 1998; 158: 741-751.
Disease	Hypertension.
Purpose	a. To evaluate the efficacy of antihypertensive drug therapy to reduce the risk of stroke in patients with isolated systolic hypertension. b. To determine the effect of diuretic-based stepped-care antihypertensive therapy on the development of heart failure in older patients with isolated systolic hypertension.

c. To determine the ability of antihypertensive drugs to reduce left ventricular mass in older patients with isolated systolic hypertension.

d. To determine the effect of diuretic-based antihypertensive treatment on major cardiovascular disease event rates in older patients with isolated systolic hypertension with noninsulin treated diabetic patients vs nondiabetic patients.

e. Retrospective analysis to determine development of diabetes in SHEP participants, including changes in serum chemistries over 3 years.

Design	a. Randomized, double blind, placebo-controlled, multicenter.
	b. Further analysis of data from multicenter randomized, double blind placebo-controlled clinical trial.
	c. Echocardiographic substudy of SHEP trial.
	d. Additional analysis from SHEP trial.
Patients	a. 4736 patients, ≥60 years old, with systolic blood pressure 160-219 and diastolic blood pressure <90 mm Hg. Patients with major cardiovascular diseases or other serious illnesses were excluded.
	b. 4736 patients aged 60 years and older with systolic blood pressure between 160-219 mmHg and diastolic pressure below 90 mmHg.
	c. 104 patients at St. Louis SHEP site who had echocardiograms; 94 had 3 year follow-up.
	d. 583 noninsulin dependent diabetic patients and 4149 nondiabetic patients.
Follow-up	a. Average 4.5 years.
	b. Average 4.5 years.
	c. Minimum follow-up was 3 years.
	d. 5 years.

SHEP

Systolic Hypertension in the Elderly Program

(continued)

Treatment regimen	a. The goal of blood pressure reduction was <160 mmHg systolic blood pressure for those with initial pressure >180 mmHg, and by at least 20 mmHg for those with initial pressure 160-179 mmHg. Patients were randomized to placebo or chlorthalidone 12.5 mg/d. Dose was doubled if the pressure goal was not reached and then atenolol 25 mg/d or placebo was added. If contraindications existed, reserpine 0.05 mg/d was given. b. As described in SHEP. c. As described in SHEP. d. As per SHEP protocol.
Additional therapy	a. Potassium supplements to all patients with serum K <3.5 mmol/l.
Results	a. After 5 years 44% of the placebo group received active antihypertensive therapy. During the trial, the goal blood pressure was reached by 65%-72% of the active drug therapy vs 32%-40% of the placebo group. Mean systolic blood pressure was lower in the active treatment than the placebo group throughout the protocol. By life table analysis, 5 year cumulative stroke rates were 5.2% vs 8.2% for the active therapy and placebo groups, respectively (RR 0.64, 95% CI 0.50-0.82, p=0.0003). After a mean of 4.5 years follow-up the mortality was 9.0% vs 10.2% (RR 0.87 (0.73-1.05)), myocardial infarction occurred in 2.1% vs 3.1% (RR 0.67 (0.47-0.96)), left ventricular failure in 2.0% vs 4.3% (RR 0.46 (0.33-0.65)), and total major cardiovascular events in 12.2% vs 17.5% (RR 0.68 (0.58-0.79)). b. Fatal or nonfatal heart failure occurred in 55 of 2365 patients randomized to therapy and 105 of 2371 patients that received placebo [relative risk (RR) .51; 95% CI 0.37 - 0.71, p <.001]. Heart failure was more likely to develop in older patients, in men, those with higher systolic blood pressures and history or ECG evidence of myocardial infarction. Among patients with history or ECG evidence of myocardial infarction treatment reduced the relative risk of developing heart failure substantially (RR = 0.19; 95% CI 0.06 - 0.13; p=.002). c. LV mass index was 93 g/m2 in active therapy group and 100g/m2 in placebo group (p<.001). LV mass index

declined by 13% with therapy and increased by 6% in the placebo group over 3 years (p=.01). 8% of subjects were receiving chlorthalidone alone by the end of year 3.

d. The 5 year rate of all outcomes and major cardiovascular disease events, [nonfatal or fatal myocardial infarction, sudden or rapid cardiac death, CABG , PTCA, stroke, transient ischemic attack, aortic aneurysm, endarterectomy] was 34% lower with active therapy vs placebo for both diabetics (95% C.I. 6% - 54%) and nondiabetics (95% C.I. 21% - 45%). Absolute reduction in risk with active therapy was twice as great in diabetics (101/1000) vs nondiabetics (51/1000) which reflects the higher risk of developing vascular events in diabetic patients.

e. New cases of diabetes occurred in 8.6% of patients receiving active treatment and 7.5% of patients on placebo (p = NS). Active treatment was associated with small increases in fasting blood glucose levels (+3.6 mg/dL, p <.01) and total cholesterol (+3.5 mg/dL, p <.01); small decreases in HDL cholesterol (-0.77 mg/dL); and small increases in creatinine (+0.03 mg/dL, p<.001). Active therapy was associated with larger increases in fasting triglyceride levels (+17 mg/dL; p <.001) and a decrease in potassium (-0.3 mmol/L, p <.001). Active therapy was associated with an increase in uric acid, +.06 mg/dL, p<.001).

Conclusions   a. Stepped-care drug therapy for isolated systolic hypertension in patients ≥60 years old reduced the incidence of major cardiovascular events and stroke.

b. In older patients with isolated systolic hypertension, stepped-care therapy based on low dose chlorthalidone reduced the incidence of heart failure. Treatment was especially dramatic among patients with prior myocardial infarctions.

c. Treatment of isolated systolic hypertension in older patients with chlorthalidone-based regimen reduces LV mass.

d. Treating older diabetic patients with isolated systolic hypertension with diuretic based therapy (chlorthalidone) is effective in prevention of major cardiovascular and cerebrovascular events.

e. Low dose chlorthalidone lowered isolated systolic hypertension and had relatively mild effects on other cardiovascular risk factors.

TOMHS

Treatment of Mild Hypertension Study

Title	a. Characteristics of participants in the treatment of mild hypertension study (TOMHS). b. The treatment of mild hypertension study. A randomized, placebo-controlled trial of a nutritional hygienic regimen along with various drug monotherapies. c. Treatment of mild hypertension study. Final results. d. Comparison of 5 antihypertensive monotherapies and placebo for change in left ventricular mass in patients receiving nutritional hygienic therapy in the treatment of mild hypertension study (TOMHS). e. Long-term effects on plasma lipids of diet and drugs to treat hypertension. f. Comparison of 5 antihypertensive monotherapies and placebo for change in left ventricular mass in patients receiving nutritional hygienic therapy in the treatment of mild hypertension study (TOMHS).
Authors	a. Masciolo SR, Grimm RH, Neaton JD, et al. b. TOMHS Research Group. c. Neaton JD, Grimm RH Jr, Prineas RJ, et al. d. Liebson PR, Grandits GA, Dianzumba S, et al. e. Grimm RH, Flack JM, Grandits GA, et al. f. Liebson, PR, Grandits GA, Dianzumba S, et al.
Reference	a. Am J Cardiol 1990;66:32C-35C. b. Arch Intern Med 1991;151:1413-1423. c. JAMA 1993;270:713-724. d. Circulation 1995;91:698-706. e. JAMA 1996;275:1549-1556. f. Circulation 1995; 91:698-706.
Disease	Hypertension.
Purpose	To assess the relative efficacy and safety of a combination of non-pharmacological therapy alone with those of nonpharmacological therapy and 5 pharmacological monotherapy regimens.
Design	Randomized, double blind, multicenter.

TOMHS

Treatment of Mild Hypertension Study

(continued)

Patients	902 patients, age 45-69 years, with mild hypertension (diastolic blood pressure 90-99 mmHg, or if they were previously treated with antihypertensive drugs, 85-99 mm Hg). Patients with cardiovascular disease or life-threatening illness were excluded.
Follow-up	>4 years (mean 4.4 years).
Treatment regimen	Randomization to: 1. Acebutalol 400 mg/d; 2. amlodipine 5 mg/d; 3. chlorthalidone 15 mg/d; 4. Doxazosin 1 mg/d for 1 month and then 2 mg/d; 5. enalapril 5 mg/d; 6. Placebo. For a participant with diastolic blood pressure ≥95 mmHg on 3 visits, or ≥105 mmHg at a single visit, medication dose was doubled. If blood pressure remained high, a second drug was added. For all groups, except the diuretic group, chlorothalidone 15 mg/d was added. In the chlorthalidone group, enalapril 2.5 mg was given.
Additional therapy	Behavior change, 10% weight loss, lowering sodium intake to ≤70 mmol/d, lowering alcohol intake, and increasing activity

TOMHS

Treatment of Mild Hypertension Study
(continued)

Results   a - e. After 12 months, weight loss averaged 4.5 kg, urinary sodium excretion declined by 23%, and physical activity was almost doubled. After 12 months blood pressure was decreased by 20.1±1.4/13.7±0.7, 17.5±1.1/12.9±0.7, 21.8±1.3/13.1±0.7, 16.1±1.2/ 12.0±0.7, 17.6±1.2/12.2± 0.7, and 10.6±1.0/8.1±0.5 mm Hg in groups 1-6, respectively (P<0.01 for each drug compared to placebo). Overall the compliance and tolerance were good for all groups and side effects were acceptable. After 4 years, 59% of the placebo and 72% of the active drug groups continued their initial drug as monotherapy. Major clinical events occurred in 7.3% of the placebo vs 5.1% of the active drug groups (p=0.21), and major cardiovascular event in 5.1% vs 3.9%, respectively (p=0.42). 844 patients underwent serial echocardiographic assessment of left ventricular mass. Average decrease in LV mass was 24, 25, 34, 24, 23, and 27 grams for groups 1-6 (p=0.53 for the difference among groups). The only significant difference vs placebo for reduction in LV mass was with chlorthalidone (p=0.03). In all treatment groups, there was a favorable change in the serum lipid profile. After 4 years total cholesterol decreased by 11.7±2.0 mg/dl in the acebutolol; 3.9±2.9 mg/dl in the amlodipine; 5.9±2.5 mg/dl in the chlorthalidone; 16.1±2.7 mg/dl in the doxazosin; 11.2±2.4 mg/dl in the enalapril; and 6.0±1.9 mg/dl in the placebo group (p=0.002 for the difference among groups). LDL-cholesterol decreased by 11.5±2.4 mg/dl in the acebutolol; 2.9±2.7 mg/dl in the amlodipine; 4.9±2.4 mg/dl in the chlorthalidone; 13.0±2.5 mg/dl in the doxazosin; 9.5±2.4 mg/dl in the enalapril; and 5.1±1.5 mg/dl in the placebo group (p=0.002 for the difference among groups). HDL-cholesterol decreased by 0.6±0.7 mg/dl in the acebutolol; increased by 0.2±0.7 mg/dl in the amlodipine; increased by 0.6±0.8 mg/dl in the chlorthalidone; increased by 0.9±0.7 mg/dl in the doxazosin; increased by 0.8±0.7 mg/dl in the enalapril; and decreased by 0.3±0.5 mg/dl in the placebo group (p=0.57 for the difference among groups). Triglycerides increased by 1.3±5.0 mg/dl in the acebutolol; decreased by 5.4±5.0 mg/dl in the amlodipine; decreased by 7.3±5.6 mg/dl in the chlorthalidone; decreased by 20.0±5.2 mg/dl in the doxazosin; decreased by 12.6±7.1 mg/dl in the enalapril; and decreased by 2.8±4.6 mg/dl in the placebo group (p=0.03 for the difference among groups). Decreases in plasma

Treatment of Mild Hypertension Study
(continued)

total cholesterol, LDL cholesterol, and triglycerides were greater with doxazosin

f. Echocardiographic assessment revealed that all groups showed significant decreases (10-15%) in left ventricular mass from baseline, that appeared by 3 months continuing for 48 months. The greatest reduction was in the chlorthalidone group. Reduction even occurred in the placebo group. Change in weight, urinary sodium restriction, and systolic blood pressure moderately correlated with changes in left ventricular mass.

Conclusions   Adding 1 of the 5 different classes of drugs resulted in significant additional decrease of blood pressure with minimal side effects. Differences among the 5 drug groups did not consistently favor one over the others concerning clinical outcomes. However, these drugs affect serum lipid profile and left ventricular mass differently, with doxazosin having the greater reduction in total cholesterol, LDL cholesterol and triglycerides, and chlorthalidone having the greater effect on reducing left ventricular hypertrophy.

STOP-Hypertension

Swedish Trial in Old Patients With Hypertension

Title	a. Morbidity and mortality in the Swedish Trial in Old Patients with Hypertension (STOP-Hypertension). b. Swedish trial in old patients with hypertension (STOP-Hypertension). Analyses performed up to 1992.
Authors	Dahlöf B, Lindholm LH, Hansson L, et al.
Reference	a. Lancet 1991;338:1281-1285. b. Clin Exper Hypertension 1993;15:925-939.
Disease	Hypertension.
Purpose	To evaluate the efficacy of pharmacological treatment of hypertension in patients 70-84 years old.
Design	Randomized, double blind, placebo controlled, multicenter.
Patients	1627 patients, age 70-84 years, with blood pressure ≥180/90 mmHg, or diastolic blood pressure >105 mmHg. Patients with blood pressure above 230/120 mmHg, orthostatic hypotension, myocardial infarction, or stroke within the previous 12 months were excluded.
Follow-up	1-4 years (average of 25 months).
Treatment regimen	Patients were randomized to either active therapy or placebo. The centers were free to chose 1 of the 4 following agents: atenolol 50 mg/d, hydrochlorothiazide 25 mg/d + amiloride 2.5 mg/d, metoprolol 100 mg/d, or pindolol 5 mg/d. If blood pressure was >160/95 mm Hg after 2 months of therapy, diuretic therapy was added to the ß blocker, and vice versa. If blood pressure exceeded 230/120 mmHg on 2 subsequent visits, open antihypertensive therapy was given.

STOP-Hypertension

Swedish Trial in Old Patients With Hypertension

(continued)

Results   a. Compared with placebo, active therapy reduced the number of myocardial infarctions (16.5 vs 14.4 per 1000 patient-years, RR 0.87, 95% CI 0.49-1.56), stroke (31.3 vs 16.8 per 1000 patient-years, RR 0.53, 95% CI 0.33-0.86, p=0.0081), total mortality (35.4 vs 20.2 per 1000 patient-years, RR 0.57, 95% CI 0.37-0.87, p=0.0079), and the occurrence of the primary endpoints (stroke, myocardial infarction or cardiovascular death) (55.5 vs 33.5 per 1000 patient-years, RR 0.60, 95% CI 0.43-0.85, p=0.0031).

b. A majority of the patients needed combined treatment to reach the goal blood pressure (160/95 mmHg). The impact on mortality and morbidity was greater than previously seen in middle-aged patients. Women benefited from treatment at least as much as men.

Conclusions   Antihypertensive therapy in hypertensive patients aged 70-84 reduced cardiovascular morbidity and mortality.

TAIM

Trial of Antihypertensive Interventions and Management

Title	a. Effect of drug and diet treatment of mild hypertension on diastolic blood pressure. b. The Trial of Antihypertensive Interventions and Management (TAIM) study. Adequate weight loss, alone and combined with drug therapy in the treatment of mild hypertension. c. Effect of antihypertensives on sexual function and quality of life: the TAIM study.
Authors	a. Langford HG, Davis BR, Blaufox D, et al. b. Wassertheil-Smoller S, Blaufox MD, Oberman AS, et al. c. Wassertheil-Smoller S, Blaufox D, Oberman A, et al.
Reference	a. Hypertension 1991;17:210-217. b. Arch Intern Med 1992;152:131-136. c. Ann Intern Med 1991;114:613-620.
Disease	Hypertension.
Purpose	To evaluate the relative efficacy of various combinations of the commonly used approaches to drug and diet therapy for hypertension.
Design	Randomized, double blind (drug therapy), placebo-controlled, 3X3 factorial, 3 centers.
Patients	787 patients, age 21-65 years, with diastolic blood pressure 90-100 mmHg without medications, and body weight of 110-160% of the ideal body weight. Patients with prior stroke, myocardial infarction, asthma, insulin treated diabetes mellitus, and renal failure were excluded.
Follow-up	6 months.
Treatment regimen	9 groups of treatment combinations of 1 out of 3 drug regimens with 1 out of 3 diet interventions. The drugs were: placebo, chlorthalidone 25 mg, or atenolol 50 mg. The diet interventions were: usual, a weight reduction (goal 10% of basal body weight or 4.54 kg), or low in sodium (52-100 mmol/d) and high in potassium (62-115 mmol/d) diets. Patients who failed to

achieve blood pressure control were given additional therapy in a double blind fashion (chlorthalidone or atenolol for the placebo and combination of atenolol and chlorthalidone to the other 2 drug groups.) If diastolic blood pressure remained ≥100 mmHg, the doses were increased, and if it did not help open-label therapy was added.

Results

a. Among the placebo drug-assigned patients 20.0%, 10.0%, and 16.5% of the usual, weight loss, and low sodium diet received additional medications to control blood pressure over the 6 months of follow-up. Only 2.7% and 3.0% of the chlorthalidone and atenolol treated patients needed an additional medication. The mean weight reduction in the weight loss diet group was 4.7 kg. The low Na/high K group had an average decrease in urinary sodium of 27.4 mmol/d and increase of potassium excretion of 10.9 mmol/d. The mean reduction of diastolic blood pressure in patients on usual diet was 7.96, 10.78, and 12.43 mmHg for placebo, chlorthalidone and atenolol groups. For patients in the weight loss diet it was 8.78, 15.06 and 14.81 mmHg, respectively, and for the low Na/high K diet it was 7.91, 12.18 and 12.76 mmHg, respectively. Atenolol as a single therapy achieved the greatest reduction of blood pressure (p=0.001 vs low Na/high K diet alone, and p=0.006 vs weight loss alone. Adding weight loss diet to chlorthalidone enhanced the blood pressure lowering response significantly (p=0.002).
b. Among the patients assigned to placebo drug and weight loss diet, diastolic blood pressure reduction after 6 months was greater among patients who lost ≥4.5 kg than among those who achieved only <2.25 kg reduction (11.6 vs 7.0 mmHg; p<0.046). The effect of ≥4.5 kg body weight reduction was comparable to that of chlorthalidone or atenolol. The weight loss diet benefited quality of life most, reducing total physical complaints (p<0.001) and increasing satisfaction with health (p<0.001). Low dose chlorthalidone and atenolol produced few side effects, except in men. Sexual problems developed in 29%, 13% and 3% of men receiving usual diet and chlorthalidone, atenolol and placebo, respectively (p=0.006 for the difference among groups). The low Na/high K diet was associated with increased fatigue.

Conclusions

Drug therapy was more efficient than diet intervention in reducing diastolic blood pressure. Weight loss of ≥4.5 kg is beneficial, especially in combination with diuretics.

TOHP-1

Trial of Hypertension Prevention (Phase I)

Title	a. The effects of nonpharmacologic interventions on blood pressure of persons with high normal levels. Results of the trials of hypertension prevention, phase I. b. The effect of potassium supplementation in persons with a high-normal blood pressure. Results from phase I of the Trials of Hypertension Prevention (TOHP). c. Lack of blood pressure effect with calcium and magnesium supplementation in adults with high-normal blood pressure. Results from phase I of the Trials of Hypertension Prevention (TOHP).
Authors	a. The Trials of Hypertension Prevention Collaborative Research Group. b. Whelton PK, Buring J, Borhani NO, et al. c. Yamamoto ME, Applegate WB, Klag MJ, et al.
Reference	a. JAMA 1992;267:1213-1220. b. Ann Epidemiol 1995;5:85-95. c. Ann Epidemiol 1995;5:96-107.
Disease	Hypertension.
Purpose	To evaluate the short-term feasibility and efficacy of 7 non-pharmacologic interventions to reduce diastolic blood pressure.
Design	3 randomized, parallel-group trials, multicenter.
Patients	2182 patients, 30-54 years old, with diastolic blood pressure of 80-89 mmHg, who were not taking medications in the prior 2 months.
Follow-up	18 months.

TOHP-1

Trial of Hypertension Prevention (Phase I)

(continued)

Treatment regimen	3 life-style change groups (weight reduction, sodium intake reduction, and stress management) were each compared with unmasked nonintervention control over 18 months. 4 nutritional supplement groups (calcium, magnesium, potassium, and fish oil) were each compared in a double blind fashion with placebo controls over 6 months.
Results	Weight reduction intervention resulted in 3.9 kg weight loss ($p<0.01$, compared to baseline), diastolic blood pressure reduction of 2.3 mmHg ($p<0.01$), and systolic blood pressure reduction of 2.9 mmHg ($p<0.01$). Sodium restriction intervention resulted in 44 mmol/24 h decrease of urinary sodium excretion ($p<0.01$), diastolic and systolic blood pressure reduction of 0.9 ($p<0.05$) and 1.7 mmHg ($p<0.01$). Potassium supplementation resulted in 1.8 mmHg ($p=0.04$) reduction in diastolic blood pressure after 3 months. However, the effect disappeared after 6 months (mean reduction 0.3 mmHg). Neither stress management nor nutritional supplements reduced blood pressure significantly.
Conclusions	Weight reduction was the most effective of the strategies in reducing blood pressure in normotensive persons. Sodium restriction was also effective.

MRC

Medical Research Council Trial of Treatment of Hypertension in Older Adults

Title	Medical Research Council trial of treatment of hypertension in older adults: Principal results.
Authors	MRC Working Party.
Reference	Br Med J 1992;304:405-412.
Disease	Hypertension.
Purpose	To evaluate the efficacy of ß blockers and diuretic therapy to reduce cardiovascular mortality and morbidity in hypertensive older adults.
Design	Randomized, single blind, placebo-controlled, multicenter.
Patients	4396 patients, age 65-74 years, with systolic blood pressure 160-209 mmHg, and diastolic blood pressure <115 mmHg. Patients on antihypertensive medications, or with secondary hypertension, heart failure, angina pectoris, myocardial infarction or stroke within 3 months, impaired renal function, diabetes mellitus, asthma, or other serious intercurrent disease were excluded.
Follow-up	Mean follow-up 5.8 years (25,355 patients-years of observation).
Treatment regimen	1. Amiloride 2.5 mg/d+ hydrochlorothiazide 25 mg/d or placebo. 2. Atenolol 50 mg/d or placebo. Drug doses were modified to reach the target blood pressure of 150-160 mm Hg.
Additional therapy	Additional therapy was started if mean blood pressure was >115 mm Hg or systolic blood pressure >210 mm Hg.

Results | Both treatment arms reduced systolic blood pressure compared with the placebo group. After 3 months, the diuretic therapy reduced blood pressure more than atenolol. However, after 2 years, systolic and diastolic blood pressures were similar in the diuretics and atenolol groups. More patients randomized to atenolol required supplementary drugs to control hypertension than the diuretic group (52% vs 38%). The atenolol group had significantly more withdrawals from the study compared to diuretics for both suspected major side effects and inadequate blood pressure control (345 vs 161 patients, respectively). In the placebo group 257 patients were withdrawn. The number of strokes was reduced with active therapy 7.3%, 9.0% and 10.8% in the diuretics, atenolol, and placebo groups (25% reduction of risk (active therapy vs placebo), 95% CI 3-42%, p=0.04). Coronary events occurred in 7.7%, 12.8%, and 12.7%, respectively (19% reduction of risk (active therapy vs placebo), 95% CI -2% to 36%, p=0.08). Total mortality was not different among the groups (21.3%, 26.4% and 24.7%, respectively). After adjusting for baseline characteristics the diuretic group had reduced risks of stroke (31%, 95% CI 3%-51%, p=0.04), coronary events (44%, 95% CI 21%-60%, p=0.0009), and all cardiovascular events (35%, 95% CI 17%-49%, p=0.0005), compared with placebo. The atenolol group showed no significant reduction in these end points. Reduction of stroke was mainly in nonsmokers taking diuretics.

Conclusions | Hydrochlorothiazide and amiloride are better than atenolol in reducing the incidence of stroke and coronary events in older hypertensive patients.

Title	Safety and efficacy of metoprolol in the treatment of hypertension in the elderly.
Authors	LaPalio L, Schork A, Glasser S, Tifft C.
Reference	J Am Geriatr Soc 1992;40:354-358.
Disease	Hypertension.
Purpose	To evaluate the short-term efficacy and safety of metoprolol in the treatment of hypertension in patients 50-75 years old.
Design	Open label, surveillance, multicenter.
Patients	21,692 patients, 50-75 years old, with hypertension (systolic blood pressure ≤200 mmHg and diastolic blood pressure 90-104 mmHg for patients that had not been under therapy before and ≤95 mmHg for those who were previously treated). Patients who needed ß blockers for angina, patients with heart block or bradycardia <55 bpm, congestive heart failure, or intolerance to ß blockers were excluded.
Follow-up	8 week clinical follow-up.
Treatment regimen	Metoprolol 100 mg/d. If diastolic blood pressure remained >90 mmHg after 4 weeks, hydrochlorothiazide 25 mg/d was added.

Results

After 4 weeks mean systolic and diastolic blood pressure were reduced from 162/95 to 148/87 mmHg (p<0.001). 58% of the patients had adequate blood pressure control with 100 mg/d metoprolol. After 8 weeks blood pressure decreased to 143/84 mmHg. At the termination of the study 50% of the patients continued with metoprolol as monotherapy and 27% needed combined therapy. There was <5% incidence of medical problems. Excellent or good tolerability was noted for 94% of the patients.

Conclusions

Metoprolol administered either as monotherapy or in combination with diuretic was an effective and safe therapy for elderly hypertensive patients.

Veterans Affairs Cooperative Study Group on Antihypertensive Agents

Title	Single-drug therapy for hypertension in men. A comparison of six antihypertensive agents with placebo.
Authors	Materson BJ, Reda DJ, Cushman WC, et al.
Reference	N Engl J Med 1993;328:914-921.
Disease	Hypertension.
Purpose	To compare the efficacy of different classes of antihypertensive agents as monotherapy for hypertension according to age and race.
Design	Randomized, double blind, placebo controlled, multicenter.
Patients	1292 men, age ≥21 years, and diastolic blood pressure 95-109 mm Hg on placebo.
Follow-up	For at least 1 year.
Treatment regimen	Randomization to: 1. placebo; 2. hydrochlorothiazide 12.5-50 mg/d; 3. atenolol 25-100 mg/d; 4. clonidine 0.2-0.6 mg/d; 5. captopril 25-100 mg/d; 6. prazosin 4-20 mg/d; and 7. sustained-release diltiazem 120-360 mg/d. Patients who reached diastolic blood pressure <90 mmHg on 2 visits entered a maintenance phase for ≥1 year.

Results   At the end of the titration phase 33%, 57%, 65%, 65%, 54%, 56%, and 75% of the patients in groups 1-7 reached diastolic blood pressure <90 mmHg. 745 patients reached diastolic blood pressure <90 mmHg without intolerable side effects during the titration phase and entered the maintenance phase. The percentage of patients with initial control of blood pressure in whom diastolic blood pressure remained <95 mmHg over 1 year was similar among groups (p=0.93). However, by intention to treat analysis, 25%, 46%, 51%, 50%, 42%, 42%, and 59% of the patients in groups 1-7 had reached diastolic blood pressure <90 mmHg during the titration phase and <95 mmHg during the maintenance phase (p<0.001 for a difference among the groups). The most effective drug was diltiazem. Diltiazem was the most effective drug in young and old blacks, while captopril was the most effective in young whites and atenolol in old whites. The least effective drug in young and old blacks was captopril, while hydrochlorothiazide was the least effective in young whites and prazosin in old whites. Intolerance to medication during the titration phase was more common with clonidine and prazosin than the other drugs.

Conclusions   Among men, age and race are important determinants of the response to monotherapy for hypertension.

BBB

Behandla Blodtryck Bättre (Treat Blood Pressure Better)

Title	The BBB study: the effect of intensified antihypertensive treatment on the level of blood pressure, side-effects, morbidity, and mortality in "well-treated" hypertensive patients.
Authors	Hansson L, for the BBB study group.
Reference	Blood Press 1994;3:248-254.
Disease	Hypertension.
Purpose	To investigate whether it is feasible to lower the diastolic blood pressure further through intensified therapy without an increase in side effects, and whether such intensified therapy will reduce morbidity and mortality.
Design	Randomized, open label, multicenter.
Patients	2127 patients, age 46-71 years, with essential hypertension (diastolic blood pressure 90-100 mmHg).
Follow-up	>4 years.
Treatment regimen	Intensified therapy (use of pharmacologic and nonpharmacologic means to reduce diastolic blood pressure ≤80 mm Hg) or unchanged therapy (maintain diastolic blood pressure 90-100 mmHg).
Additional therapy	No restriction on medications.

BBB

(continued)

Results
With intensified therapy blood pressure fell from 155/95 to 141/83 mmHg (a difference of 14/12 mmHg, $p<0.001/0.001$). In the conventional therapy, blood pressure declined from 155/94 to 152/91 mmHg (a difference of 3/3 mmHg, $p<0.05/0.05$). A difference in diastolic blood pressure of 7-8.5 mmHg between the groups persisted for more than 4 years. In both groups there was no difference in heart rate between baseline and at the end of the study. Fewer adverse effects were reported in the intensified than conventional therapy group. There was no significant difference between the intensified and conventional therapy groups in the rates of stroke (8 vs 11 patients), myocardial infarction (20 vs 18 patients). No data on mortality was provided.

Conclusions
Blood pressure can be further reduced in intensified therapy without increment of adverse effects. However, it was not associated with improved outcome.

ACCT

Amlodipine Cardiovascular Community Trial

Title	Sex and age-related antihypertensive effects of amlodipine.
Authors	Kloner RA, Sowers JR, DiBona GF, et al.
Reference	Am J Cardiol 1996;77:713-722.
Disease	Hypertension.
Purpose	To assess whether there are age, sex, or racial differences in the response to amlodipine 5-10 mg/d in patients with mild to moderate hypertension.
Design	Open label, multicenter.
Patients	1084 patients, age 21-80 years, with mild to moderate hypertension (diastolic blood pressure 95-110 mmHg on 2 visits). Patients with history of stroke or transient ischemic attack, myocardial infarction within 6 months, angina pectoris, ventricular ejection fraction <40%, NYHA class ≥II heart failure, arrhythmias, or other systemic diseases were excluded.
Follow-up	18 weeks.
Treatment regimen	A 2 week placebo run-in phase, a 4 week titration/efficacy phase- amlodipine 5-10 mg/d was administered once daily, a 12 week maintenance phase, and an optional long-term follow-up phase.
Additional therapy	All other antihypertensive medications were not permitted.

ACCT

Amlodipine Cardiovascular Community Trial

(continued)

Results
: At the end of the titration/efficacy phase, mean decrease in blood pressure was 16.3±12.3/12.5±5.9 mmHg (p<0.0001). 86% of the patients achieved diastolic blood pressure ≤90 mmHg and/or a 10 mmHg decrease in diastolic blood pressure. The blood pressure response was greater in women (91.4%) than men (83.0%, p<0.001), and in those ≥65 years (91.5%) than those <65 years old (84.1%, p<0.01). 86.0% and 85.9% of the whites and blacks responded (p=NS). Amlodipine was well tolerated. Mild to moderate edema was the most common adverse effect. 14.6% discontinued therapy during the titration phase. Discontinuation due to adverse effects related to the drug occurred in 2.4%. During the maintenance phase 5.9% discontinued medication due to adverse effects (5.1% due to adverse effects possibly related to amlodipine).

Conclusions
: Amlodipine was effective and relatively safe as a once-a-day monotherapy for mild to moderate hypertension in a community-based population. The response rate in women was greater than in men.

Title	Evaluation of blood pressure response to the combination of enalapril (single dose) and diltiazem ER (4 different doses) in systemic hypertension.
Authors	Applegate WB, Cohen JD, Wolfson P, et al.
Reference	Am J Cardiol 1996;78:51-55.
Disease	Hypertension.
Purpose	To assess the efficacy, safety, and dose response of a combination of enalapril with a new once-daily formulation of diltiazem.
Design	Randomized, double blind, placebo-controlled, multicenter.
Patients	336 patients, 21-75 years of age, with essential hypertension (diastolic blood pressure 95-115 mmHg). Patients with myocardial infarction within 2 years, secondary hypertension, previous cerebrovascular event, congestive heart failure, serious cardiac arrhythmias, or angina pectoris were excluded.
Follow-up	6 weeks.
Treatment regimen	After 7 day washout period, patients underwent 4 week single blind placebo baseline phase. Then, patients entered the 6 week double blind treatment phase: randomization to 1 of 6 groups. 1. Placebo; 2. Enalapril 5 mg/d (E5); 3. Enalapril 5 mg/d and diltiazem ER 60 mg/d (E5/D60); 4. Enalapril 5 mg/d and diltiazem ER 120 mg/d (E5/D120); 5. Enalapril 5 mg/d and diltiazem ER 180 mg/d (E5/D180); 6. Enalapril 5 mg/d and diltiazem ER 240 mg/d (E5/D240).
Additional therapy	β blockers, digitalis, any medication that could lower blood pressure, psychotropic agents, and cimetidine were prohibited.

Results

By the end of the 6 week treatment period, diastolic blood pressure was reduced by 3.2 mmHg in the placebo; 5.6 mmHg in the E5; 6.8 mmHg in the E5/D60; 8.3 mmHg in the E5/D120; 10.1 mmHg in the E5/D180; and 10.3 mmHg in the E5/D240 group ($p<0.05$ for each group vs placebo). There was a significant linear dose-response relation ($p<0.001$). Diastolic blood pressure <90 mmHg was found in 25.5% of the E5/D60, 43.1% of the E5/D120, 40.0% of the E5/D180, and 49.1% of the E5/D240 groups. Only the enalapril alone (8.2 mmHg) and the 3 higher diltiazem doses (7.9, 12.8, and 13.8 mmHg in the E5/D120, E5/D180, and E5/D240 groups) resulted in a significant reduction of systolic blood pressure ($p<0.05$), whereas systolic blood pressure was reduced by only 2.0 and 6.5 mmHg in the placebo and E5/D60 groups, respectively. Drug related adverse effects were noted in 8.6% of the placebo group, 14.3% of the E5 group, and in 8.9% to 19.0% of the 4 combination groups.

Conclusions

A combination of low dose of enalapril and diltiazem ER was effective in lowering blood pressure in mild to moderately hypertensive patients. The combination of E5/D180 appeared to be the optimal dosage for reduction of blood pressure with acceptable rate of adverse events.

Enalapril Felodipine ER Factorial Study

Title	Combined enalapril and felodipine extended release (ER) for systemic hypertension.
Authors	Gradman AH, Cutler NR, Davis PJ, et al.
Reference	Am J Cardiol 1997;79:431-435.
Disease	Hypertension.
Purpose	To investigate the efficacy and safety of combination treatment with enalapril, an angiotensin-converting enzyme inhibitor, and felodipine extended release, a vascular selective calcium antagonist, in patients with essential hypertension.
Design	Randomized, double blind, placebo-controlled, multicenter.
Patients	707 patients (65% men), mean age 53.5 years, with essential hypertension and sitting diastolic blood pressure 95-115 mmHg. Patients with creatinine clearance <60 ml/min, hepatic dysfunction, recent myocardial infarction, or congestive heart failure were not included.
Follow-up	8 weeks.
Treatment regimen	Randomization to 12 groups in a 3X4 factorial design: placebo, enalapril 5 or 20 mg/d, felodipine ER (2.5, 5, or 10 mg/d), and their combination.
Results	Data were available for 705 patients for efficacy analysis. After 8 weeks of therapy, trough sitting diastolic blood pressure decreased by 4.4 mmHg in the placebo group, 7.3 mmHg in the felodipine 5 mg/d, 11.7 mmHg in the felodipine 10 mg/d, 6.0 mmHg in the enalapril 5 mg/d, 8.9 mmHg in the enalapril 5 mg/d+ felodipine 2.5 mg/d, 10.8 mmHg in the enalapril 5 mg/d+ felodipine 5 mg/d, 13.3

mmHg in the enalapril 5 mg/d+ felodipine 10 mg/d, 8.1 mmHg in the enalapril 20 mg/d, 11.0 mmHg in the enalapril 20 mg/d+ felodipine 2.5 mg/d, 12.9 mmHg in the enalapril 20 mg/d+ felodipine 5 mg/d, and 15.4 mmHg in the enalapril 20 mg/d+ felodipine 10 mg/d. Systolic blood pressure had the same trend. In both medications, dose increment resulted in greater reduction in trough sitting systolic blood pressure and the combination of the drugs had a synergistic effect. Trough systolic blood pressure decreased by 4.0 mmHg in the placebo group, 15.0 mmHg in the felodipine 10 mg/d, 10.0 mmHg in the enalapril 20 mg/d, and 21.0 mmHg in the combination of enalapril 20 mg/d+ felodipine 10 mg/d. The estimated trough to peak ratios for sitting diastolic blood pressure ranged from 0.63 to 0.79 in the different combination groups and were consistent with effective blood pressure reduction with a once a day dose. Heart rate did not significantly change with enalapril, felodipine, or their combinations. Excellent or good blood pressure reduction was achieved in 24.0% of the placebo group, 39.8%, 54.0%, and 66.3% of the felodipine 2.5, 5, and 10 mg/d, respectively; in 36.5%, 52.1%, 66.5% and 79.8% in the enalapril 5 mg/d combined with felodipine 0, 2.5, 5, and 10 mg/d; and 44.4%, 60.0%, 74.4%, and 86.7% of the enalapril 20 mg/d combined with felodipine 0, 2.5, 5, and 10 mg/d. Thus the combination of enalapril 20 mg/d with felodipine 10 mg/d achieved excellent or good response in the majority of the patients. The average sitting diastolic blood pressure reduction was 9.3 mmHg for patients <50 years (n=249), 9.6 mmHg for patients 50-64 years old (n=337), and 11.7 mmHg for patients older than 65 (n=119). No serious drug related adverse effects were reported. Patients receiving combination therapy had less peripheral edema (4.1%) than patients receiving felodipine alone (10.8%). 641 (91%) completed the 8 week study period. Only 3% dropped out because of a clinical adverse event.

Conclusions   The combination therapy of felodipine ER and enalapril was highly effective in diastolic and systolic blood pressure reduction and was well tolerated and safe.

Low Dose Reserpine-Thiazide Combination vs Nitrendipine Monotherapy

Title	Different concepts in first-line treatment of essential hypertension. Comparison of a low dose reserpine-thiazide combination with nitrendipine monotherapy.
Authors	Krönig B, Pittrow DB, Kirch W, et al.
Reference	Hypertension 1997;29:651-658.
Disease	Hypertension.
Purpose	To compare the efficacy and tolerability of reserpine, clopamid, their combination, and nitrendipine.
Design	Randomized, double blind, parallel, multicenter.
Patients	273 patients, ≥18 years old, with essential hypertension (diastolic blood pressure 100-114 mmHg). Patients with drug or alcohol abuse, history of allergy, contraindications to one of the study medications, mental impairment, secondary hypertension, cerebrovascular event within 6 weeks, unstable angina or myocardial infarction within 3 months, severe heart failure or valvular heart disease, colitis, severe gastroenteritis, hepatic or renal impairment, depression, electrolyte disorders, and hyperlipidemia were excluded.
Follow-up	12 weeks.
Treatment regimen	4 week wash-out period followed by a 2 week single blind placebo run-in phase and then, randomization to 1 of 4 groups: 1. Reserpine 0.1 to 0.2 mg/d; 2. Clopamid 5 to 10 mg/d; 3. Reserpine 0.1 mg/d + clopamid 5 mg/d; and 4. Nitrendipine 20 to 40 mg/d. If diastolic blood pressure remained ≥90 mmHg after 6 weeks, the medication dose was doubled.

Additional therapy	The use of digitalis and nitroglycerin was permitted. Nonsteroidal anti-inflammatory agents, steroids, psychotropic, or antidepressant drugs were prohibited.
Results	Compliance was not less than 95.4% in all study groups at any visit. After 6 weeks of therapy with 1 capsule daily, mean reductions in sitting systolic/diastolic blood pressure from baseline was 14.0/11.7 mmHg in the reserpine, 13.6/11.9 mmHg in the clopamid, 11.6/12.3 mmHg in the nitrendipine, and 23.0/17.1 mmHg in the reserpine-clopamid combination group ($p<0.01$). 39.7% of the reserpine, 36.2% of the clopamid, 33.3% of the nitrendipine, and 55.2% of the combination therapy group achieved diastolic blood pressure <90 mmHg. Doubling of the respective medication dosage in the patients in whom diastolic blood pressure remained $\geq$90 mmHg after the 6th week resulted in normalization of diastolic blood pressure in 35.3% of the reserpine, 39.1% of the clopamid, 44.9% of the nitrendipine, and 65.7% of the combination therapy group ($p<0.0001$). Linear regression modeling indicated that the combination of reserpine and clopamid acted more than additively. 28% of the reserpine, 29% of the clopamid, 48% of the nitrendipine, and 27% of the combination therapy group had one or more adverse effects ($p<0.05$). Serious adverse effects were found in 0, 1%, 1%, and 0, respectively. Withdrawal from the study because of adverse effects occurred in 3%, 7%, 13%, and 3%, respectively ($p=0.06$). The percentage of patients whose diastolic blood pressure was normalized and remained free of any adverse event was 40% in the combination therapy group, 19% in the reserpine group, 20% in the clopamid group, and 12% in the nitrendipine group ($p<0.0001$).
Conclusions	A low dose combination therapy with reserpine and clopamid was more effective than either drug alone or nitrendipine alone in lowering blood pressure. The combination therapy was well tolerated and safe. Reserpine, clopamid, and nitrendipine as monotherapy were associated with relatively low success rates.

Title	Fosinopril vs enalapril in the treatment of hypertension: a double blind study in 195 patients.
Authors	Hansson L, Forslund T, Höglund C, et al.
Reference	J Cardiovasc Pharmacol 1996;28:1-5.
Disease	Hypertension.
Purpose	To compare the efficacy of 2 angiotensin-converting-enzyme inhibitors, fosinopril and enalapril, in reducing blood pressure in patients with essential hypertension.
Design	Randomized, double blind, multicenter.
Patients	195 patients, 18-80 years old, with mild to moderate essential hypertension (supine diastolic blood pressure 95-110 mmHg). Patients with collagen vascular disease, significant cardiac, renal, hepatic, hematologic, or cerebrovascular disease were excluded.
Follow-up	24 weeks.
Treatment regimen	After 4 weeks of placebo period, patients were randomized to fosinopril 20 to 40 mg/d or enalapril 10 to 20 mg/d. If supine diastolic blood pressure remained >90 mmHg, hydrochlorothiazide 12.5 mg was added.

Results

After 8 weeks of therapy diastolic blood pressure had decreased by 8.3 mmHg (p<0.01) in the fosinopril group and by 7.3 mmHg (p<0.01) in the enalapril group, whereas systolic blood pressures were reduced by 10.6 mmHg in both groups. After 8 weeks, the medication dose was doubled in 42% of the fosinopril group and 49% of the enalapril group. At week 16, hydrochlorothiazide was added to 27% of the fosinopril vs 30% of the enalapril-treated patients. By the end of the 24th week, there was no difference in reduction of either diastolic (10.7 vs 10.5 mmHg) or systolic blood pressure (14.7 vs 14.5 mmHg) between the fosinopril and enalapril groups. 8 patients in the fosinopril group vs 14 in the enalapril group were withdrawn from the study due to adverse effects. Adverse effects were reported in 58% and 67%, respectively. Serum angiotensin-converting enzyme activity was significantly lower during fosinopril therapy than during enalapril therapy.

Conclusions

Fosinopril was equally effective as enalapril in reducing blood pressure in mild to moderate essential hypertension. Fosinopril was associated with better inhibition of the serum angiotensin-converting enzyme activity.

Title	Alpha-blockade and thiazide treatment of hypertension. A double blind randomized trial comparing doxazosin and hydrochlorothiazide.
Authors	Grimm RH Jr, Flack JM, Schoenberger JA, et al.
Reference	Am J Hypertension 1996;9:445-454.
Disease	Hypertension.
Purpose	To compare the effect of hydrochlorothiazide and the $\alpha 1$ blocker doxazosin in patients with hypertension.
Design	Randomized, double blind, parallel.
Patients	107 patients with hypertension.
Follow-up	1 year.
Treatment regimen	Hydrochlorothiazide (25 to 50 mg/d) or doxazosin (2 to 16 mg/d).

(continued)

Results	Both drugs were well tolerated. Only 4% of the doxazosin and 7% of the hydrochlorothiazide-treated patients were withdrawn from the study. Both drugs were equally effective in controlling hypertension. After 1 year of treatment systolic/diastolic blood pressure was reduced, compared to baseline, by 19/16 mmHg in the doxazosin and by 22/15 in the hydrochlorothiazide groups. Sitting heart rate was not affected by the drugs. There was no evidence of tolerance development to either drug. Average final doses were 7.8 mg for doxazosin and 36 mg for hydrochlorothiazide. Changes in quality of life scores were comparable between the groups.
Conclusions	Over 1 year of therapy, both hydrochlorothiazide and doxazosin were effective in treating hypertension.

Title	An in-patient trial of the safety and efficacy of losartan compared with placebo and enalapril in patients with essential hypertension.
Authors	Byyny RL, Merrill DD, Bradstreet TE, Sweet CS.
Reference	Cardiovasc Drugs Ther 1996;10:313-319.
Disease	Hypertension.
Purpose	To compare the effects of losartan, a specific and selective angiotensin II (subtype 1) receptor antagonist, and enalapril, an angiotensin-converting enzyme inhibitor, in patients with mild to moderate essential hypertension.
Design	Randomized, double blind, placebo-controlled multicenter.
Patients	100 in-patients, 21-72 years old (mean age 54 years), within 30% of their ideal body weight, with mild to moderate hypertension (supine diastolic blood pressure 95-120 mmHg). Black patients were not included. Patients with concomitant active medical problems that might have affected the antihypertensive therapy were excluded.
Follow-up	6 days.
Treatment regimen	After a 2 week outpatient single blind placebo phase, patients were hospitalized for 2 days to determine patient eligibility for randomization, then a 5 day in-patient double blind treatment phase, and a 1 day off-drug phase. Patients were randomized to placebo, losartan 50, 100, or 150 mg/d or enalapril 10 mg/d.
Additional therapy	ß blockers, digitalis, diuretics, angiotensin-converting enzyme inhibitors, nitrates, and calcium channel blockers were prohibited.

Results

Diastolic and systolic blood pressure decreased in all 5 treatment groups, as compared with the placebo group (p≤0.05). The magnitude of the blood pressure response to 50 mg/d losartan was comparable at 24 h to that achieved with enalapril 10 mg/d. There was an apparent plateauing of response with losartan, indicating no further decrease in mean diastolic blood pressure with doses >50 mg/d on the fifth day of therapy. The area under the 24 h blood pressure curve was comparable among the treatment groups on day 5. No rebound hypertension was observed after discontinuation of the study medications on day 6. Any adverse effects were noted in 48% of the placebo, 60% of the losartan 50 mg/d, 56% of the losartan 100 mg/d, 55% of the losartan 150 mg/d, and in 63% of the enalapril 10 mg/d group. Drug-related adverse effects were noted in 17%, 30%, 28%, 30%, and 42%, respectively. There were no serious clinical adverse effects.

Conclusions

Losartan was effective and safe in treating patients with mild to moderate essential hypertension.

ABCD Trial

The Appropriate Blood Pressure Control in Diabetes (ABCD)

Title	The effect of nisoldipine as compared with enalapril on cardiovascular outcomes in patients with noninsulin-dependent diabetes and hypertension.
Author	Estacio RO, Jeffers BW, Hiatt WR, et al.
Reference	New Engl J Med 1998; 338:645-652.
Disease	Hypertension and noninsulin-dependent diabetes.
Purpose	To compare the effects of moderate blood pressure control (target diastolic pressure of 80-89 mm Hg) to intensive control (75mmHg) on complications of diabetes.
Design	Prospective, randomized, double blind.
Patients	Patients 40-74 years with noninsulin dependent diabetes and diastolic pressures greater than 80 mm Hg. This study focuses on 470 patients who had hypertension (diastolic blood pressure (90 mmHg) and diabetes.
Follow-up	5 years.
Treatment regimen	Nisoldipine (235 patients) 10-60 mg per day vs enalapril (235 patients) 5-40 mg per day. Could add metoprolol and hydrochlorothiazide.

ABCD Trial

The Appropriate Blood Pressure Control in Diabetes (ABCD)

(continued)

Results	There was similar control of blood pressure in both groups. There was no difference in blood glucose levels, glycosylated hemoglobin, or cholesterol between groups. The secondary endpoint of the incidence of myocardial infarction also was examined. There was a lower incidence of fatal and nonfatal myocardial infarction in patients on enalapril (5) compared to nisoldipine (25); risk ratio, 9.5; 95% C.I. = 2.3 - 21.4. There was no statistically significant difference in cardiovascular mortality, all cause mortality, occurrence of congestive heart failure, or stroke between the nisoldipine and enalapril treated groups.
Conclusions	In the population of patients with hypertension and non-insulin-dependent diabetes both enalapril and nisoldipine were capable of controlling blood pressure to the same extent. Enalapril was associated with a lower incidence of fatal and nonfatal myocardial infarctions compared to nisoldipine. The authors pointed out that since the infarct findings were based on a secondary endpoint, confirmation will be required.

Doxazosin in Hypertension

Title	Doxazosin in hypertension: results of a general practice study in 4809 patients.
Authors	Langdon CG, Packard RS.
Reference	Br J Clin Pract 1994;48:293-298.
Disease	Hypertension.
Purpose	To evaluate the efficacy and safety of doxazosin, a selective α_1 adrenergic blocker, in hypertensive patients.
Design	Open, non comparative, multicenter.
Patients	4809 hypertensive patients, >18 years old, with a sitting diastolic blood pressure 95-114 mmHg. Pregnant patients, patients with childbearing potential, secondary hypertension, unstable angina, a recent (<3 months) myocardial infarction or cerebrovascular accident, postural hypotension, or a history of intolerance to α receptor blocking agents were excluded.
Follow-up	10 weeks.
Treatment regimen	Doxazosin. The initial dose was 1 mg/d. Dose was increased up to 8 mg/d at 2 weekly intervals to achieve diastolic blood pressure ≤90 mmHg.
Additional therapy	Patients were not consulted to change diet, lifestyle or smoking habits during the study. Patients that had received antihypertensive medications before entry continued their medications.

Results 4385 patients (91%) completed the study, including 89% of those 65 years or older. The average daily dose of doxazosin was 2.9 mg. 63% of all patients required 1-2 mg/d. The goal of diastolic blood pressure ≤90 mmHg or a decrease of ≥10 mmHg was reached by 81% of the patients. After 10 weeks of therapy, mean systolic and diastolic blood pressure decreased by 21 mmHg and 15 mmHg, respectively. There was no change in heart rate. Mean systolic and diastolic blood pressure reduction was 22.6 mmHg and 15.0 mmHg among patients ≥65 years old, and 20.7 mmHg and 14.4 mmHg among patients <65 years old. Adverse events related or possibly related to doxazosin were detected in 17% of the patients, were severe in 1.5% of the patients and led to withdrawal from the study in 5.7% of the patients. The most frequent adverse events were dizziness (6%, severe 1.1%), headache (3.8%), and fatigue (2.6%). Syncope or fainting occurred in 0.3% of the patients. Total cholesterol levels decreased by 4.1%, LDL cholesterol decreased by 5.1%, triglycerides decreased by 9.1%, and HDL cholesterol increased by 1.55%.

Conclusions Doxazosin was effective in blood pressure control, well tolerated, and associated with modest but statistically significant effect on blood lipid profile.

The effect of an endothelin-receptor antagonist, bosentan, on blood pressure in patients with essential hypertension.

Title	The effect of an endothelin-receptor antagonist, bosentan, on blood pressure in patients with essential hypertension.
Author	Krum H, Viskoper RJ, Lacourciere Y, et al.
Reference	N Engl J Med 1998; 338; 784-790.
Disease	Hypertension.
Purpose	To determine the contribution of endothelin to blood pressure elevation by studying the effects of an endothelin-receptor antagonist, bosentan.
Design	Randomized, double blind to 1 of 6 treatments as below. There was a placebo run-in phase period of 4-6 weeks followed by the randomization phase.
Patients	293 patients with mild to moderate essential hypertension.
Follow-up	4 weeks after therapy.
Treatment regimen	Randomization was to 1 of 4 oral dose of bosentan, (100, 500, or 1000 mg x1/d, or 1000mg x2/d, placebo), or enalapril (20 mg once daily).

The effect of an endothelin-receptor antagonist, bosentan, on blood pressure in patients with essential hypertension.

Results   Compared to placebo the 500 or 2000 mg dose caused a significant reduction in diastolic blood pressure of 5.7 mmHg which was comparable to the reduction observed with enalapril 5.8 mmHg. Bosentan did not alter heart rate or activate the renin-angiotensin system or increase plasma norepinephrine levels.

Conclusions   Bosentan, an endothelial receptor antagonist, significantly lowered blood pressure in patients with essential hypertension suggesting that endothelin may contribute to hypertension.

HALT

Hypertension and Lipid Trial Study

Title	Principal results of the hypertension and lipid trial (HALT): a multicenter study of doxazosin in patients with hypertension.
Authors	Levy D, Walmsley P, Levenstein M, for the Hypertension and Lipid Trial Study Group.
Reference	Am Heart J 1996;131:966-973.
Disease	Hypertension.
Purpose	To evaluate the efficacy and safety of doxazosin, a selective α_1 adrenergic blocker, in hypertensive patients.
Design	Open, noncomparative, multicenter.
Patients	851 patients (60% men), >35 years old, with essential hypertension and a mean sitting diastolic blood pressure 96-110 mmHg. Patients with malignant or secondary form of hypertension, pregnant or lactating, hypersensitivity to α blockers, orthostatic hypotension, drug or alcohol abuse, or other medical conditions that might interfere with completion of the study were excluded. Patients on lipid lowering therapy and those who had donated blood within 30 days of the study were not included.
Follow-up	A 2 week baseline period without anti-hypertensive medications, a 6 week titration period, and 8 weeks of maintenance phase.
Treatment regimen	Doxazosin once daily.

HALT

Hypertension and Lipid Trial Study

(continued)

Results
650 patients completed the study. 103 (12.1%) patients discontinued therapy because of side effects and 98 (11.5% of patients, because of other reasons). Final mean doxazosin dose was 7.8 mg/d. Doxazosin significantly did decreased mean sitting and standing systolic blood pressure by 15.2 and 16.1 mmHg, respectively, and mean sitting and standing diastolic blood pressure by 12.5 and 12.7 mmHg, respectively (p=0.0001 compared with baseline). Mean sitting systolic and diastolic blood pressure was reduced by 13.3 and 11.4 mmHg in men and by 18.1 and 14.2 mmHg in women (p=0.0001). Doxazosin was more effective in patients 65 years or older than in those younger than 65. Systolic and diastolic blood pressure were reduced by 14.4 and 11.9 mmHg in the young patients (p=0.0001 compared with baseline) vs 18.3 and 14.6 mmHg in patients 65 years or older (p=0.0001 compared with baseline). There was no significant difference in the magnitude of blood pressure reduction when patients were stratified by race. Doxazosin had no significant effect on heart rate. Doxazosin therapy resulted in 8.3 mg/dl reduction in total cholesterol (p<0.001 compared with baseline), 6.9 mg/dl reduction in LDL cholesterol (p<0.001 compared with baseline), 8.9 mg/dl reduction in triglycerides (p<0.05 compared with baseline), and 0.4 mg/dl increase in HDL cholesterol (p=NS). The drug was well tolerated and major side effects were infrequent.

Conclusions
Doxazosin is effective therapy for patients with essential hypertension, with good efficacy in young and elderly patients, in both women and men, and in all races. The drug was well tolerated and was associated with a favorable effects on plasma lipid levels.

MIDAS

Multicenter Isradipine Diuretic Atherosclerotic Study

Title	Final outcome results of the multicenter isradipine diuretic atherosclerosis study (MIDAS). A randomized controlled trial.
Author	Borhani NO, Mercuri M, Bohani PA
Reference	JAMA 1996; 276:785-791
Disease	Hypertension
Purpose	To compare rate of medial thickening of the carotid arteries in hypertensive patients on isradipine vs hydrochlorothiazide.
Design	Randomized, double blind, control, multicenter.
Patients	883 patients, 40 years or older with diastolic pressure from 90–115 mmHg and presence of intimal-medial thickness assessed by B mode ultrasound of between 1.3-3.5 mm.
Follow-up	3 years.
Treatment regimen	Isradipine 2.5-5.0 mg or hydrochlorothiazide 12.5-25mg PO x2/d.

MIDAS

Multicenter Isradipine Diuretic Atherosclerotic Study

(continued)

Results

There was no difference in rate of progression of mean maximum intimal-medial thickness between isradipine and hydrochlorothiazide over 3 years. Mean diastolic blood pressure decreased to the same level with either treatment at 6 months (-13.0 mmHg); mean systolic blood pressure decreased by 19.5 mmHg with hydrochlorothiazide compared to 16.0 mmHg with isradipine (p= 0.002). Major vascular events (myocardial infarction, stroke, congestive heart failure, angina, sudden death) occurred more frequently in the isradipine group (5.65%) than hydrochlorothiazide group (3.17%, p=0.07). There was a significant (p=0.02) increase in nonmajor vascular events and procedures in the isradipine compared to the hydrochlorothiazide group. The increased incidence of vascular events in patients treated with isradipine could not be explained by the difference in systolic blood pressure alone.

Conclusions

There was no difference in progression of the mean maximum intimal-medial thickness of the carotid arteries in isradipine vs hydrochlorothiazide treatment. The increased incidence of vascular events in the isradipine requires further study.

STONE

Shanghai Trial Of Nifedipine in the Elderly (STONE)

Title	Shanghai trial of nifedipine in the elderly (STONE).
Author	Gong L, Zhang W, Zhu Y et al.
Reference	J Hypertens 1996; 14:1237-1245.
Disease	Hypertension
Purpose	To determine whether there was a difference between nifedipine and placebo in development of cardiovascular events in elderly hypertensive patients.
Design	Single blind, randomized, multicenter. After 4 weeks physicians could reallocate some of the subjects.
Patients	1632 patients with hypertension, between ages 60-79 years. Blood pressure ≥160/90.
Follow-up	Mean of 30 months.
Treatment regimen	Placebo or slow-release retard preparation of nifedipine 10 mg x 2/day, up to 60 mg. Captopril or dihydrochlorothiazide added if blood pressure remained above 159/90.

Shanghai Trial Of Nifedipine in the Elderly (STONE)

(continued)

Results	Clinical event end-points determined prior to trial included stroke, congestive heart failure, myocardial infarction, severe arrhythmia, sudden death, and others. 77 events occurred in placebo vs 32 in the nifedipine group and this was highly significant. There was a significant decrease in risk of strokes and severe arrhythmias; relative risk decreased from 1.0-0.41 on therapy; 95% confidence interval 0.27-0.61.

Conclusions	Long-acting nifedipine decreased the number of clinical events (including strokes and arrhythmias) in elderly hypertensive patients.

Syst-Eur

Systolic Hypertension-Europe

Title	Randomized double blind comparison of placebo and active treatment for older patients with isolated systolic hypertension.
Authors	Staessen JA, Fagard R, Thijs L, et al.
Reference	Lancet 1997;350:757-764.
Disease	Hypertension.
Purpose	To evaluate the effectiveness of antihypertensive therapy in prevention of cardiovascular complications in patients >60 years old with isolated systolic hypertension.
Design	Randomized, double blind, placebo-controlled, multicenter.
Patients	4695 patients, ≥60 years old, with sitting systolic blood pressure 160-219 mmHg, and diastolic blood pressure <95 mmHg when treated with masked placebo. Standing systolic blood pressure should have been ≥140 mmHg. Patients with secondary systolic hypertension that needed special medical or surgical correction, retinal hemorrhage or papilledema, congestive heart failure, aortic dissection, renal failure, stroke or myocardial infarction in the preceding year, dementia, substance abuse, or severe concomitant disease were excluded.
Follow-up	A median of 2 years (range 1-97 months).
Treatment regimen	Nitrendipine 10-40 mg/d (if necessary replaced or combined with enalapril 5-20 mg/d, hydrochlorothiazide 12.5-25 mg/d or both) or matching placebo. Goal of systolic blood pressure: <150 mmHg, with a reduction of at least 20 mmHg.

Syst-Eur

Systolic Hypertension-Europe

(continued)

Results
After 2 years, 58.9% of the patients who had been assigned to nitrendipine and 39.6% of the patients assigned to placebo still received the study drug as the only treatment. Among the patients who withdrew from the study treatment, but continued to be followed, 36.5% of the patients assigned to active treatment and 58.1% of the patients in the placebo group were on antihypertensive medications. By intention-to-treat analysis, the sitting systolic and diastolic blood pressure decreased after 2 years by 13 and 17 mmHg, respectively in the placebo group, and by 23 and 7 mmHg in the active treatment group. Standing systolic and diastolic blood pressure decreased by 10 and 2 mmHg in the placebo group, and by 21 and 7 mmHg in the active treatment group. At median follow-up, more patients from the active treatment group (43.5%) than the placebo group (21.4%) had reached the target blood pressure (p<0.001). The between-group differences in sitting blood pressure (the mean change from baseline in the active treatment group minus the mean change in the placebo group) were 10.1 mmHg (95% CI 8.8-11.4) systolic and 4.5 mmHg (95% CI 3.9-5.1) diastolic at 2 years, and 10.7 mmHg (95% CI 8.8-12.5) and 4.7 mmHg (95% CI 3.7-5.6) at 4 years. Heart rate was not changed with active treatment. Withdrawal from the study due to uncontrolled hypertension occurred in 5.5% of the placebo group vs 0.5% of the active treatment group (p<0.001). Total mortality per 1000 patient-years was 24.0 in the placebo and 20.5 in the active treatment group (-14% difference; 95% CI -33-+9%; p=0.22). Cardiovascular mortality was 13.5 vs 9.8, respectively (-27% difference; 95% CI -48-+2%; p=0.07). Fatal myocardial infarction occurred at a rate of 2.6 and 1.2 per 1000 patient-years in the placebo and active treatment, respectively (-56% difference; 95% CI -82-9%; p=0.08). Non cardiovascular and cancer mortality were comparable between the 2 groups. The cumulative stroke rates were 13.7 and 7.9 per 1000 patient-years (-42% difference, 95% CI -60-17%; p=0.003). Non fatal cardiac endpoints (heart failure, fatal and non fatal myocardial infarction, and sudden death) occurred at a rate of 20.5 per 1000 patient-years in the placebo group vs 15.1 in the active treatment group (-26% difference; 95% CI -44-3%; p=0.03). The rate of all cerebrovascular events was 18.0

and 11.8 per 1000 patient-years in the placebo and active treatment group, respectively (-34% difference; 95% CI -51-11%; p=0.006). Angina pectoris occurred less frequently in the active treatment group (18.1 vs 23.9 per 1000 patient-years; -24% difference; 95% CI -41-2%; p=0.04). The cumulative rate of all fatal and nonfatal cardiovascular endpoints was 33.9 per 1000 patient-years in the placebo group and 23.3 in the active treatment group (-31% difference; 95% CI -45-14%; p<0.001).

Conclusions

Nitrendipine therapy reduced the rate of cardiovascular complications and cerebrovascular events in patients ≥60 years old with isolated systolic hypertension. However, the decrease in total mortality was not statistically significant.

TONE

Trial Of Nonpharmacologic interventions in the Elderly

Title	Sodium reduction and weight loss in the treatment of hypertension in older persons. A randomized controlled trial of nonpharmacologic interventions in the elderly (TONE).
Author	Whelton PK, Appel LJ, Espeland MA et al.
Reference	JAMA 1998; 279:839-846.
Disease	Hypertension.
Purpose	To determine the efficacy of weight loss and sodium restriction as therapy for hypertension in older patients.
Design	Randomized, controlled, multicenter.
Patients	875 men and women, 60-80 years old with systolic blood pressure lower than 145mmHg and diastolic blood pressure lower than 85mmHg on a single anti-hypertensive medication.
Follow-up	Median was 29 months; range 15-36 months.
Treatment regimen	585 obese patients randomized to reduced sodium intake, weight loss, both vs usual care. 390 non obese patients randomized to reduced sodium intake or usual care. After 3 months of intervention withdrawal of anti-hypertensive medicines was attempted.

TONE

Trial Of Nonpharmacologic interventions in the Elderly

(continued)

Results   The combined outcome measures (occurrence of hypertension at 1 or more study visits following attempted withdrawal of anti-hypertensive medication, treatment with an anti-hypertensvie medicine, or occurrence of a clinical cardiovascular event (myocardial infarction, angina, congestive heart failure, stroke, coronary artery bypass grafting, or percutaneous transluminal coronary angioplasty) was less frequent among those assigned to reduced sodium intake vs not assigned to reduced sodium intake; relative hazard ratio 0.69; 95% CI 0.59-0.81, p<.001). The combined outcome measures was less frequent in obese patients assigned to weight loss vs not assigned to weight loss; relative hazard ratio 0.70; 95% CI 0.57 - 0.87, p<.001). For obese patients the hazard ratios were reduced compared to usual care for reduced sodium intake alone, weight loss and combined sodium intake, and weight loss. There were no differences in the frequency of cardiovascular events during follow-up among the groups.

Conclusions   Weight loss and reduction in sodium intake are feasible, effective, and safe non pharmacologic therapies of hypertension in the elderly.

6. Congestive Heart Failure

Title	Xamoterol in severe heart failure.
Authors	The Xamoterol in Severe Heart Failure Study Group.
Reference	Lancet 1990;336:1-6.
Disease	Congestive heart failure.
Purpose	To evaluate the efficacy and safety of xamoterol therapy for heart failure.
Design	Randomized, double blind, placebo-controlled, multicenter.
Patients	516 patients, >18 years old, with NYHA class III and IV heart failure despite therapy with diuretics and an angiotensin-converting enzyme inhibitor. Patients with myocardial infarction within 8 weeks, and premenopausal women were excluded.
Follow-up	Clinical evaluation and exercise test at baseline and after an average of 86 days for the placebo and 87 days for the xamoterol.
Treatment regimen	Xamoterol 200 mg X2/d or placebo.
Additional therapy	Any drug that influenced the ß adrenoreceptors was not permitted. Digitalis was allowed.

Results

There was no significant change in body weight at the end of the protocol for either group. Except for heart rate (79 vs 83 bpm, p<0.01) there was no difference in clinical signs between the groups. Visual analogue scale (11% vs 0%, p<0.02) and Likert scale (8% vs 2%, p=0.02) indicated that breathlessness improved with xamoterol. However, there was no difference in either the symptoms of fatigue, or exercise duration or total work done. Xamoterol did not affect the number of ventricular premature beats after exercise and had no proarrhythmogenic activity. More patients in the xamoterol group withdrew from the study (19% vs 12%). On intention to treat analysis 9.2% of the xamoterol and 3.7% of the placebo died within 100 days (hazard ratio 2.54, 95% CI 1.04-6.18, p=0.02). Death due to progression of heart failure occurred in 1.2% and 4.8% of the placebo and xamoterol groups, while sudden death in 1.8% and 3.7%, respectively.

Conclusions

Xamoterol therapy resulted in excess of mortality and was not associated with objective measures of improvement of exercise capacity. The study was terminated prematurely by the safety committee.

PROMISE

Prospective Randomized Milrinone Survival Evaluation Trial

Title	Effect of milrinone on mortality in severe chronic heart failure.
Authors	Packer M, Carver JR, Rodeheffer RJ, et al.
Reference	N Engl J Med 1991;325:1468-1475.
Disease	Congestive heart failure.
Purpose	To investigate the effects of milrinone on survival of patients with severe chronic heart failure.
Design	Randomized, double blind, placebo-controlled, multicenter.
Patients	1088 patients with chronic heart failure NYHA class III-IV, with left ventricular ejection fraction ≤0.35. Patients who received ß blockers, calcium channel blockers, disopyramide, flecainide, encainide, dopamine, or dobutamine were excluded.
Follow-up	1 day to 20 months (median 6.1 months).
Treatment regimen	Milrinone 10 mg X4/d or placebo PO.
Additional therapy	All patients received digoxin, diuretics, and angiotensin-converting enzyme inhibitors. Nitrates, hydralazine, prazosin, and other vasodilators were permitted.

PROMISE

Prospective Randomized Milrinone Survival Evaluation Trial

(continued)

Results   Mortality was 30% in the milrinone and 24% in the place-bo group. Milrinone was associated with a 28% increase in total mortality (95% CI 1-61%, p=0.038), and with 34% increase in cardiovascular mortality (95% CI 6-69%, p=0.016). The adverse effect of milrinone was more pronounced in patients with NYHA class IV (53% increase in mortality, 95% CI 13-107%, p=0.006) than in patients with class III (3% increase, 95% CI -28% to 48%, p=0.86). Milrinone did not have a beneficial effect on survival of any subgroup. Patients treated with milrinone had more hospitalization (44% vs 39%, p=0.041) and more serious adverse cardiovascular reactions, including hypotension (11.4% vs 6.5% ,p=0.006) and syncope (8.0% vs 3.8%, p=0.002).

Conclusions   Long-term therapy with milrinone increased the mortality and morbidity of patients with severe heart failure.

SOLVD - Treatment Study

Studies of Left Ventricular Dysfunction

Title	a. Studies of left ventricular dysfunction (SOLVD): rationale, design, and methods. 2 trials that evaluate the effect of enalapril in patients with reduced ejection fraction. b. Effect of enalapril on survival in patients with reduced left ventricular ejection fractions and congestive heart failure.
Authors	The SOLVD Investigators.
Reference	a. Am J Cardiol 1990;66:315-322. b. N Engl J Med 1991;325:293-302.
Disease	Congestive heart failure, left ventricular dysfunction.
Purpose	To investigate whether enalapril therapy will reduce mortality and morbidity in patients with chronic heart failure and left ventricular ejection fraction ≤ 0.35.
Design	Randomized, double blind, placebo-controlled, multicenter.
Patients	2569 Patients, age 21-80, with chronic heart failure and left ventricular ejection fraction ≤ 0.35. Patients with active angina pectoris requiring surgery, unstable angina, myocardial infarction within 1 month, renal failure, or pulmonary disease were excluded. Patients already on angiotensin-converting enzyme inhibitor therapy were excluded. Only patients that could tolerate enalapril 2.5 mg X2/d for 2-7 days were included.
Follow-up	22-55 months (average 41.4 months).
Treatment regimen	Enalapril (2.5 or 5mg X2/d initially, with gradual increase to 10 mg X2/d) or placebo.
Additional therapy	No restriction, except for other angiotensin-converting enzyme inhibitors.

SOLVD - Treatment Study

Studies of Left Ventricular Dysfunction

(continued)

Results
39.7% of the placebo and 35.2% of the enalapril patients died (risk reduction 16%, 95% CI 5-26%, p=0.0036). Cardiovascular deaths occurred in 35.9% and 31.1%, respectively (risk reduction 18% (6-28%), p<0.002). The major difference was in death due to progressive heart failure (19.5% vs 16.3%, risk reduction 22% (6-35%), p=0.0045). 57.3% and 47.7% of the placebo and enalapril patients died or were hospitalized due to heart failure (risk reduction 26% (18-34%), p<0.0001). After 1 year there were 31.2% such events in the placebo and 20.4% in the enalapril (risk reduction 40% (30-48%)). 74% of the placebo and 69% of the enalapril patients were hospitalized at least once (p=0.006), 63% and 57% of the patients were hospitalized for primarily cardiovascular reasons (p<0.001).

Conclusions
Enalapril added to conventional therapy significantly reduced mortality and hospitalizations in patients with chronic heart failure due to systolic dysfunction.

V-HeFT II

Vasodilator Heart Failure Trial II

Title	A comparison of enalapril with hydralazine-isosorbide dinitrate in the treatment of chronic congestive heart failure.
Authors	Cohn JN, Johnson G, Zeische S, et al.
Reference	N Engl J Med 1991;325:303-310.
Disease	Congestive heart failure.
Purpose	To compare the effects of hydralazine-isosorbide dinitrate and enalapril in the treatment of congestive heart failure.
Design	Randomized, double blind, multicenter.
Patients	804 men, age 18-75 years, with chronic congestive heart failure (cardiothoracic ratio$\geq$0.55 on chest radiography, LV internal diameter at diastole >2.7 cm/m2 body surface area on echocardiography, or LVEF<0.45 on radionuclide scan) and reduced exercise tolerance. Patients with active angina were excluded.
Follow-up	0.5-5.7 years (mean 2.5 years).
Treatment regimen	1. Enalapril 10 mg X2/d. 2. Hydralazine 75 mg X4/d and isosorbide dinitrate 40 mg X4/d.
Additional therapy	Digoxin and diuretics.

Results	2 year mortality was lower in the enalapril arm (18%) than the hydralazine arm (25%, p=0.016) which was attributed to a reduction of sudden death, especially in patients with NYHA class I or II. The reduction in mortality with enalapril was 33.6%, 28.2%, 14.0%, and 10.3% after 1, 2, 3, and 4 years. Body oxygen consumption at peak exercise was increased after 13 weeks and after 6 months only in the hydralazine-isosorbide dinitrate group (p<0.05). However, after 1 year, oxygen consumption began to decline in both groups. Left ventricular ejection fraction increased more during the first 13 weeks in the hydralazine-isosorbide dinitrate group (0.033 vs. 0.021, p<0.03). However, after 3 years there was no difference between the groups. An increase in the incidence of cough and symptomatic hypotension was noted in the enalapril group and of headache in the hydralazine-isosorbide dinitrate group.
Conclusions	While enalapril improved survival better than hydralazine-isosorbide dinitrate, the improvement of left ventricular ejection fraction and exercise capacity was greater with hydralazine-isosorbide dinitrate. A combination of these drugs may enhance their efficacy.

SOLVD - Prevention Study

Studies of Left Ventricular Dysfunction

Title	a. Studies of left ventricular dysfunction (SOLVD): rationale, design, and methods. 2 trials that evaluate the effect of enalapril in patients with reduced ejection fraction. b. Effect of enalapril on mortality and the development of heart failure in asymptomatic patients with reduced left ventricular ejection fractions.
Authors	The SOLVD Investigators.
Reference	a. Am J Cardiol 1990;66:315-322. b. N Engl J Med 1992;327:685-691.
Disease	Congestive heart failure, left ventricular dysfunction.
Purpose	To investigate whether enalapril therapy will reduce mortality and morbidity in asymptomatic patients with left ventricular dysfunction.
Design	Randomized, double blind, placebo-controlled, multicenter.
Patients	4228 patients, age 21-80, with left ventricular ejection fraction ≤0.35, who did not receive therapy for heart failure. However, diuretic therapy for hypertension and digoxin for atrial fibrillation were permitted.
Follow-up	Clinical follow-up for an average of 37.4 months (range 14.6-62.0 months).
Treatment regimen	Enalapril (2.5 mg X2/d initially, with gradual increase to 10 mg X2/d) or placebo.
Additional therapy	No restriction, except for other angiotensin-converting enzyme inhibitors.

SOLVD - Prevention Study

Studies of Left Ventricular Dysfunction

(continued)

Results
: Total mortality was 15.8% and 14.8% in the placebo and enalapril groups (reduction of risk 8%, 95% CI -8% to 21%, p=0.30). The difference was entirely due to a reduction in cardiovascular death (14.1% vs 12.6%, respectively, risk reduction 12%, 95% CI -3% to 26%, p=0.12). Heart failure developed in 30.2% vs 20.7% of the placebo and enalapril patients (risk reduction 37%, 95% CI 28% to 44%, p<0.001). The median length of time to development of heart failure was 8.3 vs 22.3 months, respectively. Hospitalization due to heart failure occurred in 12.9% vs 8.7%, respectively (p<0.001). The median length of time to the first hospitalization for heart failure was 13.2 vs 27.8 months, respectively.

Conclusions
: Enalapril therapy delayed the development of heart failure and reduced the rate of related hospitalizations among patients with asymptomatic left ventricular dysfunction. There was also a trend toward decreased cardiovascular mortality in the enalapril group.

MDC

Metoprolol in Dilated Cardiomyopathy

Title	Beneficial effects of metoprolol in idiopathic dilated cardiomyopathy.
Authors	Waagstein F, Bristow MR, Swedberg K, et al.
Reference	Lancet 1993;342:1441-1446.
Disease	Congestive heart failure, dilated cardiomyopathy.
Purpose	To evaluate the effect of metoprolol therapy upon survival and morbidity in patients with dilated cardiomyopathy.
Design	Randomized, double blind, placebo-controlled, multicenter.
Patients	383 patients, 16-75 years old, with dilated cardiomyopathy (ejection fraction <0.40). Patients treated with ß blockers, calcium channel blockers, inotropic drugs (except digoxin), or high doses of tricyclic antidepressant drugs were excluded. Patients with significant coronary artery disease, active myocarditis, chronic obstructive lung disease, insulin dependent diabetes, and alcoholism were not included. Only patients that could tolerate metoprolol 5 mg X2/d for 2-7 days were included.
Follow-up	Clinical follow-up for 12-18 months. Exercise test, right heart catheterization, and radionuclide ventriculography at baseline, 6 and 12 months.
Treatment regimen	Placebo or metoprolol. The target dose was 100-150 mg/d for 12-18 months.
Additional therapy	Digitalis, diuretics, angiotensin-converting enzyme inhibitors, and nitrates were permitted.

Metoprolol in Dilated Cardiomyopathy

(continued)

Results

The primary end point of death or need for cardiac transplantation was reached by 20.1% of the placebo and
12.9% of the metoprolol group (34% risk reduction, 95%
CI -6-62%, p=0.058). 10.1% vs 1.0% of the placebo and
metoprolol patients needed cardiac transplantation
(p=0.0001). However, there was no difference in mortality alone (10.0% vs 11.9%, respectively). Mean ejection fraction was similar at baseline (0.22±0.09 vs 0.22±0.08).
However, ejection fraction increased more in the metoprolol group after 6 months (0.26±0.11 vs 0.32±0.13 (p
<0.0001)) and after 12 months (0.28±0.12 vs 0.34±0.14
(p<0.0001)). The improvement in ejection fraction was
independent of the use of other medications and on the
initial ejection fraction. Quality of life improved more in
the metoprolol group (p=0.01). Exercise time at 12
months was significantly longer (p=0.046) in the metoprolol group. Heart rate and pulmonary wedge pressure
decreased significantly more in the metoprolol than in the
placebo group, whereas systolic pressure, stroke volume,
and stroke work index increased more with metoprolol.

Conclusions

Metoprolol reduced clinical deterioration, improved
symptoms and cardiac function, and was well tolerated.
However, mortality was not reduced.

FACET

Flosequinan-ACE Inhibitor Trial

Title	Can further benefit be achieved by adding flosequinan to patients with congestive heart failure who remain symptomatic on diuretic, digoxin, and an angiotensin converting enzyme inhibitor? Results of the Flosequinan-ACE Inhibitor Trial (FACET).
Authors	Massie BM, Berk MR, Brozena SC, et al.
Reference	Circulation 1993;88:492-501.
Disease	Congestive heart failure.
Purpose	To evaluate whether the addition of flosequinan to angiotensin-converting enzyme inhibitors, diuretics and digoxin will improve exercise tolerance and quality of life of patients with congestive heart failure.
Design	Randomized, double blind, placebo-controlled, multicenter.
Patients	322 patients, ≥18 years old, with congestive heart failure ≥12 weeks, left ventricular ejection fraction ≤35%, and were able to exercise to an end point of dyspnea or fatigue. All patients were on angiotensin-converting enzyme inhibitor and diuretic therapy for ≥12 weeks.
Follow-up	Clinical follow-up, 24 h ECG monitoring, and repeated exercise test for 16 weeks.
Treatment regimen	Placebo, flosequinan 100 mg X1/d, or flosequinan 75 mg X2/d. If the heart rate increased by ≥15 bpm, the dose was reduced to 75 mg X1/d or 50 mg X2/d.

FACET

Flosequinan-ACE Inhibitor Trial

(continued)

Additional therapy	Calcium channel blockers, ß or α blockers, long acting nitrates, disopyramide or other class Ic antiarrhythmic agents, theophylline, bronchodilators, or other investigational drugs were not permitted.
Results	After 16 weeks, exercise time increased by 64 seconds in the 100 mg/d flosequinan group compared with only 5 seconds in the placebo group (p<0.05), whereas the higher dose did not reach statistical significant improvement. Flosequinan 100 mg/d resulted in improvement of the Minnesota Living With Heart Failure Questionnaire (LWHF) score compared with placebo. Both flosequinan doses were associated with improvement of the physical score, whereas the 75 mg X2/d was associated with worsening of the emotional component. NYHA class was improved in 22.0% and worsened in 14.7% of the placebo group, while the corresponding rates for flosequinan 100 mg/d were 30.9% and 16.4%, and for flosequinan 75 mg X2/d 39.3% and 15.7%, respectively. There was no significant difference in mortality, hospitalization for all causes, hospitalization for heart failure, or withdrawal for worsening of heart failure among the groups. There was no increase in ventricular arrhythmias with flosequinan.
Conclusions	Flosequinan resulted in symptomatic benefit when added to angiotensin-converting enzyme inhibitor and diuretic therapy for heart failure. However, in another study, the same dose resulted in an adverse effect on survival.

REFLECT

Randomized Evaluation of Flosequinan on Exercise Tolerance

Title	Double blind, placebo-controlled study of the efficacy of flosequinan in patients with chronic heart failure.
Authors	Packer M, Narahara KA, Elkayam U, et al.
Reference	J Am Coll Cardiol 1993;22:65-72.
Disease	Congestive heart failure.
Purpose	To evaluate the effects of flosequinan on symptoms and exercise capacity in patients with chronic heart failure who remained symptomatic despite therapy with digitalis and diuretics.
Design	Randomized, double blind, placebo-controlled, multicenter.
Patients	193 patients, ≥18 years old, with dyspnea or fatigue on exertion (NYHA II or III), left ventricular ejection fraction ≤40% and cardiothoracic ratio ≥50%. All patients were symptomatic despite therapy with digitalis and diuretics for ≥2 months. Patients with hypotension, angina, pulmonary renal or hepatic disease, claudication, or myocardial infarction within 3 months were excluded.
Follow-up	12 weeks of clinical follow-up and repeated exercise test and radionuclide ventriculography.
Treatment regimen	Flosequinan 100 mg/d or placebo in addition to diuretic agent and digoxin. If the dose was not tolerated, a dose of 75 mg/d was permitted.
Additional therapy	Use of other vasodilators was not permitted. Use of antiarrhythmic agents, except ß blockers, was permitted.

REFLECT

Randomized Evaluation of Flosequinan on Exercise Tolerance
(continued)

Results | After 12 weeks, maximal exercise time increased by 96 seconds in the flosequinan vs 47 seconds in the placebo group (p=0.22). Maximal oxygen consumption increased by 1.7 vs 0.6 ml/kg/min, respectively (p=0.05). By 12 weeks, 55% of the flosequinan vs 36% of the placebo treated patients improved their heart failure symptoms (p=0.018), while 10% vs 19% had worsening heart failure (p=0.07). Flosequinan did not change the functional class, cardiothoracic ratio, or ejection fraction. 7 vs 2 deaths occurred in the flosequinan and placebo groups, respectively (p>0.10).

Conclusions | Flosequinan therapy resulted in symptomatic improvement and an increase in exercise time. However, the effect on survival remains to be determined.

GESICA

Grupo de Estudio de la Sobrevida en la
Insuficiencia Cardiaca en Argentina

Title	Randomized trial of low dose amiodarone in severe congestive heart failure.
Authors	Doval HC, Nul DR, Grancelli HO, et al.
Reference	Lancet 1994;344:493-498.
Disease	Congestive heart failure, arrhythmia.
Purpose	To evaluate the effect of low dose amiodarone on survival of patients with severe heart failure.
Design	Randomized, multicenter.
Patients	516 patients with severe heart failure NYHA class II-IV with evidence of cardiac enlargement or reduced ejection fraction ≤ 0.35. Patients with thyroid dysfunction, concomitant serious disease, valvular heart disease, hypertrophic or restrictive cardiomyopathy, angina pectoris, or history of sustained ventricular arrhythmias were excluded.
Follow-up	2 years.
Treatment regimen	Amiodarone 600 mg/d for 14 d and then 300 mg/d for 2 years.
Additional therapy	Low sodium diet, diuretics, digitalis, and vasodilators. Antiarrhythmic agents were not permitted.

GESICA

Grupo de Estudio de la Sobrevida en la Insuficiencia Cardiaca en Argentina
(continued)

Results
Mortality was 41.4% in the control and 33.5% in the amiodarone group (risk reduction 28%, 95% CI 4-45%, p=0.024). Both sudden death and death due to progressive heart failure were reduced. Fewer patients in the amiodarone group died or were hospitalized due to worsening of heart failure (45.8% vs 58.2%, RR 31%, 95% CI 13-46%, p=0.0024). The beneficial effect was evident in all subgroups examined and was independent of the presence of nonsustained ventricular tachycardia. Side effects were reported in 6.1% of the amiodarone group and lead to drug withdrawal in 4.6%.

Conclusions
Low dose amiodarone is a safe and effective treatment for reduction of mortality and morbidity in patients with severe heart failure.

CIBIS

The Cardiac Insufficiency Bisoprolol Study

Title	A randomized trial of ß blockade in heart failure. The Cardiac Insufficiency Bisoprolol Study (CIBIS).
Authors	CIBIS Investigators and Committees.
Reference	Circulation 1994;90:1765-1773.
Disease	Congestive heart failure.
Purpose	To assess the effects of bisoprolol therapy on mortality in patients with heart failure.
Design	Randomized, double blind, placebo-controlled, multicenter.
Patients	641 patients, 18-75 years of age, with chronic heart failure (NYHA class III or IV) treated with diuretics and vasodilators, and left ventricular ejection fraction <40%. Patients with heart failure due to hypertrophic or restrictive cardiomyopathy, or due to mitral or aortic valve disease, or within 3 months of myocardial infarction were excluded. Patients awaiting for coronary artery bypass grafting or cardiac transplantation were not included.
Follow-up	Mean follow-up 1.9±0.1 years.
Treatment regimen	Placebo or bisoprolol. Initial dose was 1.25 mg/d with gradual increase to 5 mg/d.
Additional therapy	Diuretics and a vasodilator therapy. Digitalis and amiodarone were permitted. ß blockers or mimetic agents and phosphodiesterase inhibitors were prohibited. Only calcium channel blockers of the dihydropyridine type were allowed.

CIBIS

The Cardiac Insufficiency Bisoprolol Study

(continued)

Results
Bisoprolol was well tolerated. Premature withdrawal from treatment occurred in 25.5% of the placebo and 23.4% of the bisoprolol group (p=NS). Bisoprolol did not significantly reduce mortality (20.9% vs 16.6% in the placebo and bisoprolol group, RR 0.80, 95% CI 0.56-1.15, p=0.22). No significant difference was found in sudden death rate (5.3% vs 4.7%, respectively), death due to documented ventricular tachycardia, or fibrillation (2.2% vs 1.3%). However, bisoprolol improved the functional status of the patients. Hospitalization for cardiac decompensation occurred in 28.0% vs 19.1% (p<0.01), and improvement by >1 NYHA class was noted in 15.0% vs 21.3%, respectively (p<0.03).

Conclusions
ß blockers conferred functional improvement in patients with severe heart failure. However, there was no improvement in survival.

Title	Long-term evaluation of treatment for chronic heart failure: a 1 year comparative trial of flosequinan and captopril.
Authors	Cowley AJ, McEntegart DJ, Hampton JR, et al.
Reference	Cardiovasc Drugs Ther 1994;8:829-836.
Disease	Congestive heart failure.
Purpose	To compare the efficacy of flosequinan and captopril in patients with moderate to severe heart failure who remained symptomatic despite optimal diuretic therapy.
Design	Randomized, double blind, multicenter.
Patients	209 patients with moderate to severe heart failure (NYHA class III-IV) despite ≥80 mg frusemide/d or an equivalent diuretic, and a cardiothoracic ratio >50% on a standard chest x-ray. Patients treated with vasodilators were excluded.
Follow-up	12 months of clinical follow-up and either repeated exercise test or corridor walk test.
Treatment regimen	Flosequinan (50 mg/d for 2 weeks and then 100 mg/d for 2 weeks and 150 mg/d thereafter) or captopril 12.5 mg X3/d for 2 weeks, 25 mg X3/d for additional 2 weeks and then, 50 mg X3/d.
Additional therapy	Other vasodilators were not permitted.

Results

64% of the flosequinan vs 40% of the captopril groups failed to complete the study due to death or withdrawal (p<0.001). There was no statistically significant difference in mortality (18.6% in the flosequinan vs 14.0% in the captopril groups, 38% increase risk of death with flosequinan, 95% CI -30% to 172%, p=0.29). Worsening of heart failure occurred in 12.7% vs 10.3%, respectively. There were more adverse effects in the flosequinan treated patients. Both medications had similar effects on treadmill exercise test. The mean increase in exercise time at 52 weeks was 117 vs 156 seconds in the flosequinan and captopril groups (p=0.57). The increase in corridor walk distance was 40 vs 62 meters, respectively (p=0.015).

Conclusions

Flosequinan had comparable long-term efficacy to captopril. However, it is associated with a higher incidence of adverse events.

Carvedilol in Congestive Heart Failure Due to Ischemic Heart Disease

Title	a. Effects of carvedilol, a vasodilator-ß blocker, in patients with congestive heart failure due to ischemic heart disease. b. Randomized, placebo-controlled trial of carvedilol in patients with congestive heart failure due to ischaemic heart disease.
Authors	a. Australia-New Zealand Heart Failure Research Collaborative Group.
Reference	a. Circulation 1995;92:212-218. b. Lancet 1997;349:375-380.
Disease	Congestive heart failure.
Purpose	To evaluate the effects of carvedilol on symptoms, exercise performance, and left ventricular function in patients with heart failure due to coronary artery disease.
Design	Randomized, double blind, placebo-controlled, multicenter.
Patients	415 patients, with chronic stable heart failure NYHA class II or III due to ischemic heart disease, left ventricular ejection fraction of <45%. Patients with systolic blood pressure <90 mmHg, heart rate of <50 /min, heart block, coronary event or procedure within 4 weeks, primary myocardial or valvular disease, insulin dependent diabetes, chronic obstructive airway disease, renal impairment, current therapy with verapamil, β blockers, or agonists were excluded.
Follow-up	a. Clinical follow-up for 6 months and repeated exercise test, radionuclide ventriculography, and echocardiography at 6 months have been reported. b. Left ventricular radionuclide ventriculography, echocardiography, treadmill exercise duration, and clinical follow-up at baseline, 6 and 12 months. Average follow-up of 19 months.
Treatment regimen	2-3 weeks of open label carvedilol, started at 3.125 mgX2/d and increased to 6.25 mgX2/d. Patients who could tolerate the dose were randomized to placebo or carvedilol with gradual increments of the dose towards 25 mgX2/d
Additional therapy	Patients were treated with conventional therapy including angiotensin-converting enzyme inhibitors, diuretics, and digoxin.

Results   a. A total of 30 patients in the carvedilol vs 13 in the placebo group withdrew from the study (p=0.01), but no single cause accounted for the difference. After 6 months, left ventricular ejection fraction increased by 5.2% in the carvedilol group compared with placebo (95% CI 3.7%-6.8%, p<0.0001). Left ventricular end diastolic diameter did not change from baseline to 6 months of follow-up in the placebo group (68.1 vs 68.3 mm, respectively), whereas it decreased in the carvedilol group (69.5 mm at baseline vs 68.3 mm at 6 months, p=0.048 for the difference between the groups). Left ventricular end systolic diameter did not change in the placebo group (56.1 vs 56.1 mm, respectively) whereas it decreased in the carvedilol group (57.3 mm at baseline vs 55.0 mm at follow-up, p=0.0005 for the difference between the groups). There was no change in exercise time between the groups after 6 months (mean difference -22 seconds, 95% CI -59-15 seconds). There was no difference in 6 min walk distance between the groups (mean difference -6 meter, 95% CI -18-6 meter). The severity of symptoms was unchanged in 67% of the of the placebo vs 65% of the carvedilol-treated patients. However, 28% of the placebo vs 23% of the carvedilol patients were improved according to NYHA classification, while 5% vs 12% were worsened (p=0.05). The same trend was present using the Specific Activity Scale (p=0.02).

b. By the end of the follow-up, the numbers of withdrawals from the 2 groups were comparable (41 vs 30 in the carvedilol and placebo groups, respectively, p>0.1). After 12 months, left ventricular ejection fraction increased from 28.4% at baseline to 33.5% among the carvedilol assigned patients, whereas left ventricular ejection fraction did not change much in the placebo treated group. Therefore, at 12 months, left ventricular ejection fraction was 5.3% higher in the carvedilol than placebo group (p<0.0001). After 12 months, left ventricular end-diastolic and end-systolic dimensions were 1.7 mm (p=0.06) and 3.2 mm (p=0.001) smaller in the carvedilol compared with the placebo group. There was no clear differences between the groups in 6 min walk distance, treadmill exercise duration, NYHA class, or Specific Activity Scale. After 19 months, there was no difference between the groups in the incidence of worsening of heart failure (82 vs 75 of the carvedilol and placebo groups ; relative risk 1.12; 95% CI 0.82-1.53) and mortality (20 vs 26, respectively; relative risk 0.76; 95% CI 0.42-1.36; p>0.1). However, the rate of death or hospitalization was lower in the carvedilol group (104 vs 131; relative risk 0.74; 95% CI 0.57-0.95; p=0.02).

Conclusion   a. In patients with heart failure due to coronary artery disease, 6 month therapy with carvedilol improved left ventricular function, but symptoms were slightly worsened.
b. 12 months of carvedilol therapy resulted in improvement in left ventricular ejection fraction and a decrease in end-systolic and end-diastolic dimensions. There was an overall reduction in the combined end-point of death or hospitalization. However, there was no effect on mortality, exercise performance, symptoms, or episodes of worsening of heart failure.

Amiodarone in Patients with Congestive Heart Failure and Asymptomatic Ventricular Arrhythmia

Title	a. Amiodarone in patients with congestive heart failure and asymptomatic ventricular arrhythmia. b. Effect of amiodarone on clinical status and left ventricular function in patients with congestive heart failure.
Authors	a. Singh SN, Fletcher RD, Fisher SG, et al. b. Massie BM, Fisher SG, Deedwania PC, et al.
Reference	a. N Engl J Med 1995;333:77-82. b. Circulation 1996;93:2128-2134.
Disease	Congestive heart failure, arrhythmia.
Purpose	To evaluate the efficacy of amiodarone to reduce mortality in patients with heart failure and asymptomatic ventricular arrhythmias.
Design	Randomized, double blind, placebo-controlled, multicenter
Patients	674 patients with congestive heart failure, left ventricular ejection fraction of ≤0.40, and ≥10 PVCs/h, unaccompanied by symptoms.
Follow-up	Clinical follow-up and repeated 24 h ambulatory ECG monitoring for >1 year (median follow-up 45 months, range 0-54 months).
Treatment regimen	Placebo or amiodarone 800 mg/d for 14 days, then 400 mg/d for 50 weeks, and then 300 mg/d until the end of the study.
Additional treatment	All patients received vasodilator therapy. Digoxin and diuretics were permitted.

Results	During follow-up 39% of the amiodarone vs 42% of the placebo patients died (p=NS). The overall actuarial survival at 2 years was 69.4% vs 70.8%, respectively (p=0.6). At 2 years the rate of sudden death was 15% vs 19% in amiodarone and placebo (p=0.43). Amiodarone had no effect on mortality among patients with ischemic heart disease. However, there was a trend toward less mortality with amiodarone therapy among the 193 patients with nonischemic heart disease (p=0.07). Survival without cardiac death or hospitalization for heart failure was significantly reduced in amiodarone treated patients with nonischemic heart disease (relative risk 0.56 (95% CI 0.36-0.87); p=0.01), but not in patients with ischemic heart disease (relative risk 0.95 (0.73-1.24); p=0.69). Amiodarone was effective in suppressing ventricular arrhythmias. While left ventricular ejection fraction was comparable at baseline (24.9±8.3% in the amiodarone vs 25.7±8.2% in the placebo), ejection fraction was significantly improved in the amiodarone group (at 24 months 35.4±11.5% vs 29.8±12.2, p<0.001). However, this increase in ejection fraction was not associated with greater clinical improvement, less diuretic requirements, or fewer hospitalization for heart failure.
Conclusions	Although amiodarone therapy suppressed ventricular tachyarrhythmias and improved left ventricular function, it was not associated with improved outcome, except for reduction of cardiac mortality and hospitalization for heart failure among patients with nonischemic cardiomyopathy.

MEXIS

Metoprolol and Xamoterol Infarction Study

Title	a. Effects of ß receptor antagonists in patients with clinical evidence of heart failure after myocardial infarction: double blind comparison of metoprolol and xamoterol. b. Effects of β receptor antagonists on left ventricular function in patients with clinical evidence of heart failure after myocardial infarction. A double blind comparison of metoprolol and xamoterol. Echocardiographic results from the metoprolol and xamoterol infarction study (MEXIS).
Authors	a. Persson H, Rythe'n-Alder E, Melcher A, Erhardt L b. Persson H, Eriksson SV, Erhardt L.
Reference	a. Br Heart J 1995;74:140-148. b. Eur Heart J 1996;17:741-749.
Disease	Congestive heart failure.
Purpose	To compare the effects of xamoterol and metoprolol on exercise time in patients with mild to moderate heart failure after myocardial infarction.
Design	Randomized, double blind, single center.
Patients	210 patients, age 40-80 years, with evidence of heart failure at any time during the 5-7 days after myocardial infarction. patients with NYHA class IV, hypertrophic cardiomyopathy, aortic stenosis, pulmonary disease, or unstable angina were excluded.
Follow-up	12 months of clinical follow-up and repeated exercise test and echocardiography.
Treatment regimen	Metoprolol 50 mgX2/d or xamoterol 100 mgX2/d for 1 day, and then the dose was doubled. The lowest dose allowed was 50 mg/d metoprolol and 100 mg/d xamoterol.

Additional therapy	Diuretics, digitalis, nitrates, and angiotensin-converting enzyme inhibitors were allowed. Calcium channel blockers were not permitted.

Results	a. Exercise time increased at 3 months by 22% in the metoprolol and 29% in the xamoterol groups (p=NS). Improvements in quality of life, clinical signs of heart failure, and NYHA class were seen in both groups over 1 year. Breathlessness improved only with xamoterol (p=0.003 and p=0.046 vs metoprolol after 3 and 6 months, however, there was no difference at 12 months). 18 vs 22 patients of the metoprolol and xamoterol groups withdrew from the study during 1 year. 5 and 6 patients of the metoprolol and xamoterol patients died.
	b. In the xamoterol-treated patients, there was an increase in E-point septal separation from 12.2 mm at baseline to 13.2 mm after 12 months, whereas in the metoprolol group it decreased from 12.4 mm to 11.1 mm (p<0.005). Fractional shortening decreased in the xamoterol group (from 26.0% to 25.0%) and increased in the metoprolol group (from 25.8% to 26.9%) (p<0.05). There were no significant differences between the groups concerning left ventricular end systolic and end diastolic dimensions.

Conclusions	a. The efficacy of xamoterol and metoprolol in improving exercise tolerance, quality of life, and signs of heart failure were comparable.
	b. In contrast to metoprolol, xamoterol therapy was associated with impairment of left ventricualr systolic function in patients with heart failure after myocardial infarction.

Carvedilol Heart Failure Study

Title	The effect of carvedilol on morbidity and mortality in patients with chronic heart failure.
Authors	Packer M, Bristow MR, Cohn JN, et al.
Reference	N Engl J Med 1996;334:1349-1355.
Disease	Congestive heart failure.
Purpose	To evaluate the effects of carvedilol, a nonselective ß-blocker that also blocks α1-receptors and has antioxidant properties, on survival and hospitalization of patients with chronic heart failure.
Design	Randomized, double blind, placebo-controlled, multicenter.
Patients	1094 patients with symptomatic heart failure for ≥3 months and left ventricular ejection fraction ≤0.35, despite ≥2 months of treatment with diuretics and an angiotensin-converting enzyme inhibitor. Patients with primary valvular heart disease, active myocarditis, ventricular tachycardia or advanced heart block not controlled by antiarrhythmic intervention, or a pacemaker were excluded. Patients with systolic blood pressure >160 or <85 mmHg, heart rate <68 bpm, major cardiovascular event or surgery within 3 months, comorbidity that could affect survival or limit exercise capacity, or patients treated with ß blocker, calcium channel antagonist or class IC or III antiarrhythmics were not included.
Follow-up	6 months (12 months for the group with mild heart failure).

Treatment regimen	During the open-label phase, all patients received carvedilol 6.25 mgX2/d for 2 weeks. Patients who tolerated the drug were randomized on the basis of their baseline exercise capacity to 1 of 4 treatment protocols. Within each of the 4 protocols patients with mild, moderate, or severe heart failure were randomized to either carvedilol 12.5-50 mgX2/d or placebo.
Additional therapy	Treatment with digoxin, hydralazine, or nitrate were permitted.
Results	Of the 1197 patients that had entered the open-label phase, 5.6% failed to complete the period due to adverse effects. Another 3.0% violated the protocol. 1094 patients were randomized to the double blind stage. The overall mortality was 7.8% in the placebo and 3.2% in the carvedilol group (65% reduction of risk, 95% CI 39-80%; p<0.001). Death from progressive heart failure was 3.3% in the placebo vs 0.7% in the carvedilol group. Sudden death occurred in 3.8% vs 1.7% of the placebo and carvedilol groups. The reduction in mortality was similar regardless of age, sex, the cause of heart failure, ejection fraction, exercise tolerance, systolic blood pressure, or heart rate. During the follow-up 19.6% vs 14.1% of the placebo and carvedilol groups were hospitalized at least once for cardiovascular causes (27% reduction of risk, 95% CI 3-45%; p=0.036). The combined end-point of hospitalization for cardiovascular causes or death was reduced by 38% (24.6% vs 15.8% in the placebo and carvedilol group; 95% CI 18-53%, p<0.001).
Conclusions	Carvedilol reduces the risk of death and the risk of hospitalization for cardiovascular causes in patients with heart failure who are receiving treatment with digoxin, diuretics, and angiotensin-converting enzyme inhibitor.

MOCHA

Multicenter Oral Carvedilol Heart failure Assessment

Title	Carvedilol produces dose related improvements in left ventricular function and survival in subjects with chronic heart failure.
Authors	Bristow MR, Gilbert EM, Abraham WT, et al.
Reference	Circulation 1996;94:2807-2816.
Disease	Congestive heart failure.
Purpose	To assess the dose response characteristics of carvedilol in patients with chronic heart failure.
Design	Randomized, double blind, placebo-controlled, dose response evaluation, multicenter.
Patients	345 patients, aged 18 to 85 years, with left ventricular ejection fraction ≤0.35 and symptoms of stable heart failure for ≥3 months. All patients had to be treated with diuretics and angiotensin-converting enzyme inhibitor for ≥1 month before entry. Patients had to be able to walk 150 to 450 m on the 6 min walk test. Patients with heart rate <68 bpm, uncorrected valvular disease, hypertrophic cardiomyopathy, uncontrolled ventricular tachycardia, sick sinus syndrome, advanced AV block, symptomatic peripheral vascular disease, severe concomitant disease, a stroke or myocardial infarction within 3 months, hypertension or hypotension were excluded. A PTCA, CABG or transplantation could not be planned or be likely for the 6 months after entry. Only patients that completed a 2 to 4 week challenge phase of open-label carvedilol 6.25 mgX2/d were included.
Follow-up	6 months.

MOCHA

Multicenter Oral Carvedilol Heart failure Assessment
(continued)

Treatment regimen	Randomization to: 1. Placebo; 2. Carvedilol 6.25 mgX2/d; 3. Carvedilol 12.5 mgX2/d; or 4. Carvedilol 25 mgX2/d.
Additional therapy	Diuretic therapy was mandatory. Angiotensin-converting enzyme inhibitors were recommended. Digoxin, hydralazine and nitrates were permitted, if they had been started ≥ 2 months before entry. Calcium channel blockers, flosequinan, α or ß blockers, anti-arrhythmic agents, and monoamine oxidase inhibitors were not permitted.
Results	92% of subjects tolerated the open-label challenge period. Carvedilol therapy was not associated with an improvement in either the 6 min corridor walk test or the 9 min self-powered treadmill test. Similarly, there was no difference in the Minnesota Living With Heart Failure Questionnaire scores among the groups. However, carvedilol therapy resulted in a dose related increase in left ventricular ejection fraction (by 5, 6, and 8% ejection fraction units in the low, medium, and high dose carvedilol, compared with only 2 units in the placebo group; $p<0.001$ for the linear dose response). Carvedilol improved ejection fraction both in patients with ischemic and with nonischemic cardiomyopathy. Carvedilol therapy was associated with lower cardiovascular hospitalization rate (mean number of hospitalization per patient 0.36, 0.14, 0.15, and 0.13, for the placebo, lower, medium and high carvedilol dose, respectively; $p=0.003$ for linear trend). Moreover, carvedilol reduced mortality (from 15.5% in the placebo group to 6.0% ($p<0.05$), 6.7% ($p=0.07$), and 1.1% ($p<0.001$) in the low, medium and high carvedilol dose; $p<0.001$ for the linear trend). The reduction in mortality occurred both in patients with ischemic and nonischemic cardiomyopathy. When the 3 carvedilol groups were combined, mortality risk was 73% lower than in the placebo group (relative risk 0.272; 95% CI 0.124 to 0.597; $p<0.001$).
Conclusions	In subjects with mild to moderate heart failure due to systolic dysfunction and who can tolerate carvedilol therapy, carvedilol treatment resulted in dose related improvement in LV function and reduction in mortality and hospitalization rates.

US Carvedilol Heart Failure Study

Title	Carvedilol inhibits clinical progression in patients with mild symptoms of heart failure.
Authors	Colucci WS, Packer M, Bristow MR, et al.
Reference	Circulation 1996;94:2800-2806.
Disease	Congestive heart failure.
Purpose	To evaluate the effect of carvedilol in patients with mildly symptomatic heart failure.
Design	Randomized, double blind, placebo-controlled, dose response evaluation, multicenter.
Patients	366 patients, 18-85 years old, with chronic stable symptomatic heart failure despite treatment with diuretics and an angiotensin-converting enzyme inhibitor, and left ventricular ejection fraction ≤ 0.35. Patients with primary valvular disease; hypertrophic cardiomyopathy; symptomatic ventricular arrhythmias; myocardial infarction, unstable angina or CABG within 3 months; likelihood for revascularization or transplantation within 12 months; sick sinus syndrome or high degree AV block; hypotension or hypertension; or serious concomitant disease were excluded. Only patients who were able to walk 450-550 m on a 6 min walk test and tolerated a carvedilol 6.25 mgX2/d during a 2 week challenge open label phase were included in this protocol.
Follow-up	12 months of maintenance phase.

Treatment regimen	Randomization in a 2:1 ratio to carvedilol (n=232) or placebo (n=134). There was an initial 2–6 week double blind up-titration phase, beginning at 12.5 mgX2/d (maximum 25 mgX2/d for patients <85 kg; 50 mgX2/d for heavier patients).
Additional therapy	Diuretics and an angiotesnin converting enzyme inhibitor. Digoxin, hydralazine, and nitrates were allowed. Antiarrhythmic drugs, calcium channel blockers, α or ß blockers, flosequinan, and monoamine oxidase inhibitors were prohibited.
Results	Clinical progression of heart failure (defined as death due to heart failure, hospitalization for heart failure, or the need for a sustained increase in heart failure medications) occurred in 21% of the placebo group and in 11% of the carvedilol group (relative risk 0.52; 95% CI 0.32 to 0.85; p=0.008). This favorable effect was not influenced by gender, age, race, etiology of heart failure, or baseline left ventricular ejection fraction. 4.0% vs 0.9% of the placebo and carvedilol treated patients died (risk ratio 0.231; 95% CI 0.045 to 1.174; p=0.048). NYHA functional class improved in 12% of the carvedilol-treated patients vs 9% of the placebo-treated patients, whereas it worsened in 4% vs 15%, respectively (p=0.003). During the study more carvedilol than placebo treated patients stated that their symptoms improved (75% vs 60%; p=0.013). Similarly, the physician global assessment rated improvement in 69% vs 47% of the patients, respectively (p=0.001). However, there was no difference in the quality of life scores and the distance walked in 9 min treadmill test between the groups. At follow-up, the mean increase in left ventricular ejection fraction was larger in the carvedilol (0.10) than in the placebo (0.03) patients (p<0.001). The drug was well tolerated.
Conclusions	In patients with mildly symptomatic stable heart failure due to systolic dysfunction and who could tolerate carvedilol treatment, carvedilol reduced clinical progression of heart failure and mortality.

PRECISE

Prospective Randomized Evaluation of Carvedilol on Symptoms and Exercise

Title	Double blind, placebo-controlled study of the effects of carvedilol in patients with moderate to severe heart failure. The Precise Trial.
Authors	Packer M, Colucci WS, Sackner-Bernstein JD, et al.
Reference	Circulation 1996;94:2793-2799.
Disease	Congestive heart failure.
Purpose	To evaluate the effect of carvedilol in patients with moderate to severe heart failure.
Design	Randomized, double blind, placebo-controlled, dose response evaluation, multicenter.
Patients	278 patients, with chronic stable symptomatic heart failure despite treatment with diuretics and an angiotensin-converting enzyme inhibitor for ≥2 months, and left ventricular ejection fraction ≤0.35. Patients with primary valvular disease; active myocarditis; restrictive or hypertrophic cardiomyopathy; symptomatic ventricular arrhythmias; myocardial infarction, unstable angina or CABG within 3 months; angina that limits exercise capacity; sick sinus syndrome or high degree AV block; hypotension or hypertension; stroke; peripheral vascular or pulmonary disease; or serious concomitant disease were excluded. Patients receiving antiarrhythmic drugs, calcium channel blockers, or α or ß blockers or agonists, were not included. Only patients who were able to walk 150–450 m on a 6 min walk test and tolerated carvedilol 6.25 mgX2/d during a 2 week challenge open label phase were included in this protocol.
Follow-up	Maintenance phase of 6 months.

PRECISE

Prospective Randomized Evaluation of Carvedilol on Symptoms and Exercise

(continued)

Treatment regimen	Randomization to placebo or carvedilol 12.5 mgX2/d. The dose was increased gradually to 25 mgX2/d (50 mgX2/d for patients >85 kg)
Additional therapy	Diuretics and an angiotensin-converting enzyme inhibitor. Digoxin, hydralazine, and nitrates were allowed. Anti-arrhythmic drugs, calcium channel blockers, α or ß blockers, or agonists were prohibited.
Results	Of the 301 patients entering the open-label phase, 23 (8%) did not complete it (17 patients due to adverse effects). By intention-to-treat analysis, the 6 min walk distance increased by 9 meters in the carvedilol and decreased by 3 meters in the placebo group (p=0.048). There was no difference between the groups on the 9 min treadmill test and in quality of life scores. Carvedilol was associated with greater improvement in NYHA class (p=0.014). Whereas the proportion of patients with NYHA class III or IV remains unchanged in the placebo group (from 58% to 51%), it decreased in the carvedilol treated patients (from 64% to 41%). A deterioration in NYHA class was observed in 3% of the carvedilol group vs 15% of the placebo group (p=0.001). Global assessment of disease severity by the patients and by the physicians revealed greater improvement with carvedilol than placebo. Left ventricular ejection fraction increased by 0.08 and 0.03 U with carvedilol and placebo therapy (p<0.001). 16.5% of the carvedilol-treated patients vs 25.5% of the placebo group had a cardiovascular hospitalization (p=0.06), and 4.5% vs 7.6% died (p=0.26). Death or cardiovascular hospitalization occurred in 19.6% of the carvedilol group vs 31.0% of the placebo group (p=0.029). The effects of carvedilol were similar in patients with ischemic or nonischemic cardiomyopathy.
Conclusions	In patients with moderate to severe stable heart failure due to systolic dysfunction who are treated with diuretics, angiotensin-converting enzyme inhibitors and digoxin, and can tolerate carvedilol treatment, carvedilol produces clinical benefits.

DiDi

Diltiazem in Dilated Cardiomyopathy

Title	Diltiazem improves cardiac function and exercise capacity in patients with idiopathic dilated cardiomyopathy. Results of the diltiazem in dilated cardiomyopathy trial.
Authors	Figulla HR, Gietzen F, Zeymer U, et al.
Reference	Circulation 1996;94:346-352.
Disease	Dilated cardiomyopathy.
Purpose	To evaluate whether diltiazem in addition to conventional therapy improves survival, hemodynamics, and well-being in patients with idiopathic dilated cardiomyopathy.
Design	Randomized, double blind, placebo-controlled, multicenter.
Patients	186 patients, 18-70 years old, with idiopathic dilated cardiomyopathy (LVEF<0.50). Patients with hypertension, 2nd or 3rd degree AV block, valvular or congenital heart disease, coronary artery disease, active myocarditis, insulin dependent diabetes, or systemic disease were excluded. Patients with previous treatment with any calcium antagonist or ß-blocker for >3 months were not included.
Follow-up	Coronary angiography with left heart catheterization, pulmonary artery catheterization at rest and during supine ergometry, 24 h ambulatory ECG monitoring, echocardiography, radionuclide ventriculography, endomyocardial biopsy, plasma norepinephrine and ergorespirometry at baseline. Patients were followed every 6 months for 2 years.
Treatment regimen	Placebo or diltiazem started at 30 mgX3/d. Target dose was 90 mgX3/d or 60 mgX3/d (for patients weighing ≤50 kg).

DiDi

Diltiazem in Dilated Cardiomyopathy

(continued)

Additional therapy	Any other calcium antagonist or ß blocker was prohibited. ACE inhibitors, digitalis, diuretics, and nitrates were prescribed as needed.
Results	33 patients dropped out of the study (13 receiving placebo and 20 receiving diltiazem). 24 month survival was 80.6% for the placebo vs 83.3% for the diltiazem group (p=0.78). Of the 153 patients that finished the protocol, 27 died or had a listing for heart transplantation (16 in the placebo and 11 in the diltiazem). The transplant listing-free survival was 85% for diltiazem vs 80% for the placebo (p=0.44). After 2 years, only the diltiazem group had an increase in cardiac index at rest (0.37±1.40 vs 0.33±1.14 L/min in the placebo, p=0.011), cardiac index at workload (0.57±1.52 vs 0.33±1.81 L/min, p=0.017), stroke volume index (8±24 vs 3±18 mL/m2, p=0.003), and stroke work index (15±31 vs 5±20 g • min • m-2, p=0.000), and decreased pulmonary artery pressure under workload (-5.2±12.2 vs -3.4±10.9 mmHg, p=0.007). Diltiazem increased exercise capacity (180±450 vs 60±325 W • min, p=0.002), and subjective well being (p= 0.01). Adverse effects were minor and evenly distributed in both groups.
Conclusions	Diltiazem improves cardiac function, exercise capacity, and subjective status in patients with idiopathic dilated cardiomyopathy without deleterious effects on transplant listing-free survival.

PRAISE

Prospective Randomized Amlodipine Survival Evaluation trial

Title	Effect of amlodipine on morbidity and mortality in severe chronic heart failure.
Authors	Packer M, O'Connor CM, Ghali JK, et al.
Reference	N Engl J Med 1996;335:1107-1114.
Disease	Congestive Heart failure.
Purpose	To evaluate the long-term effect of amlodipine, a calcium channel blocker, on mortality and morbidity in patients with advanced congestive heart failure.
Design	Randomized, double blind, placebo-controlled, multicenter.
Patients	1153 patients with congestive heart failure (NYHA class IIIB or IV) and left ventricular ejection fraction <0.30, despite therapy with digoxin, diuretics, and an angiotensin-converting-enzyme inhibitor. Patients with uncorrected primary valvular disease, active myocarditis, constrictive pericarditis, history of cardiac arrest or who had sustained ventricular fibrillation or tachycardia within the previous year, unstable angina or acute myocardial infarction within the previous month, cardiac revascularization or stroke within 3 months, severe concomitant disease, hypotension or hypertension, or serum creatinine >3.0 mg/dL were excluded.
Follow-up	6 to 33 months (median 13.8 months).
Treatment regimen	Randomization to amlodipine or placebo. The initial dose of amlodipine was 5 mg X1/d for two weeks and than increased to 10 mg/d.
Additional therapy	Diuretics, digoxin, and an angiotensin-converting-enzyme inhibitor. Nitrates were permitted, but other vasodilators, β blockers, calcium channel blockers, and, class IC antiarrhythmic agents were prohibited.

PRAISE

Prospective Randomized Amlodipine Survival Evaluation trial (continued)

Results	Of the patients with ischemic heart disease, 370 were assigned to placebo and 362 to amlodipine. Of the patients with nonischemic cardiomyopathy, 212 were assigned to placebo and 209 patients to amlodipine. A primary end point of the study (mortality from all causes or cardiovascular morbidity, defined as hospitalization for $\geq$24 h for pulmonary edema, severe hypoperfusion, acute myocardial infarction, or ventricular tachycardia/ fibrillation) was reached by 39% of the amlodipine-treated patients and in 42% of the placebo group. Amlodipine therapy was associated with insignificant risk reduction of primary end-points (9%; 95% CI 24% reduction to 10% increase; p=0.31). 33% vs 38% of the amlodipine and control groups died, respectively (16% risk reduction; 95% CI 31% reduction to 2% increase; p=0.07). Among patients with ischemic etiology, amlodipine therapy did not affect mortality or the combined end-point of mortality and cardiovascular morbidity. 45% of the patients in both groups had a fatal or non fatal event, and 40% of the patients in both groups died. However, in patients with nonischemic cardiomyopathy amlodipine was associated with better outcome. Primary endpoint was reached by 36.8% of the placebo, but in only 27.8% of the amlodipine group (31% risk reduction; 95% CI 2% to 51% reduction; p=0.04). Mortality was 34.9% vs 21.5% in the placebo and amlodipine group, respectively (46% risk reduction; 95% CI 21% to 63% reduction; p<0.001). Subgroup analysis revealed that amlodipine therapy was not associated with adverse effects in any of the subgroups. A favorable effect on survival was found only in patients without a history of angina. Total adverse effects that mandated discontinuation of double blind therapy was comparable between the groups. However, peripheral edema (27% vs 18%, p<0.001) and pulmonary edema (15% vs 10%, p=0.01) occurred more frequently in the amlodipine group, while uncontrolled hypertension (2% vs <1%, p=0.03) and symptomatic cardiac ischemia (31% vs 25% among patients with ischemic heart disease, p=0.07) was more frequent in the placebo than amlodipine group. The frequencies of myocardial infarction, arrhythmias, and worsening of heart failure were similar.
Conclusions	Amlodipine was not associated with increased mortality and morbidity among patients with severe congestive heart failure. Amlodipine was associated with better outcome in patients with nonischemic cardiomyopathy, whereas in patients with ischemic heart disease there was no difference in outcome.

Note: Amlodipine is not indicated for CHF.

PICO

Pimobendan In COngestive heart failure

Title	Effect of pimobendan on exercise capacity in patients with heart failure: main results from the pimobendan in congestive heart failure (PICO) trial.
Authors	The Pimobendan in Congestive Heart Failure (PICO) Investigators.
Reference	Heart 1996;76:223-231.
Disease	Congestive heart failure.
Purpose	To assess the effects of pimobendan, a positive inotropic agent, on exercise capacity in patients with congestive heart failure.
Design	Randomized, double blind, placebo-controlled, multicenter.
Patients	317 patients, ≥18 years old, with stable chronic heart failure (NYHA class II-III), and left ventricular ejection fraction of ≤0.45. Patients with stenotic, obstructive, or infectious cardiac disease, exercise capacity limited by angina, on waiting list for transplantation, acute myocardial infarction, coronary revascularization, episodes of syncope or cardiac arrest within 3 months, AICD implantation, or severe concomitant disease were excluded. Patients in whom a first testing dose of pimobendan caused significant intolerance were excluded.
Follow-up	24 weeks of therapy with repeated exercise tests (efficacy phase). Clinical follow-up for a mean of 11 months.
Treatment regimen	Randomized to placebo or pimobendan 1.25 or 2.5 mg twice a day.

PICO

Pimobendan In COngestive heart failure

(continued)

Additional therapy	An angiotensin-converting enzyme inhibitor and a diuretic were mandatory. Digitalis, nitrates, and molsidomine were permitted. Other inotropic agents, phosphodiesterase inhibitors, ibopamine, antiarrhythmic agents (except amiodarone), ß blockers, calcium antagonists, and other vasodilators were prohibited.
Results	Exercise duration on bicycle ergometry of the 2.5 mg/d pimobendan-treated patients was 13, 27, and 29 sec longer than that of the placebo-treated patients, after 4, 12, and 24 weeks of therapy, respectively (p=0.03), and in the 5 mg/d treated patients it was 19, 17, and 28 sec longer than that of the placebo group (p=0.05). After 24 weeks of therapy there was no difference in the percent of patients still alive and able to exercise to at least the baseline level (63% of the pimobendan group vs 59% of the placebo group; p=0.5). Pimobendan did not affect oxygen consumption or quality of life (assessed by questionnaire). 4% of the placebo vs 10% of the pimobendan-treated patients did not worsen or die and were in better NYHA class at least once during follow-up than at baseline (p=0.06). Double blind therapy was stopped or reduced more often in the pimobendan than placebo treated group (p=0.04). All cause mortality after a mean of 11 months of follow-up was lower in the placebo group (10.8 per 100 person-years) than in the pimobendan treated patients (21.3 and 17.4 per 100 person-years in the 2.5 mg/d and 5 mg/d groups) (Hazard ratio of the pimobendan 2.5 mg/d 2.0; 95% CI 0.9 to 4.1; and that of the 5.0 mg/d 1.6; 95% CI 0.7 to 3.4). When both pimobendan groups were combined, the hazard ratio of death was 1.8 (95% CI 0.9–3.5) times higher than in the placebo group.
Conclusions	Pimobendan therapy in patients with congestive heart failure and left ventricular ejection fraction ≤0.45 was associated with an increase in exercise capacity. However, there was a trend towards an increased mortality in the treated patients.

DIG

The Digitalis Investigation Group study

Title	The effect of digoxin on mortality and morbidity in patients with heart failure.
Authors	The Digitalis Investigation Group.
Reference	N Engl J Med 1997;336:525-533.
Disease	Congestive heart failure
Purpose	To assess the effects of digoxin on morbidity and mortality in patients with heart failure and normal sinus rhythm.
Design	Randomized, double blind, placebo-controlled, multicenter.
Patients	6800 patients with left ventricular ejection fraction of ≤0.45 and 988 patients with left ventricular ejection fraction of >0.45. All patients had heart failure and were in sinus rhythm.
Follow-up	The mean duration of follow-up was 37 months (28 to 58 months).
Treatment regimen	Digoxin or placebo.
Additional therapy	Angiotensin-converting-enzyme inhibitors were encouraged. If patients remained symptomatic despite efforts to optimize other forms of therapy, open-label digoxin therapy was allowed and the study drug was discontinued.

DIG

The Digitalis Investigation Group study
(continued)

Results   In patients with ejection fraction ≤0.45, the mortality was similar (34.8% with digoxin and 35.1% with placebo, risk ratio 0.99; 95% CI 0.91-1.07, p=0.80). Cardiovascular mortality was similar (29.9% vs 29.5% in the digoxin and placebo group, respectively). There was a trend toward lower mortality ascribed to worsening of heart failure among the digoxin treated patients (11.6% vs 13.2%; risk ratio 0.88; 95% CI 0.77-1.01; p=0.06). Hospitalization rate due to cardiovascular reasons was lower in the digoxin treated group (49.9% vs 54.4%, risk ratio 0.87; 95% CI 0.81-0.93; p<0.001). Hospitalization rate due to worsening of heart failure was lower in the digoxin group (26.8% vs 34.7%, respectively; risk ratio 0.72; 95% CI 0.66-0.79; p<0.001). There was no significant difference between the 2 groups in hospitalization rate for ventricular arrhythmia or cardiac arrest (4.2% vs 4.3%). In all, 64.3% of the digoxin and 67.1% of the placebo group were hospitalized (risk ratio 0.92; 95% CI 0.87-0.98; p=0.006). There was no difference in hospitalization rate for myocardial infarction or unstable angina and for non cardiovascular reasons. At 1 year, 85.6% and 82.9% of the digoxin and placebo treated patients were taking the study medication. At the final study visit, 70.8% of the surviving digoxin-treated patients were taking study medication and an additional 10.3% received open-label digoxin. In the placebo-group, 67.9% of the patients that were alive were taking placebo and 15.6% received open-label digoxin. In the cohort of patients with left ventricular ejection fraction >0.45, mortality was 23.4% in both groups. The combined end-point of death or hospitalization for worsening of heart failure occurred less in the digoxin-treated patients (risk ratio 0.82; 95% CI 0.63-1.07).

Conclusions   Digoxin therapy in patients with heart failure and left ventricular ejection fraction ≤0.45 was associated with lower rates of overall hospitalization and hospitalization due worsening of heart failure. There was no difference in mortality and occurrence of myocardial ischemia or arrhythmia between the digoxin and placebo groups.

ELITE

Evaluation of Losartan In The Elderly

Title	Randomized trial of losartan vs captopril in patients ≥65 with heart failure (Evaluation of Losartan in the Elderly study, ELITE).
Authors	Pitt B, Martinez FA, Meurers GG, et al.
Reference	Lancet 1997;349:747-752.
Disease	Congestive heart failure.
Purpose	To compare the efficacy and safety of losartan (a specific angiotensin II receptor blocker) and captopril (an angiotensin-converting enzyme inhibitor) in the treatment of elderly patients with heart failure.
Patients	722 patients, ≥65 years old, with symptomatic heart failure (NYHA class II-IV), left ventricular ejection fraction ≤0.40, and no history of prior angiotensin-converting enzyme inhibitor therapy. Patients with systolic blood pressure <90 mmHg or diastolic blood pressure >95 mmHg, significant obstructive valvular heart disease, symptomatic arrhythmias, pericarditis or myocarditis, PTCA within 72h, CABG within 2 weeks, ICD within 2 weeks, likelihood for cardiac surgery during the study period, acute myocardial infarction within 72 h, unstable angina within 3 months, stable angina, stroke or transient ischemic attack within 3 months, concomitant severe disease, creatinine ≥2.5 mg/dl, anemia, leukopenia, and electrolyte disturbances were excluded.
Follow-up	48 weeks.
Treatment regimen	A 2 week placebo run-in phase, and then randomization to captopril (6.25 mg-50 mgX3/d) plus placebo losartan, or placebo captopril plus losartan (12.5-50 mgX1/d).

ELITE

Evaluation of Losartan In The Elderly
(continued)

Additional therapy	Treatment with all other cardiovascular medications (except open-label angiotensin-converting enzyme inhibitors) was permitted.
Results	352 patients were randomized to losartan and 370 to captopril. Persisting increases in serum creatinine (≥ 0.3 mg/dl) occurred in 10.5% in each group (risk reduction 2%; 95% CI -51% to 36%; p=0.63). Death and/or admissions for heart failure occurred in 9.4% in the losartan group vs 13.2% in the captopril group (risk reduction 32%; 95% CI -4% to 55%; p=0.075). Mortality was 4.8% in the losartan group vs 8.7% in the captopril group (risk reduction 46%; 95% CI 5% to 69%; p=0.035). Sudden death occurred in 1.4% vs 3.8%, respectively (risk reduction 64%; 95% CI 3% to 86%). The cumulative survival curves separated early and remained separated throughout the study. 22.2% of the losartan group vs 29.7% of the captopril group were admitted to the hospital for any reason (risk reduction 26%; 95% CI 5% to 43%; p=0.014). However, there was no difference in admission for heart failure (5.7% in each group; p=0.89). NYHA class improved in both treatment groups. The percentage of patients in NYHA class I or II was increased from 66% at baseline to 80% at the end of the study in the losartan group, and from 64%-81% in the captopril group. 18.5% of the losartan group vs 30% of the captopril group discontinued the study medication or died (p$\leq$0.001). 12.2% vs 20.8% of the patients, respectively, discontinued the study medication because of adverse effects (p$\leq$0.002). Cough leading to discontinuation of therapy was reported in 0 vs 3.8%, respectively. Persistent (≥ 0.5 mmol/L) increases in serum potassium was observed in 18.8% of the losartan group vs 22.7% of the captopril group (p=0.069).
Conclusions	Losartan therapy was associated with lower mortality and hospitalization rate than captopril therapy in elderly patients with symptomatic heart failure. Losartan was better tolerated than captopril.

NETWORK

Clinical Outcome with Enalapril in Symptomatic Chronic Heart Failure

Title	a. The NETWORK study: rationale, design, and methods of a trial evaluating the dose of enalapril in patients with heart failure. b. Clinical outcome with enalapril in symptomatic chronic heart failure; a dose comparison.
Authors	a. Long C, on behalf of the Steering Committee of the Network Study. b. The NETWORK investigators
Reference	a. B J Clin Res 1995;6:179-189. b. Eur Heart J 1998;481-489.
Disease	Congestive heart failure.
Purpose	To study the relationship between enalapril dose and the incidence of mortality, heart failure related hospitalizations and progression of disease in patients with symptomatic heart failure.
Design	Randomized, double blind, parallel group, multicenter.
Patients	1532 patients, aged 18-85 years, with symptomatic heart failure (NYHA class II-IV). Patients with significant valvular disease, unstable angina, recent myocardial infarction, uncontrolled hypertension, hypotension, severe pulmonary disease, hypokalemia, renal failure, previous ACE inhibitor therapy, or contraindications to ACE inhibition were excluded.
Follow-up	6 months.

Clinical Outcome with Enalapril in Symptomatic Chronic Heart Failure

(continued)

Treatment regimen	Randomization to enalapril 2.5 mg BID (group I), 5 mg BID (group II) and 10 mg BID (group III).
Results	99.8%, 95.9%, and 84.7% reached the target dose level in group I, II and III, respectively. Less patients in group III were on study drug at the end of 24 weeks follow-up period (73%) than in group II (81%) or group I (81%). There was no relationship between enalapril dose and clinical event rates. The primary end-point (death, heart failure related hospitalizations, and progression of heart failure) occurred in 12.3%, 12.9% and 14.7% of group I, II and III, respectively. Worsening of heart failure in 7.7%, 7.8% and 7.8%, respectively; hospitalization due to heart failure in 5.1%, 5.5% and 7.0%, respectively; and death in 4.2%, 3.3% and 2.9%, respectively. The percentages of patients with improvement in NYHA class were 34%, 33% and 31%, respectively. Deterioration by 1 NYHA grade occurred in 5.3%, 4.9% and 2.7%.
Conclusions	Increasing the enalapril dose from 2.5 mg BID to 10 mg BID did not result in better clinical outcome in patients with heart failure.

PRIME II

The Second Prospective Randomized Study of Ibopamine on Mortality and Efficacy

Title	Randomized study of effect of ibopamine on survival in patients with advanced severe heart failure.
Authors	Hampton, JR, van Veldhuisen DJ, Kleber FX, et al.
Reference	Lancet 1997;349:971-977.
Disease	Congestive heart failure.
Purpose	To investigate the efficacy of ibopamine, an agonist of dopaminergic DA-1 and DA-2 receptors that causes peripheral and renal vasodilatation, on survival in patients with advanced heart failure.
Design	Randomized, placebo-controlled, multicenter.
Patients	1906 patients, aged 18-80 years, with advanced severe heart failure (NYHA class III or IV), despite therapy with angiotensin-converting enzyme inhibitor, diuretics, digoxin or other vasodilators. Patients with obstructive valve disease, obstructive or restrictive cardiomyopathy, any potential transient cause of heart failure, myocardial infarction within 3 months, unstable angina, uncontrolled arrhythmias, current need for intravenous inotropic agents, pregnancy or lactation, intolerance to dopamine or dobutamine, and concomitant therapy with agents that interact with ibopamine were excluded.
Follow-up	An average of 363 days in the placebo group and 347 days in the ibopamine group.
Treatment regimen	Oral ibopamine 100 mg TID or placebo for >6 months.

PRIME II

The Second Prospective Randomized Study of Ibopamine on Mortality and Efficacy

(continued)

Results   The study was terminated prematurely by the safety committee due to a significantly higher mortality rate among the ibopamine-treated patients than among the placebo-treated group. The interim analysis revealed that 24.3% of the ibopamine vs 20.3% of the placebo group died (relative risk 1.26; 95% CI 1.04 to 1.53; p=0.017). Kaplan-Meier survival curve revealed that survival was similar in both groups for the first 3 months of therapy, and then diverged. Sudden death tended to be more common in the ibopamine group (29.8% of all fatality cases) than in the placebo group (23.8%). However, death due to progression of heart failure was comparable (47.0% vs 45.6%, respectively). In contrast, death due to acute myocardial infarction tended to occur less in the ibopamine group (6.5%) than in the placebo group (10.9%). Admission to the hospital was comparable (46% vs 44% in the ibopamine and placebo groups, respectively; relative risk 1.13; 95% CI 0.99 to 1.29). The patients' self-assessment scores of symptoms in the 2 groups were similar. There was no difference between the groups in the distribution between the NYHA classes. In multivariate analysis, only the use of antiarrhythmic drugs at baseline was independently associated with increased fatality with ibopamine therapy.

Conclusions   Ibopamine therapy increased mortality without improvement in NYHA class or the patients' self-assessment scores among patients with advanced congestive heart failure. Antiarrhythmic therapy was the only independent predictor of adverse outcome with ibopamine treatment.

V-HeFT III

Vasodilator - Heart Failure Trial III

Title	Effect of the calcium antagonist felodipine as supplementary vasodilator therapy in patients with chronic heart failure treated with enalapril.
Author	Cohn JN, Ziesche S, Smith R, et al.
Reference	Circulation 1997; 96:856-863.
Disease	Chronic heart failure.
Purpose	1. To determine whether addition of the calcium channel blocker felodipine extended release (ER) to enalapril could improve short-term symptoms and exercise capacity over 3 months. 2. To determine with felodipine (ER) could slow the progression of heart failure and improve long-term morbidity and mortality.
Design	Randomized, double blind, multicenter.
Patients	450 male patients with chronic heart failure, average age 63-64.
Follow-up	Average 18 months (range 3 - 39 months).
Treatment regimen	97% of patients were on enalapril, 89% on diuretics. Patients were randomized to felodipine ER (5 mg bid) or placebo.

V-HeFT III

Vasodilator - Heart Failure Trial III

(continued)

Results   There was no difference in long-term mortality in the felodipine (13.8%) vs placebo group (12.8%). At 3 months felodipine increased ejection fraction (+2.1%) compared to placebo (-0.1%, p=.001), but did not improve exercise tolerance, quality of life, or frequency of hospitalizations. There was a trend toward better exercise tolerance and quality of life in the second year of treatment. At 27 months exercise times were significantly better with felodipine than placebo (p=.01). At 12 months there was no significant difference in ejection fraction between the 2 groups. Edema was more common with felodipine.

Conclusions   Felodipine resulted in a trend toward better exercise tolerance and less depression of quality of life in the second year of treatment. It was well tolerated in heart failure patients but not effective in reducing mortality or improving ejection fraction long term.

7. Lipid Lowering Studies

POSCH

Program On the Surgical Control of the Hyperlipidemias

Title	Effect of partial ileal bypass surgery on mortality and morbidity from coronary heart disease in patients with hypercholesterolemia. Report of the Program on the Surgical Control of the Hyperlipidemias (POSCH).
Authors	Buchwald H, Varco RL, Matts JP, et al.
Reference	N Engl J Med 1990;323:946-955.
Disease	Hyperlipidemia, coronary artery disease.
Purpose	To evaluate whether cholesterol lowering induced by the partial ileal bypass operation would reduce mortality or morbidity due to coronary heart disease.
Design	Randomized, open label.
Patients	838 patients, 30-64 years of age, 6-60 months after a single myocardial infarction with total plasma cholesterol> 5.69 mmol/l or LDL cholesterol> 3.62 mmol/l. Patients with hypertension, diabetes mellitus, or obesity were excluded.
Follow-up	7-14.8 years (mean 9.7 years).
Treatment regimen	Partial ileal bypass of either the distal 200 cm or 1/3 of the small intestine, whichever was greater.
Additional therapy	American Heart Association Phase II diet. Hypocholesterolemic medications were discontinued.

POSCH

Program On the Surgical Control of the Hyperlipidemias

(continued)

Results
: 5 years after randomization the surgical group had lower total plasma cholesterol (4.71±0.91 vs 6.14±0.89 mmol/l; p<0.0001) and LDL-cholesterol (2.68±0.78 vs 4.30±0.89 mmol/l; p<0.0001); while HDL-cholesterol was higher (1.08±0.26 vs. 1.04±0.25 mmol/l; p=0.02). There was a trend towards lower overall mortality and mortality due to coronary artery disease in the surgical group, however, without statistical significance. The combined end point of cardiovascular death or nonfatal myocardial infarction was 35% lower in the surgical group (82 vs 125 events; p<0.001). The surgical group had less disease progression on follow-up angiograms (p<0.001 at 5 and 7 years). During follow-up, 52 and 137 patients of the surgical and control groups underwent coronary artery bypass grafting surgery (p<0.0001), while 15 and 33 of the surgical and control group patients underwent angioplasty (p=0.005).

Conclusions
: Partial ileal bypass surgery induced a sustained reduction in plasma cholesterol levels and reduced the morbidity due to coronary artery disease.

FATS

Familial Atherosclerosis Treatment Study

Title	Regression of coronary artery disease as a result of intensive lipid lowering therapy in men with high levels of apolipoprotein B.
Authors	Brown G, Alberts JJ, Fisher LD, et al.
Reference	N Engl J Med 1990;323:1289-1298.
Disease	Hyperlipidemia, coronary artery disease.
Purpose	To assess the effect of intensive lipid lowering therapy on coronary atherosclerosis among high risk men.
Design	Randomized, double blind, placebo (or colestipol) controlled, multicenter.
Patients	146 men, ≤62 years of age, with plasma levels of apolipoprotein ß ≥125 mg/dl, documented coronary artery disease (≥1 lesion of ≥50% stenosis, or ≥3 lesions of ≥30% stenosis), and a positive family history of vascular disease.
Follow-up	Clinical evaluation, plasma lipid levels, and coronary angiography at baseline and at 30 months.
Treatment regimen	1. Lovastatin 20 mg X2/d, and colestipol 10gX3/d. 2. Niacin 1gX4/d, and colestipol 10gX3/d. 3. Placebo or colestipol (if LDL cholesterol exceeded the 90th percentile for age).
Additional therapy	American Heart Association Phase I and II diet.

FATS

Familial Atherosclerosis Treatment Study

(continued)

Results   The levels of LDL and HDL cholesterol changed only slightly in the control group (mean change -7% and +5%, respectively). However they were improved with the lovastatin+colestipol (-46% and +15%) or niacin+colestipol (-32% and +43%) arms. In the control group 46% of the patients had definite lesion progression, while 11% had regression. Progression was observed in only 21% and 25% of the lovastatin+ colestipol and niacin+colestipol patients, while regression was observed in 32% and 39%, respectively (p for trend=0.005). Multivariate regression analysis revealed that reduction in the apolipoprotein ß levels, and in systolic blood pressure, and an increase in HDL cholesterol were associated with regression of coronary lesions. Death, myocardial infarction, or revascularization due to worsening symptoms occurred in 10 of the 52 patients with conventional therapy, as compared to 3 of 46 and 2 of 48 of the lovastatin+colestipol and niacin+colestipol treated patients (p=0.01). Overall, intensive lipid lowering therapy reduces the incidence of clinical events by 73% (95% CI 23-90%).

Conclusions   In men with coronary artery disease who are at high risk, intensive lipid lowering therapy reduced the frequency of progression and increases regression of atherosclerotic coronary lesions, and reduced the incidence of cardiovascular events.

EXCEL

Expanded Clinical Evaluation of Lovastatin

Title	a. Expanded Clinical Evaluation of Lovastatin (EXCEL) study: design and patient characteristics of a double blind, placebo-controlled study in patients with moderate hyper-cholesterolemia.
	b. Expanded Clinical Evaluation of Lovastatin (EXCEL) study results. I. Efficacy in modifying plasma lipoproteins and adverse event profile in 8245 patients with moderate hypercholesterolemia.
	c. Expanded Clinical Evaluation of Lovastatin (EXCEL) study results: III. Efficacy in modifying lipoproteins and implications for managing patients with moderate hyper-cholesterolemia.
	d. Expanded Clinical Evaluation of Lovastatin (EXCEL) study results: IV. Additional perspectives on the tolerabili-ty of lovastatin.
Authors	a-c. Bradford RH, Shear CL, Chremos AN, et al.
	d. Dujovne CA, Chermos AN, Pool JL, et al.
Reference	a. Am J Cardiol 1990;66:44B-55B.
	b. Arch Intern Med 1991;151:43-49.
	c. Am J Med 1991;91(suppl 1B):18S-24S.
	d. Am J Med 1991;91(suppl 1B):25S-30S.
Disease	Hypercholesterolemia.
Purpose	To evaluate dose response relation of lovastatin in lipid/lipoprotein modifying efficacy and of drug related adverse effects in patients with moderate hypercholes-terolemia.
Design	Randomized, double blind, multicenter.

EXCEL

Expanded Clinical Evaluation of Lovastatin

(continued)

Patients	8245 patients, age 18-70 years, with primary type II hyper-lipidemia (fasting total plasma cholesterol 6.21-7.76 mmol/l, LDL cholesterol ≥4.14 mmol/l, and triglyceride <3.95 mmol/l). Patients with diabetes mellitus requiring medications, secondary hypercholesterolemia, and pre-menopausal women were excluded.
Follow-up	48 weeks.
Treatment regimen	One of the following regimens for 48 weeks: 1. lovastatin 20 mg X1/d; 2. lovastatin 40 mg X1/d; 3. lovastatin 20mg X2/d; 4. lovastatin 40mg X2/d; and 5. placebo.
Additional therapy	American Heart Association phase I diet.
Results	Lovastatin therapy resulted in a sustained, dose related decrease of total cholesterol (-17%, -22%, -24%, and -29% for groups 1-4, while it increased by +0.7% in the placebo group, p<0.001 for dose trend), of LDL-cholesterol (-24%, -30%, -34%, and -40% for groups 1-4, while it increased by +0.4% in the placebo group, p<0.001 for dose trend), and of triglyceride (-10%, -14%, -16%, and -19%, respectively, while in the placebo it increased by 3.6%, p<0.001 for dose trend). HDL cholesterol increased by 6.6%, 7.2%, 8.6%, and 9.5%, respectively, while in the placebo it increased in only 2.0%. (p<0.001 for dose trend). Patients withdrawal due to adverse effects occurred in 6% of the placebo and 7-9% of the lovastatin groups. Increases in serum transam-inase occurred in 0.1%, 0.1%, 0.9%, 0.9%, and 1.5% of groups 1-5, p<0.001 for trend). Myopathy was rare.
Conclusions	Lovastatin is a safe and highly effective and well tolerated therapy for hypercholesterolemia.

MAAS

Multicentre Anti-Atheroma Study

Title	Effect of simvastatin on coronary atheroma: the Multicentre Anti-Atheroma Study (MAAS).
Authors	MAAS Investigators.
Reference	Lancet 1994;344:633-638.
Disease	Coronary artery disease.
Purpose	To evaluate the effects of simvastatin on coronary atheroma in patients with moderate hypercholesterolemia and coronary artery disease.
Design	Randomized, double blind, placebo-controlled, multicenter.
Patients	381 patients, age 30-67 years, with documented coronary artery disease, serum cholesterol 5.5-8.0 mmol/l and triglyceride <4.0 mmol/l. Patients with unstable angina or myocardial infarction within 6 weeks, angioplasty or surgery within 3 months, treated diabetes mellitus, or patients with congestive heart failure or ejection fraction <30% were excluded.
Follow-up	Clinical follow-up for 4 years. Coronary angiography before therapy was started and after 2 and 4 years.
Treatment regimen	Simvastatin 20 mg/d or placebo.
Additional therapy	Lipid lowering diet.

MAAS

Multicentre Anti-Atheroma Study

(continued)

Results

Patients receiving simvastatin had 23% reduction of serum cholesterol, 31% reduction of LDL cholesterol, and a 9% increase in HDL cholesterol compared with placebo after 4 years. 345 patients had repeated angiograms after 4 years. Mean luminal diameter was reduced by 0.08±0.26 mm vs 0.02±0.23 mm in the placebo and simvastatin groups (treatment effect 0.06, 95% CI 0.02-0.10), and minimal luminal diameter was reduced by 0.13±0.27 mm vs 0.04±0.25 mm (treatment effect 0.08, 95% CI 0.03-0.14) (combined p=0.006). Diameter stenosis was increased by 3.6±9.0% vs 1.0±7.9%, respectively (treatment effect -2.6%, 95% CI -4.4% to -0.8%). The beneficial effect of simvastatin was observed regardless of the initial diameter stenosis. Angiographic progression occurred in 32.3% vs 23.0% of the placebo and simvastatin groups, and regression in 12.0% vs 18.6%, respectively (combined p=0.02). New lesions developed in 3.7% vs 2.0% of the segments studied, respectively. There was no difference in clinical outcome. However, more patients in the placebo than simvastatin group (34 vs 23 patients) underwent coronary revascularization.

Conclusions

Simvastatin 20 mg/d reduced hyperlipidemia and slowed the progression of diffuse and focal coronary artery disease.

Scandinavian Simvastatin Survival Study

Title	a. Randomized trial of cholesterol lowering in 4444 patients with coronary heart disease: the Scandinavian Simvastatin Survival Study (4S). b. Baseline serum cholesterol and treatment effect in the Scandinavian Simvastatin Survival Study (4S). c. Reducing the risk of coronary events: evidence from the Scandinavian Simvastatin Survival Study (4S). d. Cholesterol lowering therapy in women and elderly patients with myocardial infarction or angina pectoris. Findings from the Scandinavian Simvastatin Survival Trial (4S). e. Cost effectiveness of simvastatin treatment to lower cholesterol levels in patients with coronary heart disease. f. Lipoprotein changes and reduction in the incidence of major coronary heart disease events in the Scandinavian Simvastatin Survival Study (4S) g. Effect of simvastatin on ischemic signs and symptoms in the Scandinavian Simvastatin Survival Study (4S).
Authors	a + b. Scandinavian Simvastatin Survival Study Group. c. Kjekshus J, Pedersen TR, for the Scandinavian Simvastatin Survival Study Group d. Miettinen TA, Pyorala K, Olsson AG, et al. e. Johannesson M, Jonsson B, Kjekshus J, et al. f. Pederson TR, Olsson AG, Faergeman O, et al. g. Pedersen TR, Kjekshus J, Pyorala K et al.
Reference	a. Lancet 1994;344:1383-1389. b. Lancet 1995;345:1274-1275. c. Am J Cardiol 1995;76:64C-68C. d. Circulation 1997;96:4211-4218. e. N Engl J Med 1997;336:332-336. f. Circulation 1998;97:1453-1460. g. Am J Cardiol 1998;81:333-335.
Disease	Coronary artery disease, hyperlipidemia.

Scandinavian Simvastatin Survival Study

(continued)

Purpose	To assess the effect of simvastatin therapy on mortality and morbidity of patients with coronary artery disease and serum cholesterol 5.5-8.0 mmol/l. e. To determine the cost effectiveness of lowering cholesterol in relationship to age, sex, and the cholesterol level from the 4S study. f. To determine which baseline lipoproteins are predictive of coronary events. To determine which changes in lipoproteins accounted for the reduction in coronary events in the 4S. g. To determine effect of lipid intervention with simvastatin on noncoronary ischemic symptoms and signs over 5.4 years.
Design	Randomized, double blind, placebo-controlled, multicenter. e. As per 4S trial. Estimation of cost per year of life gained with simvastatin therapy.
Patients	4444 patients, aged 35-70 years, with a history of angina pectoris or myocardial infarction, and serum cholesterol 5.5-8.0 mmol/l, (213–209 mg per deciliter) and serum triglyceride ≤2.5 mmol/l. Premenopausal women and patients with secondary hypercholesterolemia were excluded. Patients with myocardial infarction within 6 months, congestive heart failure, planned coronary artery surgery, or angioplasty were not included.
Follow-up	Clinical follow-up for 4.9-6.3 years (median 5.4 years). e. 5 years. f. 5.4 years

Scandinavian Simvastatin Survival Study

(continued)

Treatment regimen	Simvastatin 20 mg/d or placebo. If serum cholesterol did not reach the target range of 3.0-5.2 mmol/l by simvastatin 20 mg/d, the dose was increased to 40 mg/d, or decreased to 10 mg/d. f. Placebo vs simvastatin 20 mg/day with titration to 40 mg. Target serum total cholesterol 116–201 mg/dL.
Additional therapy	Dietary advice.
Results	Lipid concentrations changed only little in the placebo group, whereas simvastatin resulted in -25%, -35%, +8%, and -10% change from baseline of total-, LDL-, and HDL-cholesterol, and triglycerides. After 1 year, 72% of the simvastatin group had achieved total cholesterol <5.2 mmol/l. During the follow-up mortality was 12% in the placebo and 8% in the simvastatin group (RR 0.70, 95% CI 0.58-0.85, p=0.0003). The Kaplan-Meier 6 year probability of survival was 87.7% in the placebo vs 91.3% in the simvastatin group. Coronary mortality was 8.5% vs 5.0%, respectively (RR 0.58, 95% CI 0.46-0.73). There was no difference in noncardiovascular death. 28% of the placebo and 19% of the simvastatin group had 1 or more major coronary events (coronary death, myocardial infarction, or resuscitated cardiac arrest (RR 0.66, 95% CI 0.59-0.75, p<0.00001). The relative risk of having any coronary event in the simvastatin group was 0.73 (95% CI 0.66-0.80, p<0.00001). Simvastatin also reduced the risk of undergoing coronary artery bypass surgery or angioplasty (RR 0.63, 95% CI 0.54-0.74, p<0.00001). The overall rates of adverse effects were not different between the groups. Simvastatin significantly reduced the risk of major coronary events in all quartiles of baseline total, HDL, and LDL cholesterol, by a similar amount in each quartile. d. A recent post-hoc analysis showed that patients ≥65 years of age who received simvastatin had a reduced relative risk (RR) for clinical events. The RRs (95% confidence intervals) were 0.66 (0.40-0.90) for all-cause mortality; 0.57 (0.39-0.83) for coronary heart disease mortality; and 0.66 (0.52-0.84) for major coronary

events. The RR was also reduced for any atherosclerotic-related events and revascularization procedures. In women the RRs were 1.16 (0.68–1.99), 0.86 (0.42–1.74), and 0.66 (0.48–0.91) for all cause mortality, coronary heart disease mortality, and major coronary events. Any atherosclerotic-related event and revascularization procedures also were reduced in women on simvastatin.

e. The cost of each year of life gained ranged from $3,800 for 70 year old men with cholesterol levels of 309 mg/dL to $27,400 for 35 year old women with 213 mg/dL. With indirect costs included, the costs ranged from youngest patients exhibiting a savings in money while 70 year old women with 213 cholesterol levels cost $13,300 per year of life gained.

f. Simvastatin reduced cholesterol by 25% and LDL cholesterol by 34%. Three fourths of patients on simvastatin had reduction of LDL cholesterol by 30%; a quarter had reduction by > 45%. Reduction in coronary events on simvastatin correlated with on-treatment levels and changes in total, LDL cholesterol, and apolipoprotein B. There was less of a correlation with triglyceride levels. Each 1% reduction in LDL cholesterol reduced coronary risk by 1.7%. There was no evidence for any % reduction or on-treatment threshold below which further reduction of LDL cholesterol did not have benefit.

g. Risk of claudication, bruits, and angina were decreased by simvastatin. The risk of new or worsening carotid bruits was significantly decreased. Fatal plus nonfatal cerebral events (stroke or transient ischemic attacks) was reduced by 28% with simvastatin. New or worsening intermittent claudication was decreased by 38% with the statin; new or worsening angina was decreased by 26%.

Conclusions	Long-term therapy with simvastatin is safe and effective in improvement of survival and reduction of the rate of coronary events.

d. Simvastatin produced similar reductions in relative risk for major coronary events in women vs men and in elderly vs younger patients.

e. In patients with coronary artery disease, simvastatin is cost effective.

f. The beneficial effect of simvastatin on major coronary events was dependent upon the magnitude of reduction in LDL cholesterol, without a threshold below which reduction was no longer beneficial.

g. Cholesterol lowering with simvastatin 20–40 mg/day retards progression of atherosclerosis throughout the vascular system.

PLAC I and II

Pravastatin Limitation of Atherosclerosis in the Coronary Arteries

Title	a. Design and recruitment in the United States of a multi-center quantitative angiographic trial of pravastatin to limit atherosclerosis in the coronary arteries (PLAC I). b. Pravastatin, lipids, and atherosclerosis in the carotid arteries (PLAC-II). c. Reduction in coronary events during treatment with pravastatin.
Authors	a. Pitt B, Ellis SG, Mancini GBJ, et al. b. Crouse JR III, Byington RP, Bond MG, et al. c. Furberg CD, Pitt B, Byington RP, et al.
Reference	a. Am J Cardiol 1993;72:31-35. b. Am J Cardiol 1995;75:455-459. c. Am J Cardiol 1995;76:60C-63C.
Disease	Hyperlipidemia.
Purpose	To assess the effects of pravastatin on progression and regression of coronary artery disease in patients with moderate hypercholesterolemia.
Design	Randomized, double blind, placebo-controlled, multicenter.
Patients	559 patients (PLAC I: 408 patients, age ≤75 years, with documented ≥1 stenosis ≥50% in a major epicardial coronary artery, LDL cholesterol 130-189 mg/dl, and triglycerides ≤350 mg/dl. Patients with secondary hyperlipidemia, diabetes mellitus, congestive heart failure, and other serious concomitant diseases were excluded. PLAC II: 151 patients with coronary artery disease and extracranial carotid lesion. Same criteria as above.
Follow-up	Clinical follow-up for 3 years. Coronary angiography at baseline and after 36 months (PLAC I).

PLAC I and II

Pravastatin Limitation of Atherosclerosis in the Coronary Arteries

(continued)

Treatment regimen	Pravastatin 40 mg X1/d or placebo for 3 years in PLAC-I, 20-40 mg/d in PLAC-II.
Additional therapy	Patients whose LDL cholesterol remained ≥190 mg/dl received cholestyramine, and then 5-10 mg open label pravastatin or placebo. If these measures failed, the patient was withdrawn from the study.
Results	The incidence of coronary events was 4.0%/year in the placebo vs 1.8%/year in the pravastatin patients (55% risk reduction, 95% CI 19-79%, p=0.014). A similar effect was seen in patients <65 years and ≥65 years of age. 11 patients vs 7 patients in the placebo and pravastatin groups died (40% risk reduction, 95% CI -65% to 85%, p=0.31). Nonfatal myocardial infarction occurred in 24 patients of the placebo vs 9 of the pravastatin group (67% risk reduction, 95% CI 32%-88%, p=0.006). The angiographic results have not been published yet.
Conclusions	Pravastatin therapy was associated with reduction of clinical events in coronary patients with mild to moderate hyperlipidemia.

WOSCOPS

Prevention of Coronary Heart Disease With Pravastatin in Men With Hypercholesterolemia. The West of Scotland Coronary Prevention Study

Title	a. Prevention of coronary heart disease with pravastatin in men with hypercholesterolemia. b. Influence of pravastatin and plasma lipids on clinical events in the West of Scotland Coronary Prevention Study (WOSCOPS).
Authors	a. Shepherd J, Cobbe SM, Ford I, et al. b. West of Scotland Coronary Prevention Study Group.
Reference	a. N Engl J Med 1995;333:1301-1307. b. Circulation 1998;97:1440-1445
Disease	Hypercholesterolemia, coronary artery disease.
Purpose	a. To assess whether pravastatin therapy reduces the incidence of acute myocardial infarction and mortality from coronary heart disease in hypercholesterolemic men without a history of prior myocardial infarction. b. To determine the extent to which reduction of LDL influenced coronary heart disease risk reduction in the WOSCOPS.
Design	a. Randomized, double blind, placebo-controlled, multi-center. b. Relationship between baseline lipid levels and rates of cardiovascular events; relationships between on-treatment lipid concentrations and risk reduction in patients taking pravastatin were examined by Cox regression models and division of cohorts into quintiles.

WOSCOPS

***Prevention of Coronary Heart Disease With
Pravastatin in Men With Hypercholesterolemia.
The West of Scotland Coronary Prevention Study***
(continued)

Patients	6595 men, 45-64 years of age, with fasting LDL cholesterol >252 mg per deciliter before diet and >155 mg per deciliter after 4 weeks of diet. None of the patients had a history of prior myocardial infarction. 78% of the patients were ex- or current smokers and 5% had angina pectoris.
Follow-up	a. The average follow-up was 4.9 years (32,216 subject-years of follow-up). b. 5 years.
Treatment regimen	Pravastatin (40 mg/d) or placebo.
Results	a. Compared to baseline values pravastatin reduced plasma total cholesterol levels by 20% and LDL-cholesterol by 26%, whereas no such changes were observed in the placebo-treated group. Pravastatin reduced coronary events by 31% (95% CI 17-43%; p<0.001). There were 174 (5.5%) and 248 (7.9%) coronary events in the pravastatin and control group, respectively. Pravastatin reduced the risk for nonfatal infarction by 31% (4.6% vs 6.5%; p<0.001; 95% CI 15-45%), and the risk for death from all cardiovascular causes by 32% (1.6 vs 2.3%; p=0.033; 95% CI 3-53%). There was no increase in mortality from noncardiovascular causes. b. Baseline LDL cholesterol was only a weak predictor of cardiac risk in both treated and untreated groups. The reduction in risk of a cardiac event by pravastatin was similar across all quintiles of baseline LDL levels. Baseline HDL showed a strong negative association with cardiovascular event rate, but reduction in risk with pravastatin was similar for all quintiles of HDL elevation. The fall in LDL level in the pravastatin group did not correlate with the reduction in risk of a cardiac event on multivariate regression. The maximum benefit of about a 45% risk reduction was

Prevention of Coronary Heart Disease With
Pravastatin in Men With Hypercholesterolemia.
The West of Scotland Coronary Prevention Study
(continued)

observed in the middle quintile of LDL reduction, representing a 24% fall in LDL. Further decreases in LDL, up to 39%, did not result in further reduction in coronary heart disease risk reduction. When event rates between placebo and pravastatin-treated subjects with the same LDL cholesterol level were compared, there was evidence for an LDL independent treatment benefit of pravastatin that remains to be determined.

Conclusions
a. Primary prevention in moderately hypercholesterolemic men with 5 years Pravastatin therapy reduced the incidence of myocardial infarction and death from cardiovascular causes. No excess of noncardiovascular death was observed.

b. A fall in LDL cholesterol of 24% was sufficient to produce full benefit in patients taking pravastatin. Further reduction was not associated with further reduction in coronary heart disease risk.

REGRESS

The Regression Growth Evaluation Statin Study

Title	a. Effects of lipid lowering by pravastatin on progression and regression of coronary artery disease in symptomatic men with normal to moderately elevated serum cholesterol levels. The regression Growth Evaluation Statin Study (REGRESS). b. Reduction of transient myocardial ischemia with pravastatin in addition to the conventional treatment in patients with angina pectoris.
Authors	a. Jukema JW, Bruschke AVG, van Boven AJ, et al. b. van Boven AJ, Jukema JW, Zwinderman AH, et al.
Reference	a. Circulation 1995;91:2528-2540. b. Circulation 1996;94:1503-1505.
Disease	Hyperlipidemia, coronary artery disease.
Purpose	To evaluate whether 2 years of statin therapy will affect the progression of coronary artery disease and clinical outcome of patients with coronary artery disease who have normal to moderately elevated plasma cholesterol levels.
Design	Randomized, double blind, placebo-controlled, multicenter.
Patients	a. 885 men with serum cholesterol 4-8 mmol/L and ≥1 coronary lesion with ≥50% of luminal narrowing. b. 768 men with stable angina pectoris, with serum cholesterol 4-8 mmol/L and ≥1 coronary lesion with ≥50% of luminal narrowing.
Follow-up	a. Clinical evaluation and repeated angiography after 2 years. b. Ambulatory holter ECG monitoring before randomization, and after intervention (in patients that underwent CABG or PTCA) or after 2 years (in patients treated medically).

REGRESS

The Regression Growth Evaluation Statin Study

(continued)

Treatment regimen	Pravastatin 40 mg/d or placebo.
Additional therapy	Dietary advice. Cholestyramine for patients with cholesterol >8.0 mmol/L on repeated assessments. Routine antianginal therapy.
Results	a. 778 (88%) had an evaluable final coronary angiography. Mean segment diameter decreased 0.10 mm and 0.06 mm in the placebo and pravastatin groups (mean difference 0.04 mm, 95% CI 0.01-0.07 mm, p=0.19). The median minimum obstruction diameter decreased 0.09 and 0.03 mm, respectively (difference of the medians 0.06 mm, 95% CI 0.02-0.08 mm, p=0.001). After 2 years 89% of the pravastatin and 81% of the placebo treated patients were without new cardiovascular events (p=0.002). b. In the pravastatin-assigned patients, transient myocardial ischemia was detected at baseline in 28% and after treatment in 19%. In the placebo-treated patients it was found in 20% at baseline and 23% at follow-up (odds ratio 0.62; 95% CI 0.41 to 0.93; p=0.021). The number of ischemic episodes per ambulatory ECG monitoring was reduced at follow-up by 0.53±0.25 episodes in the placebo group and by 1.23±0.25 episodes in the pravastatin group (p=0.047). Ischemic burden (the product of duration of ischemia in minutes multiplied by ST segment depression in mm) decreased from 41±5 to 22±5 mm • min in the pravastatin treated patients (p=0.0058), and from 34±6 to 26±4 mm • min in the placebo group (p=0.24). After adjustment for other independent risk factors, the effect of pravastatin on reduction of ischemia remained significant (odds ratio 0.45; 95% CI 0.22 to 0.91; p=0.026).
Conclusions	a. 2 years of pravastatin therapy, in men with coronary artery disease and normal to moderately elevated cholesterol levels, resulted in less progression of coronary atherosclerosis and fewer new cardiovascular events. b. Pravastatin ameliorated transient myocardial ischemia in patients with coronary artery disease and optimal antianginal therapy.

CARE

Cholesterol And Recurrent Events

Title	a. The effect of pravastatin on coronary events after myocardial infarction in patients with average cholesterol levels. b. Relationship between plasma LDL concentrations during treatment with pravastatin and recurrent coronary events in the cholesterol and recurrent events trial. c. Reduction of stroke incidence following myocardial infarction with pravastatin: the CARE study.
Authors	a. Sacks FM, Pfeffer MA, Moye LA, et al. b. Sacks FM, Moye LA, Davis BR, et al. c. Plehn JF et al.
Reference	a. 1. Am J Cardiol 1991;68:1436-1446. 2. Am J Cardiol 1995;75:621-623. 3. Am J Cardiol 1995;76:98C-106C. 4. N Engl J Med 1996;335:1001-1009. b. Circulation 1998; 97:1446-1452. c. Presentation at the American Heart Association's 23rd International Joint Conference on Stroke and Cerebral Circulation. February 5-7, 1998, Orlando, Florida.
Disease	a. Coronary artery disease, myocardial infarction. b. Myocardial infarction, hypercholesterolemia.
Purpose	a. To evaluate the effectiveness of lowering blood cholesterol levels with pravastatin in patients after myocardial infarction and its effect on subsequent cardiac events. b. To determine the relationship between the LDL concentration during therapy, absolute reduction in LDL, and percent reduction in LDL and outcome. c. To analyze the effect of lipid lowering with pravastatin on the risk of stroke and transient ischemic attacks in the CARE trial.
Design	Randomized, double blind, placebo-controlled, multicenter.

CARE

Cholesterol And Recurrent Events
(continued)

Patients	4159 patients, 21-75 years old, who have experienced myocardial infarction 3-20 months before randomization, had plasma total cholesterol <240 mg/dl, LDL cholesterol 115-174 mg/dl, triglycerides <350 mg/dl, fasting glucose levels ≤ 220 mg/dl, left ventricular ejection fraction ≥25%, and no symptomatic congestive heart failure.
Follow-up	Median follow-up 5 years (4-6.2 years).
Treatment regimen	Pravastatin 40 mg/d or placebo. For patients with LDL cholesterol >175 mg/dl at follow-up, dietary counseling, and then cholestyramine.
Results	a. Pravastatin therapy lowered the mean LDL cholesterol of 139 mg/dl by 32% and maintained mean levels of 98 mg/dl. During follow-up LDL cholesterol was 28% lower, total cholesterol was 20% lower, HDL 5% higher, and triglycerides level 14% lower in the pravastatin than placebo group (p< 0.001 for all comparisons). Primary endpoints (death from coronary artery disease or nonfatal myocardial infarction) occurred in 13.2% vs 10.2% in the placebo and pravastatin group, respectively (risk reduction 24%; 95% CI 9-36%; p=0.003). Cardiovascular death occurred in 5.7% in the placebo vs 4.6% in the pravastatin group (risk reduction 20%; 95% CI -5-39%; p=0.10), and non fatal myocardial infarction occurred in 8.3% vs 6.5%, respectively (risk reduction 23%; 95% CI 4-39%; p=0.02). However, total mortality was comparable (9.4% vs 8.6% in the placebo and pravastatin group, respectively; 9% risk reduction; 95% CI -12-26%; p=0.37). There was no difference in mortality from noncardiovascular causes. The risk of myocardial infarction was 25% lower in the pravastatin group (7.5% vs 10.0%; 95% CI 8-39%; p=0.006). The rate of coronary artery bypass surgery or PTCA was lower in the pravastatin group (14.1% vs 18.8%; risk reduction 27%; 95% CI 15-37%; p<0.001). The pravastatin group had also a 31% lower incidence of stroke (2.6% vs 3.8%; 95% CI 3 -52%; p=0.03). There was also a trend toward less unstablangina in the pravastatin group (15.2% vs. 17.3%; risk reduction 13%; 95% CI -1-25%; p=0.07). The effect of pravastatin was greater among women then among men (46% vs 20% risk reduction for women and men respectively).

Patients with baseline LDL cholesterol >150 mg/dl had a 35% reduction in major coronary events, as compared with a 26% reduction in those with baseline LDL cholesterol of 125–150 mg/dl, and a 3% increase in those with baseline levels < 125 mg/dl (p=0.03 for the interaction between baseline LDL cholesterol level and risk reduction). The overall incidence of fatal or nonfatal cancer was comparable (161 in the placebo vs 172 in the pravastatin group). However, breast cancer occurred in 1 patient in the placebo and in 12 in the pravastatin group (p=0.002). Of the 12 cases in the pravastatin group, 3 occurred in patients who had previously had breast cancer. There was no other significant differences between the groups in the occurrence of other types of cancer.

b. Coronary death or recurrent MI were reduced by 24% with pravastatin. Coronary event rate declined as LDL was reduced from 174 to about 125 mg/dL; however, no further decline occurred in the LDL range of 71 mg/dL–125 mg/dL. LDL concentration achieved during follow-up was a significant but nonlinear predictor of coronary event rate; the extent of LDL reduction as absolute amount or percentage of LDL reduction was not a significant predictor of event rate. Triglycerides but not HDL weakly but significantly were associated with coronary event rate.

c. The stroke incidence was 3.7% in placebo patients and 2.5% in patients on pravastatin. Stroke or transient ischemic attack occurred in 6% of patients on placebo and 4.4% of patients on pravastatin. Thus, pravastatin decreased strokes by 32%; it decreased either strokes or transient ischemic attacks by 27% over 5 years. Unlike the CARE findings for reduced risk of myocardial infarction, (whereby lowering LDL below 125 mg/dL did not further reduce myocardial infarction), the investigators did not observe a threshold effect of LDL's below 125 mg/dL for stroke. Patients with LDL's above 150 had a 44% lower rate of strokes; those between 125-150, a 28% lower stroke rate; and under 125, a 25% reduction in stroke rate with pravastatin.

Conclusions

a. Pravastatin therapy lowered cardiac mortality, the need for revascularization, and occurrence of stroke in both men and women with coronary artery disease, plasma total cholesterol of <240 mg per deciliter and plasma LDL cholesterol >125 mg per deciliter. In this study, no reduction in event rate was found in patients with LDL cholesterol <125 mg per deciliter. There was no reduction in overall mortality

b. Reduction of LDL down to a concentration of about 125mg/dL was associated with a reduction in coronary events. Further reduction to <125mg/dL with therapy was not associated with additional benefit.

c. In the population of patients in the CARE study, pravastatin reduced the rates of stroke and stroke or transient ischemic attacks.

Title	Comparison of 1 year efficacy and safety of atorvastatin vs lovastatin in primary hypercholesterolemia.
Authors	Davidson M, McKenney J, Stein E, et al.
Reference	Am J Cardiol 1997;79:1475-1481.
Disease	Hyperlipidemia.
Purpose	To compare the efficacy and safety of 2 3-hydroxy-3-methylglutaryl coenzyme A reductase inhibitors, atorvastatin and lovastatin, in patients with hypercholesterolemia.
Design	Randomized, double blind, placebo-controlled, multicenter.
Patients	1049 patients (58% men), 18–80 years old, with LDL cholesterol ≥ 3.75 mmol/L and triglycerides <4.52 mmol/L and a body mass index ≤ 32 kg/m^2. Patients with renal or hepatic disease, insulin dependent diabetes mellitus, uncontrolled type II diabetes mellitus, unstable medical conditions, elevated creatine kinase levels, $<80\%$ compliance with study medications during the placebo run in phase were excluded. Patients on immunosuppressive agents, drugs known to affect lipid levels, or medications known to be associated with rhabdomyolysis were not included.
Follow-up	1 year.
Treatment regimen	Randomization to 4 groups: 1. atorvastatin 10 mg/d for 52 weeks; 2. lovastatin 20 mg/d for 52 weeks; 3. placebo for 16 weeks followed by atorvastatin for 36 weeks; and 4. placebo for 16 weeks followed by lovastatin for 36 weeks. In patients who had not reached their LDL cholesterol goal after 22 weeks of therapy, the medication dose was doubled.

Additional therapy	NCEP step 1 diet.

Results	Throughout the study compliance was >93%. At the end of the 52 week treatment, 12% of patients had withdrawn from the study. LDL-cholesterol level at week 16 increased by 1.0±1.0% compared to the baseline in the placebo group. In contrast, it was reduced by 27±0.8% with lovastatin and by 36.0±0.5% with atorvastatin (p=0.0001 vs placebo and vs lovastatin). HDL-cholesterol at week 16 increased by 1.0±1.0% in the placebo group, by 7.0±0.9% in the lovastatin group (p<0.05 vs placebo), and by 7.0±0.5% in the atorvastatin group (p<0.05 vs placebo). Triglycerides increased by 4.0±2.3% in the placebo group, decreased by 19.0±0.6% in the lovastatin group, and decreased by 27.0±0.4% in the atorvastatin group (p<0.05 vs placebo and vs lovastatin). Apolipoprotein B increased by 3.0±1.0% in the placebo group, decreased by 20.0±0.8% in the lovastatin group, and decreased by 28.0±0.5% in the atorvastatin group (p<0.05 vs placebo and vs lovastatin). At week 16, 74% of the atorvastatin group vs 55% of the lovastatin group and 7% of the placebo group reached NCEP target. At week 52, 27% of the atorvastatin group and 49% of the lovastatin group needed to double their medication dose based on response to therapy and risk status. At the end of follow-up 78% of the atorvastatin group vs only 63% of the lovastatin group reached NCEP target. Among patients with coronary artery disease, target LDL-cholesterol levels were achieved by 37% of the atorvastatin group vs only 11% of the lovastatin group. By week 52, LDL cholesterol was reduced by 29.0±0.7% and 37.0±0.5% in the lovastatin and atorvastatin groups respectively (p<0.05), HDL cholesterol was increased by 7.0±0.9% and 7.0±0.5%, triglycerides were reduced by 8.0±2.0% and 16.0±1.3% (p<0.05), and apolipoprotein B was reduced by 22.0±0.7% and 30.0±0.4%, respectively. Adverse effects occurred in similar rates with both medications (20% with atorvastatin and 21% with lovastatin). Serious adverse effects occurred in 8% vs 7% of the atorvastatin and lovastatin groups, respectively.

Conclusions	Atorvastatin was better than lovastatin in reducing LDL cholesterol, apolipoprotein B, and triglycerides and had a similar safety profile as lovastatin.

CCAIT

The Canadian Coronary Atherosclerosis Intervention Trial

Title	Effects of monotherapy with an HMG-CoA reductase inhibitor on the progression of coronary atherosclerosis as assessed by serial quantitative arteriography. The Canadian Coronary Atherosclerosis Interventn Trial.
Authors	Waters D, Higginson L, Gladstone P, et al.
Reference	Circulation 1994;89:959-968.
Disease	Coronary artery disease, hypercholestolemia
Purpose	To evaluate whether lovastatin (an HMG-CoA reductase inhibitor) therapy will affect coronary atherosclerosis as assessed by serial quantitative coronary angiography.
Design	Randomized, double blind, placebo-controlled, multicenter.
Patients	331 patients (81% men), 27-70 years old, with angiographically proven diffuse coronary artery disease, total serum cholesterol 220-300 mg/dl, and serum triglycerides ≤500 mg/dl. Women with childbearing potential, and patients with previous coronary artery bypass surgery; previous coronary angioplasty within 6 months; ejection fraction <40%; left main coronary artery stenosis>50%; 3 vessel disease with proximal LAD stenosis >70%; coexisting severe illness; myocardial infarction or unstable angina within 6 weeks prior to randomization; concurrent use of lipid lowering drugs, corticosteroids, anticoagulants, cimetidine, or cyclosporine; liver function disturbances; or renal failure were excluded.
Follow-up	Clinical follow-up for 24 months. Coronary angiography at baseline and 24 months.
Treatment regimen	Randomization to lovastatin 20 mg/d (n=165) or placebo (n=166). The dose was increased to 40 mg/d in patients whose LDL-cholesterol was >130 mg/dl despite 4 weeks of therapy. If LDL cholesterol was still >130 mg/dl, the dose was increased to 80 mg/d.

CCAIT

The Canadian Coronary Atherosclerosis Intervention Trial
(continued)

Additional therapy	AHA phase I diet. Aspirin 325 mg on alternate days. Revascularization (CABG or PTCA) was not permitted during the 24 month study period.
Results	The mean lovastatin dose was 36 mg/d. The target LDL cholesterol ≤130 mg/dl was achieved by 69% of the lovastatin and 10% of the placebo treated patients. Total cholesterol reduced by 21±11% (p<0.001), LDL-cholesterol reduced by 29±11% (p<0.001), HDL cholesterol increased by 7.3±19% (p<0.001), and apolipoprotein B decreased by 21±12% (p<0.001) in the lovastatin-assigned patients. Angina class improved by ≥1 grade in 50 lovastatin and 43 placebo patients, and worsened by ≥1 grade in 23 lovastatin and 27 placebo patients (p=0.087). There was a trend towards less coronary events in the lovastatin group (14 vs 18 patients had ≥1 event) that was not statistically significant. A second coronary angiography was obtained in 299 patients (90%). Coronary change score (defined as the per-patient mean of the minimum lumen diameter changes (follow-up minus baseline angiogram) for all lesions measured, excluding those with <25% stenosis on both films) worsened by 0.09±0.16 mm in the placebo group and by 0.05±0.13 mm in the lovastatin group (p=0.01). Mean percent diameter stenosis increased by 2.89±5.59% in the placebo group and by 1.66±4.5% in the lovastatin group (p=0.039). Progression ≥a decrease in minimum lumen diameter of ≥1 lesion by ≥0.4 mm) with no regression at other coronary segments was observed in 33% of the lovastatin vs 50% of the placebo group (p=0.003). 6.8% vs 9.4% of the lesions in the lovastatin and placebo treated patients progressed, respectively (p=0.017). ≥15% diameter stenosis progression was noted in 5.9% and 9.6% of the lesions in the lovastatin and placebo treated patients, respectively (p=0.008). Progression to a new total occlusion was noticed in 1.6% of the lovastatin group vs 1.9% of the placebo group. New coronary lesions were detected in 16% of the lovastatin vs 32% of the placebo group (p=0.001). Lovastatin was equally effective in men and women.
Conclusions	Lovastatin slowed the progression of coronary atherosclerotic lesions and inhibited the formation of new coronary stenotic lesions.

CIS

The Multicenter Coronary Intervention Study

Title	The effect of simvastatin on progression of coronary artery disease. The multicenter Coronary Intervention Study (CIS)
Authors	Bestehorn HP, Rensing UFE, Roskamm H, et al.
Reference	Eur Heart J 1997;18:226-234.
Disease	Coronary artery disease, hyperlipidemia.
Purpose	To assess the effects of 40 mg/d simvastatin therapy on progression of coronary artery disease in young male patients with coronary artery disease and hyperlipidemia.
Design	Randomized, double blind, placebo-controlled, multicenter.
Patients	254 men, aged 30-55 years, with total plasma cholesterol 207-350 mg/dl and total triglycerides <330 mg/dl, and known coronary artery disease by angiography. Patients with hypertension, diabetes, LVEF <30%, myocardial infarction within 4 weeks, PTCA within 4 months, CABG in the past, or scheduled for coronary interventions were excluded
Follow-up	Coronary angiography at baseline and at follow-up (up to 4 years, an average of 2.3 years).
Treatment regimen	Simvastatin 20 mg/d or placebo. After 6 weeks if LDL-cholesterol >90 mg/dl, the simvastatin dose was increased to 40 mg/d.

The Multicenter Coronary Intervention Study

(continued)

Additional therapy	Lipid lowering diet. An ion-exchange resin was added after 12 weeks if LDL-cholesterol was ≥120 mg/dl or ≥250 mg/dl in the simvastatin and placebo groups, respectively.
Results	129 patients were randomized to simvastatin and 125 to placebo. Follow-up angiogram was performed in 205 patients. Mean simvastatin daily dose was 34.5 mg. Simvastatin therapy resulted in 35% reduction of LDL-cholesterol compared with placebo (p=0.0000). Coronary artery disease progressed slower in the simvastatin group. The mean global change score (visual evaluation by the method of Blankenhorn, a 7-point scale from -3 (strong regression) to +3 (strong progression)) was +0.20±0.08 in the simvastatin and +0.58±0.10 in the placebo group (p=0.02). 34.6% of the simvastatin and 53.5% of the placebo-treated patients had progression. Minimum lumen diameter decreased by 0.02±0.014 mm in the simvastatin vs 0.10±0.02 mm in the placebo group (p=0.002). In patients receiving simvastatin, there was a significant correlation between LDL-cholesterol levels during therapy and the per patient mean loss of minimum lumen diameter (r=0.29; p=0.003). There was no difference between the groups in the incidence of serious cardiac events.
Conclusions	Simvastatin therapy, 40 mg/d for an average of 2.3 years, reduced serum cholesterol and slowed the progression of coronary artery disease in young men with hypercholesterolemia and known coronary artery disease.

The CURVES Study

Comparative Dose Efficacy of Atorvastatin, Simvastatin, Pravastatin, Lovastatin and Fluvastatin

Title	Comparative dose efficacy study of atorvastatin vs simvastatin, pravastatin, lovastatin, and fluvastatin in patients with hypercholesterolemia (The CURVES Study).
Authors	Jones P, Kafonek S, Laurora I, et al.
Reference	Am J Cardiol 1998;81:582-587.
Disease	Hyperlipidemia.
Purpose	To assess comparative dose efficacy of 5 different 3-hydroxy-3-methylglutaryl coenzyme A reductase inhibitors in hypercholesterolemic patients during 8 weeks of therapy.
Design	Randomized, open label, parallel-group, multicenter.
Patients	534 patients, 18-80 years old, with plasma LDL cholesterol $\geq$160 mg/dl and triglyceride $\leq$400 mg/dl. Patients with hypothyroidism, nephrotic syndrome, insulin dependent or uncontrolled diabetes, hepatic dysfunction, elevated levels of creatine kinase, body mass index >32 kg/m2, uncontrolled hypertension, myocardial infarction, coronary revascularization, or severe or unstable angina within the preceding 3 months, or hypersensitivity to hypolipemic medications were not included.
Follow-up	8 weeks.
Treatment regimen	Atrovastatin 10, 20, 40, or 80 mg/d; simvastatin 10, 20, pravastatin 10, 20 and 40 mg/d; lovastatin 20, 40 or 80 mg/d; and fluvastatin 20 or 40 mg/d.

The CURVES Study

Comparative Dose Efficacy of Atorvastatin, Simvastatin, Pravastatin, Lovastatin and Fluvastatin

(continued)

Addtional therapy	Medications known to affect clinical laboratory parameters, anticoagulants, immunosuppressive agents, steroids, and lipid lowering agents were prohibited.

Results	518 patients completed the study. The intention to treat analysis included 522 patients (59% men). Atorvastatin, pravastatin and simvastatin 10 mg/d produced 38%, 19%, and 28% reduction in LDL cholesterol ($p \leq 0.02$ for atorvastatin vs pravastatin and vs simvastatin). Total cholesterol was reduced by 28%, 13%, and 21%, respectively ($p \leq 0.02$ for atorvastatin vs pravastatin and vs simvastatin), and HDL-cholesterol was increased by 5.5%, 9.9%, and 6.8%, respectively (p=NS). Atorvastatin, pravastatin, simvastatin, fluvastatin, and lovastatin 20 mg/d caused reduction of 46%, 24%, 35%, 17%, and 29% in LDL cholesterol ($p \leq 0.05$ for atorvastatin against each of the other 4 agents); 35%, 18%, 26%, 13%, and 21% reduction in total cholesterol levels ($p \leq 0.02$ for atorvastatin vs each of the other 4 agents); and an increase of 5.1%, 3.0%, 5.2%, 0.9%, and 7.3% in HDL-cholesterol (p=NS). Atorvastatin, pravastatin, simvastatin, fluvastatin, and lovastatin 40 mg/d caused reduction of 51%, 34%, 41%, 23%, and 31% in LDL cholesterol ($p \leq 0.05$ for atorvastatin against each of the other 4 agents); 40%, 24%, 30%, 19%, and 23% reduction in total cholesterol levels ($p \leq 0.02$ for atorvastatin vs each of the other 4 agents); and an increase of 4.8%, 6.2%, 9.6%, -3.0% and 4.6% in HDL-cholesterol ($p \leq 0.05$ for simvastatin vs atorvastatin). Atorvastatin and lovastatin 80 mg/d produced 54% and 48% decrease in LDL-cholesterol, 42% and 36% in total cholesterol, and -0.1% and 8.0% increase in HDL-cholesterol. Atorvastatin 10 mg/d was more effective in reducing LDL-cholesterol levels than simvastatin 10mg/d; pravastatin 10 and 20 mg/d; lovastatin 20 and 40 mg/d; and fluvastatin 20 and 40 mg/d ($p \leq 0.02$). Atorvastatin 20 mg/d resulted in greater reduction in LDL-cholesterol than simvastatin 10, 20, and 40 mg/d; pravastatin 10, 20, and 40 mg/d; lovastatin 20 and 40 mg/d; and fluvastatin 20 and 40 mg/d ($p \leq 0.01$). The effect on triglycerides was comparable among the groups, except for atorvastatin 40 mg/d which produced greater (32%; $p \leq 0.05$) decrease in levels. The effect of atorvastatin on HDL-cholesterol was comparable to that of the other

The CURVES Study

Comparative Dose Efficacy of Atorvastatin, Simvastatin, Pravastatin, Lovastatin and Fluvastatin
(continued)

agents, except that simvastatin 40 mg/d produced the greatest increase in levels. Adverse event rates were comparable among the groups. There were no cases of persistent elevations in serum transaminases or creatine kinase, or reports of myopathy.

Conclusions   Atorvastatin at a dose of 10, 20, and 40 mg/d produced a significantly greater reduction in LDL-cholesterol levels. All 5 agents were safe and well tolerated.

LCAS

Lipoprotein and Coronary Atherosclerosis Study

Title	Effects of fluvastatin on coronary atherosclerosis in patients with mild to moderate cholesterol elevations: (Lipoprotein and Coronary Atherosclerosis Study (LCAS).
Authors	Herd JA, Ballantyne CM, Farmer JA, et al.
Reference	Am J Cardiol 1997;80:278-286.
Disease	Coronary artery disease.
Purpose	To assess whether therapy with fluvastatin, a 3-hydroxy-3-methylglutaryl coenzyme A reductase inhibitor, would induce regression or slow the progression of coronary atherosclerosis in patients with coronary artery disease and mild to moderate hypercholesterolemia.
Design	Randomized, double blind, placebo-controlled, single center.
Patients	429 patients (19% women), 35-75 years old, with angiographically proven coronary artery disease with 30%-75% diameter stenosis, LDL cholesterol levels 115-190 mg/dl despite diet, and triglycerides ≤300 mg/dl. Patients with prior angioplasty or myocardial infarction within 6 months, >50% left main coronary artery stenosis, prior CABG, uncontrolled hypertension, diabetes mellitus, or treatment with other hypolipemic agents were excluded.
Follow-up	Coronary angiography at baseline and after 130 weeks.
Treatment regimen	Randomization to fluvastatin 20 mg BID or placebo.

LCAS

Lipoprotein and Coronary Atherosclerosis Study

Additional therapy	NCEP Step I diet. Open label cholestyramine, up to 12 g/d was given as adjunctive therapy to patients whose mean LDL levels before randomization remained ≥160 mg/dl.
Results	In 340 patients, both the baseline and follow-up angiograms were evaluable. By the end of follow-up total cholesterol levels decreased by 13.5±13.1% in the fluvastatin group and increased by 0.3±12.5% in the placebo group (p<0.0001). LDL cholesterol decreased by 22.5±17.6% and 2.2±17.1%, respectively (p<0.0001), HDL cholesterol increased by 8.7±15.2% and 3.9±15.4%, respectively (p=0.0054), and triglyceride levels decreased by 0.1±40.3% and increased by 9.5±42.1%, respectively (p=0.0297). In the fluvastatin + cholestyramine total cholesterol decreased by 18.3±12.4%, LDL cholesterol decreased by 27.9±16.9%, HDL increased by 8.0±14.9%, and triglyceride decreased by 0.3±29.2%. Final minus baseline minimal lumen diameter of qualifying lesions within each patient, adjusted for age and gender demonstrated less progression in the fluvastatin treated patients (with or without cholestyramine)(-0.028±0.021 mm) compared with the placebo treated patients (with or without cholestyramine) (-0.100±0.022 mm; p=0.005). Minimal lumen diameter decreased by 0.024 mm in the fluvastatin alone group and by 0.094 mm in the placebo alone group (p<0.02). Diameter stenosis increased by 0.6±0.7% in the fluvastatin group and by 2.8±0.8% in the placebo group (p=0.0137). Among the 84 patients with baseline LDL cholesterol <130 mg/dl, fluvastatin-treated patients had 0.021±0.040 mm increase in the minimal lumen diameter, indicating regression, whereas the placebo treated patients had a decrease of 0.062±0.040 mm in minimal lumen diameter (p=0.083). Progression was detected in 28.7% of the fluvastatin groups (with or without cholestyramine) vs 39.1% of the placebo groups (with or without cholestyramine), regression in 14.6% vs 8.3%, and mixed change or no response in 56.7% vs 52.7%, respectively (p=0.0198 for the difference in distribution between the 2 groups). New lesions appeared in 13% of the fluvastatin groups vs 22% of the placebo groups (p=0.03). Clinical event rates were lower with fluvastatin (14.5%) than with placebo (19.1%)(p=NS). Fewer fluvastatin treated patients underwent myocardial revascularization (10.7% vs 13.5%; p=NS).

LCAS

Lipoprotein and Coronary Atherosclerosis Study
(continued)

Conclusions   Fluvastatin therapy in patients with coronary artery disease and mild to moderate hypercholesterolemia reduced the rate of progression of coronary atherosclerotic lesions.

PREDICT

Prevention of Restenosis by Elisor After Transluminal Coronary Angioplasty

Title	Effect of pravastatin on angiographic restenosis after coronary balloon angioplasty.
Authors	Bertrand ME, McFadden EP, Fruchart J-C, et al.
Reference	J Am Coll Cardiol 1997;30:863-869.
Disease	Coronary artery disease, restenosis
Purpose	To assess the efficacy of pravastatin, an HMG coenzyme A reductase inhibitor, to prevent restenosis after coronary balloon angioplasty.
Design	Randomized, double blind, placebo-controlled, multicenter.
Patients	695 patients, 25-75 years old, with LVEF >40%, total cholesterol levels 200-310 mg/dl and triglyceride levels <500 mg/dl who had undergone successful uncomplicated PTCA of one or more coronary artery lesions. Patients with a recent myocardial infarction (<15 d) and patients who had undergone previous PTCA or CABG of the target vessel were excluded. Randomization within 24 h of the PTCA.
Follow-up	Clinical follow-up, repeated blood lipid measurement and coronary angiography at 6 months.
Treatment regimen	Randomization to pravastatin 40 mg/d or placebo.
Additional therapy	All patients received aspirin 100 mg/d. Fish oil and other lipid-lowering agents, corticosteroids, or immunosuppressive drugs were prohibited.

PREDICT

Prevention of Restenosis by Elisor After Transluminal Coronary Angioplasty
(continued)

Results

347 patients were randomized to pravastatin and 348 patients to placebo. 625 (90%) patients had angiographic follow-up. At baseline, the average total cholesterol levels was 231±36 mg/dl in the placebo group and 228±38 mg/dl in the pravastatin group (p=0.42). The average LDL cholesterol was 157±29 mg/dl and 155±32 mg/dl, respectively (p=0.3). After 6 months of therapy total cholesterol decreased to 195±37 mg/dl in the pravastatin group, but remained the same (239±40 mg/dl) in the placebo group (p=0.0001), and LDL cholesterol decreased to 119±31 mg/dl in the pravastatin group but did not change (159±33 mg/dl) in the placebo group (p=0.0001). HDL cholesterol levels after 6 months were 52±13 mg/d in the pravastatin group and 49±14 mg/dl in the placebo group (p=0.01). Apolipoprotein A1 at 6 months was higher in the pravastatin group (150±27 mg/dl) than in the placebo group (144±28 mg/dl)(p=0.003). At baseline average minimal lumen diameter (MLD) was similar in the 2 groups. At follow-up angiography MLD was 1.54±0.66 mm in the pravastatin group and 1.47±0.62 mm in the placebo group (p=0.21). The late loss in MLD was comparable between the pravastatin group (0.46±0.58 mm) and the placebo group (0.48±0.56 mm)(p=0.54), as was the net gain (0.71±0.62 mm and 0.62±0.59 mm, respectively; p=0.07). Percent stenosis before and immediately after PTCA was comparable between the groups. At follow-up angiography mean restenosis severity was 48.4±20% in the pravastatin and 49.7±20% in the placebo group (p=0.44). Restenosis (>50%) occurred in 39.2% of the pravastatin group vs 43.8% of the placebo group (p=0.26). Target vessel revascularization was performed in 19% of the pravastatin vs 21.6% of the placebo group during follow-up. There was no relationship between late loss in MLD and the magnitude of change in lipid blood levels with pravastatin.

Conclusions

Pravastatin 40 mg/d, started within 24 h of successful elective PTCA did not reduce restenosis after 6 months of therapy.

POST-CABG TRIAL

The Post Coronary Artery Bypass Graft Trial

Title	The effect of aggressive lowering of low density lipoprotein cholesterol levels and low dose anticoagulation on obstructive changes in saphenous-vein coronary-artery bypass grafts.
Author	The Post Coronary Artery Bypass Graft Trial Investigators.
Reference	N Engl J Med. 1997; 336:153-162.
Disease	Coronary artery disease.
Purpose	To determine whether aggressive lowering of low density lipoprotein (LDL) cholesterol levels or low dose anticoagulation would delay progression of atherosclerosis in saphenous vein coronary artery bypass grafts.
Design	A 2 x 2 factorial design to test if aggressive lowering of LDL (with a goal of 60-85 mg per deciliter) is more effective than moderate lowering (with a goal of 130-140 mg per deciliter) in delaying progression of atherosclerosis in grafts; and low dose anticoagulation as compared to placebo, in reducing obstruction of bypass grafts.
Patients	1351 patients who had undergone bypass surgery 1-11 years prior to baseline with LDL cholesterols of 130-175 mg per deciliter and at least 1 patent vein graft observed on coronary angiographic study.
Follow-up	4.3 years.

POST-CABG TRIAL

The Post Coronary Artery Bypass Graft Trial

(continued)

Treatment regimen	For aggressive lipid lowering, lovastatin was given at 40 mg per day vs 2.5 mg per day in moderate treatment group. Doses were adjusted to reach target LDL cholesterol levels of less that 85 mg per deciliter in aggressive treatment group and target of less than 140 in moderate treatment group. Cholestyramine at 8 g per day was added if needed. Warfarin or placebo started at 1 mg and then increased by 1 mg up to 4mg and adjusted to an INR of 1.8 to < 2.
Results	The percentage of grafts with progression of atherosclerosis was 27% for patients with aggressive LDL cholesterol lowering and 39% for those who received moderate treatment (p=0.001). There was no difference in angiographic findings on patients receiving warfarin vs placebo. 6.5% of patients with aggressive lipid therapy vs 9.2% with moderate therapy required additional revascularization procedures over 4 years (p=0.03).
Conclusions	Aggressive lowering of LDL cholesterol to < 100 mg per deciliter reduced progression of atherosclerosis in saphenous-vein coronary artery bypass grafts. Low dose warfarin was ineffective

Simvastatin reduced graft vessel disease and mortality after heart transplantation. A 4 year randomized trial.

Title	Simvastatin reduced graft vessel disease and mortality after heart transplantation. A 4 year randomized trial.
Author	Wenke K, Meiser B, Thiery J, et al.
Reference	Circulation 1997; 96:1398-1402.
Disease	Accelerated graft vessel disease (GVD) in heart transplant patients.
Purpose	To determine the effects of long-term antihypercholesterolemic therapy with diet and simvastatin on cholesterol levels, survival, and graft rejection.
Design	Prospective, randomized.
Patients	72 consecutive patients with heart transplant.
Follow-up	4 years.
Treatment regimen	35 patients treated with a low cholesterol diet and simvastatin and 37 with diet alone. All patients received azathioprine. Dose of simvastatin adjusted to a maximum of 20 mg/day. Target LDL cholesterol level of 110–120 mg/dL.

Simvastatin reduced graft vessel disease and mortality after heart transplantation. A 4 year randomized trial.

Results
: During therapy, mean cholesterol level was lower in the simvastatin group (198±18 mg/dL) than the control group (228±19 mg/dL, p = .03). LDL cholesterol levels were also reduced by simvastatin (115±14 vs 156±17 mg/dL, p = .002). After 4 years, survival rate was higher in the simvastatin group (88.6%) vs the control group (70.3%, p = .05). Severe graft rejection as a cause of death occurred in 1 patient in the simvastatin group and 5 in the control group. At 4 years coronary angiographic signs of GVD were 16.6% in treated vs 42.3% in controls. Intravascular ultrasound in a subgroup of patients showed less intimal thickening in patients with LDL cholesterol levels of < 110 mg/dL.

Conclusions
: Simvastatin plus diet in heart transplant patients was more effective than diet in reducing cholesterol, LDL cholesterol, and GVD; and improving survival rate.

AFCAPS/TexCAPS

The Air Force Texas Coronary Atherosclerosis Prevention Study

Title	a. Design & rationale of the airforce/Texas coronary atherosclerosis prevention study (AFCAPS/TexCAPS) b. Primary prevention of acute coronary events with lovastatin in men and women with average cholesterol levels. Results of AFCAPS/TexCAPS.
Author	a. Downs JR, Beere PA, Whitney E, et al. b. Downs JR, Clearfield M, Whitney E, et al.
Reference	a. Am J Cardiol 1997;80:287-293. b. JAMA 1998;279:1615-1622.
Disease	Coronary artery disease
Purpose	To investigate whether lovastatin therapy, in addition to a lipid lowering diet, will be associated with reduction in major coronary events in patients with normal to mildly elevated cholesterol levels and no evidence of atherosclerotic cardiovascular disease.
Design	Randomized, double blind, placebo-controlled, 2 centers.
Patients	5608 men (age 45-73 years) and 997 women (age 55-73 years), with serum total cholesterol 180-264 mg/dl, LDL cholesterol 130-190 mg/dl, HDL cholesterol ≤45 mg/dl for men and ≤47 mg/dl for women, and triglycerides ≤400 mg/dl. Patients with prior history of cardiovascular disease, secondary forms of hyperlipidemia, nephrotic syndrome, insulin-dependent or uncontrolled diabetes mellitus, or uncontrolled hypertension were excluded.
Follow-up	An average of 5.2 years (0.1-7.2 years).
Treatment regimen	Randomization placebo or lovastatin 20 mg/d, titrated to 40 mg/d in patients who had LDL cholesterol >110 mg/dl.

AFCAPS/TexCAPS

The Air Force Texas Coronary Atherosclerosis
Prevention Study
(continued)

Additional therapy	AHA step 1 diet for all patients.
Results	The study was terminated early after the second interim analysis due to a finding of statistically significant benefit for lovastatin therapy. Study drug regimens were maintained until the termination of the study by 71% of the patients assigned to lovastatin and by 63% if the patients assigned to placebo. Lovastatin theapy was associated with 25% decrease in LDL cholesterol levels (p<0.001), 18% decrease in triglyceride levels (p<0.001), and 6% increase in HDL levels (p<0.001). Changes in the lipid profile among the placebo treated patients were small and insignificant. Lovastatin was equally effective in men and women. the primary end point (myocardial infarction, unstalbe angina, or sudden cardiac death) was reached by 10.9% of the placebo group vs 6.8% of the lovastatin group (relative risk 0.63; 95% CI 0.50-0.79; p<0.001). 9.3% of the placebo vs 6.2% of the lovastatin assigned patients needed revascularization (relative risk 0.67; 95% CI 0.52-0.85; p=0.001). 5.6% of the placebo vs only 33% of the lovastatin group had myocardial infarction (relative risk 0.60; 95% CI 0.43-0.83; p=0.002). Unstable angina occurred in 5.1% of the placebo vs 3.5% of the lovastatin group 9relative risk 0.68; 95% CI 0.49-0.95; p=0.02). Life-table plots demonstrated that treatment benefit began in the first year of treatment and continued throughout the study period. The effect of lovastatin therapy on the relative risk of first acute major coronary events was 46% in women vs 37% in men (p=NS). The overal mortality (4.4 vs 4.6 per 1000 patient-years) and the incidence of cancer (15.6 vs 15.1 per 1000 patient-years) were comparable in the placebo and lovastatin groups. Lovastatin was well tolerated. Adverse events leading to discontinuation of the study medication occurred in 13.6% of the lovastatin group vs 13.8% in the placebo group.

The Air Force Texas Coronary Atherosclerosis Prevention Study

(continued)

Conclusion   Lovastatin therapy for an average of 5.2 years reduced the risk for the first acute major coronary event in men and women without prior history of coronary artery disease and with average triglyceride and LDL cholesterol levels and low HDL cholesterol levels.

8. Arrhythmia

CAST

Cardiac Arrhythmia Suppression Trial

Title	a. Preliminary report: effect of encainide and flecainide on mortality in a randomized trial of arrhythmia suppression after myocardial infarction. b. Mortality and morbidity in patients receiving encainide, flecainide, or placebo. The Cardiac Arrhythmia Suppression Trial. c. Events in the Cardiac Arrhythmia Suppression Trial (CAST): mortality in the entire population enrolled. d. Events in the Cardiac Arrhythmia Suppression Trial (CAST): mortality in patients surviving open label titration but not randomized to double blind therapy. e. Association between ease of suppression of ventricular arrhythmia and survival.
Authors	a. The CAST Investigators. b. Echt DS, Leibson PR, Mitchell LB, et al. c. Epstein AE, Bigger JT Jr, Wyse DG, et al. d. Wyse DG, Hallstrom A, McBride R, et al. e. Goldstein S, Brooks MM, Ledingham R, et al.
Reference	a. N Engl J Med 1989;321:406-412. b. N Engl J Med 1991;324:781-788. c. J Am Coll Cardiol 1991;18:14-19. d. J Am Coll Cardiol 1991;18:20-28. e. Circulation 1995;91:79-83.
Disease	Ventricular arrhythmia, coronary artery disease.
Purpose	To evaluate whether suppression of asymptomatic or mildly symptomatic ventricular arrhythmias in patients after myocardial infarction would reduce mortality from arrhythmia.
Design	Randomized, open label (titration phase), double blind (main phase), placebo-controlled, multicenter.

CAST

Cardiac Arrhythmia Suppression Trial
(continued)

Patients	2309 patients, 6 days to 2 years after myocardial infarction, with ≥6 PVCs per h, and left ventricular ejection fraction of ≤0.55 for patients with infarction within 90 days and ≤0.40 for patients with infarction 90 days to 2 years before randomization. Patients with ventricular arrhythmias that caused severe symptoms (such as presyncope or syncope) were excluded.
Follow-up	An average of 9.7 months.
Treatment regimen	An open label titration phase (average 15 days), during which up to 3 drugs (encainide, flecainide and moricizine) at 2 oral doses were tested. This phase was terminated as soon as suppression of ≥80% of the PVCs and ≥90% suppression of nonsustained ventricular tachycardia was detected by 24 h ambulatory ECG monitoring 4-10 days after each dose was begun. Flecainide was not used in patients with ejection fraction <0.30. In patients with ejection fraction ≥0.30, moricizine was used as a second drug. Patients whose arrhythmia worsened or who were intolerant were not included in the main phase. In the main phase patients were randomized to receive either the active drug that had suppressed the arrhythmia or placebo.

Cardiac Arrhythmia Suppression Trial
(continued)

Results   1727 patients (75%) had initial suppression of their arrhythmia and were included in the main phase. 1498 patients were assigned to flecainide, encainide, or placebo. After an average of 10 months total mortality was 7.7% in the encainide/flecainide groups vs 3.0% in the placebo (relative risk 2.5, 95% CI 1.6-4.5). The relative risks for death from any cause for encainide and flecainide considered separately were not different (2.7 vs 2.2 compared to placebo). Death from arrhythmia was more common in the encainide/flecainide groups (4.5%) than placebo (1.2%, relative risk 3.6, 95% CI 1.7-8.5, p=0.0004). The relative risk for encainide was 3.4 and for flecainide 4.4, compared with placebo. The relative risk for death or cardiac arrest with resuscitation was 2.38 (95% CI 1.59-3.57). Subgroup analyses revealed that in every subgroup tested, flecainide and encainide were associated with increased total mortality and arrhythmic death. The mortality in the placebo-treated patients was lower than expected. This was probably due to selection bias including only patients whose arrhythmias were suppressable in the titration phase. Nonrandomized patients had more extensive coronary disease and experienced higher mortality and arrhythmic events than the randomized placebo group.

Conclusions   Encainide and flecainide were associated with increased death rate due to arrhythmia and acute myocardial infarction complicated by shock in patients after acute myocardial infarction with asymptomatic ventricular arrhythmias, even though these drugs were effective in suppression of the arrhythmia.

BASIS

Basel Antiarrhythmic Study of Infarct Survival

Title	a. Effect of antiarrhythmic therapy on mortality in survivors of myocardial infarction with asymptomatic complex ventricular arrhythmias: Basel Antiarrhythmic Study of Infarct Survival (BASIS). b. Long-term benefit of 1 year amiodarone treatment for persistent complex ventricular arrhythmias after myocardial infarction.
Authors	a. Burkart F, Pfisterer M, Kiowski W, et al. b. Pfisterer ME, Kiowski W, Brunner H, et al.
Reference	a. J Am Coll Cardiol 1990;16:1711-1718. b. Circulation 1993;87:309-311.
Disease	Arrhythmia, acute myocardial infarction.
Purpose	To evaluate the effects of prophylactic antiarrhythmic treatment in survivors of myocardial infarction with persisting asymptomatic complex arrhythmias.
Design	Randomized, 3 centers.
Patients	312 patients, <71 years old, who survived acute myocardial infarction and had asymptomatic complex ventricular ectopic activity on a 24 h ECG recording 24 h after discontinuation of all antiarrhythmic medications.
Follow-up	a. Clinical evaluation and 24 h ECG monitoring at baseline and after 3, 6 and 12 months. b. 55-125 months (mean 72 months).

BASIS

Basel Antiarrhythmic Study of Infarct Survival

(continued)

Treatment regimen	Patients were randomized to either: 1. Individualized antiarrhythmic drugs guided by continuous ECG monitoring (quinidine and mexiletine as first line drugs and ajmaline, disopyramide, flecainide, propafenone, or sotalol as second line drugs). If none of these drugs suppressed the arrhythmias, amiodarone was given. 2. Low dose amiodarone. 1g/d for 5 days followed by 200 mg/d. If symptomatic arrhythmias developed, the therapy was changed and the patients were considered to be treatment deviators. Treatment was continued for 1 year. 3. Control without prophylactic antiarrhythmic drug. If symptoms occurred, antiarrhythmic medications were given, and they were considered as treatment deviators.
Additional therapy	No limitations on other nonantiarrhythmic medications.
Results	a. During 1 year follow-up, 10%, 5.1%, and 13.2% of groups 1, 2, and 3 died (61% reduction of mortality by amiodarone vs control; p=0.048). After exclusion of noncardiac mortality, amiodarone was still associated with 55% reduction of mortality. Sudden death or sustained ventricular tachycardia or fibrillation occurred in 5.1% of the amiodarone and 16.7% of the control group (p<0.01). The effect of individualized therapy (group 1) was less marked (40% reduction, p=NS). b. The probability of death after 84 months (Kaplan Meier) was 30% for amiodarone and 45% for control patients (p=0.03). However, this was entirely due to the first year amiodarone effect. A similar effect was observed regarding cardiac death (p=0.047).
Conclusions	Low dose amiodarone decreased mortality during the first year after acute myocardial infarction in asymptomatic patients with persistent complex ventricular arrhythmias. The beneficial effect of amiodarone lasted several years after discontinuation of amiodarone.

CASCADE

Cardiac Arrest in Seattle: Conventional Vs Amiodarone Drug Evaluation

Title	a. Cardiac Arrest in Seattle: Conventional vs Amiodarone Drug Evaluation (the CASCADE study). b. the CASCADE study: randomized antiarrhythmic drug therapy in survivors of cardiac arrest in Seattle.
Authors	a. The CASCADE Investigators. b. Greene HL, for the CASCADE Investigators.
Reference	a. Am J Cardiol 1991;67:578-584. b. Am J Cardiol 1993;72:70F-74F.
Disease	Ventricular fibrillation.
Purpose	To evaluate the efficacy of empiric amiodarone therapy and electrophysiologic testing and ambulatory ECG monitoring guided drug therapy in survivors of out-of-hospital ventricular fibrillation.
Design	Randomized, open label, multicenter.
Patients	228 patients who survived an episode of out-of-hospital ventricular fibrillation that was not associated with Q wave infarction. Only patients who were considered high risk for recurrence were included.
Follow-up	Up to 6 years.
Treatment regimen	Amiodarone or electrophysiologic testing and ambulatory ECG monitoring guided conventional drug therapy.
Additional therapy	Approximately 50% of all patients received an implanted defibrillator (since 1988).

CASCADE

Cardiac Arrest in Seattle: Conventional Vs Amiodarone Drug Evaluation
(continued)

Results

Of the 115 patients randomized to conventional therapy 33 received quinidine, 26 procainamide, 12 received flecainide, and 17 combination therapy. 82% and 69% of the amiodarone and conventional therapy groups were free from either cardiac death, resuscitated VF, or syncopal shocks from implanted defibrillator after 2 years. The corresponding numbers for 4 and 6 years are 66% vs 52% and 53% vs 40%, in the amiodarone and conventional therapy groups, respectively (p=0.007). 83% vs 78%, 65% vs 62%, and 58% vs 37% of the patients were still alive after 2, 4, and 6 years. 105 patients had automatic implantable defibrillators. 38% of the amiodarone and 60% of the conventional therapy experienced shock from the defibrillator (p=0.032). However, 29% of the amiodarone and only 17% of the conventional therapy group stopped their medications. Possible pulmonary toxicity was diagnosed in 6% of the patients over 12 months and 10% over 3 years. Thyroid dysfunction was relatively common (22.1%) in the amiodarone group.

Conclusions

Although amiodarone was associated with mild reduction of mortality, overall mortality remained high, and side effects were common.

CAST-2

Cardiac Arrhythmia Suppression Trial-2

Title	a. The Cardiac Arrhythmia Supression Trial: first CAST, then CAST-II. b. Effect of the antiarrhythmic agent moricizine on survival after myocardial infarction.
Authors	a. Greene HL, Roden DM, Katz RJ, et al. b. The Cardiac Arrhythmia Suppression Trial II investigators.
Reference	a. J Am Coll Cardiol 1992;19:894-898. b. N Engl J Med 1992;327:227-233.
Disease	Ventricular arrhythmia, coronary artery disease.
Purpose	To evaluate whether suppression of asymptomatic or mildly symptomatic ventricular premature depolarizations by moricizine would decrease mortality in patients after myocardial infarction.
Design	Randomized, double blind, placebo-controlled, multicenter.
Patients	Patients, 6-90 days after myocardial infarction, with ≥6 PVCs per h, and left ventricular ejection fraction of ≤0.40. Patients with ventricular arrhythmias that caused severe symptoms (such as presyncope or syncope), or runs ≥30 seconds at a rate of ≥120 bpm were excluded. 1325 patients (10 patients were included in CAST-I) were included in the short-term trial and 1374 patients (536 patients were included in CAST-I) in the long-term trial.
Follow-up	Short-term protocol: 2 weeks. Long-term protocol: a mean of 18 months.

CAST-2

Cardiac Arrhythmia Suppression Trial-2

(continued)

Treatment regimen	Short-term protocol: moricizine 200 mg X3/d for 14 days vs placebo or no therapy. Long-term protocol: titration phase of moricizine started with 200 mg X3/d and increased to 250 mg X3/d and then to 300 mg X3/d until arrhythmia was suppressed or adverse effects occurred. Only patients in whom suppression of ≥80% of the PVCs and ≥90% suppression of nonsustained ventricular tachycardia was detected by 24 h ambulatory ECG monitoring were entered into the long-term protocol.
Results	CAST-II was stopped early because moricizine therapy was associated with excess mortality in the first 14 day phase. The rate of death or resuscitated cardiac arrest was 2.6% (17 of 665 patients) of the moricizine group vs 0.5% (3 of 660 patients) of the no therapy group (adjusted p<0.01, relative risk 5.6, 95% CI 1.7-19.1). Other adverse effects such as recurrent myocardial infarction, new or worsened heart failure, and proarrhythmia tended to be higher in the moricizine group. Arrhythmia suppression was achieved in 1155 patients (87.2%) who were included in the long-term phase. During a mean follow-up of 18 months 8.4% of the moricizine vs 7.3% of the placebo treated group died or had cardiac arrests due to arrhythmias (p=0.4). The 2 year survival rate was 81.7% in the moricizine vs 85.6% in the placebo. Nonfatal adverse effects were more common with moricizine (p=0.03).
Conclusions	Moricizine was effective in suppression of asymptomatic or mildly symptomatic ventricular arrhythmias in patients after myocardial infarction. However, therapy with moricizine was associated with increased mortality in the short protocol and no beneficial effect in the long-term protocol.

ESVEM

The Electrophysiologic Study Vs Electrocardiographic Monitoring

Title	a. The ESVEM Trial: Electrophysiologic Study vs Electrocardiographic Monitoring for selection of antiarrhythmic therapy of ventricular tachyarrhythmias.
	b. Determinants of predicted efficacy of antiarrhythmic drugs in the electrophysiologic study vs electrocardiographic monitoring trial.
	c. A comparison of electrophysiologic testing with holter monitoring to predict antiarrhythmic-drug efficacy for ventricular tachyarrhythmias.
	d. A comparison of 7 antiarrhythmic drugs in patients with ventricular tachyarrhythmias.
	e. Cost of initial therapy in the electrophysiological study vs ECG monitoring trial (ESVEM).
	f. Significance and incidence of concordance of drug efficacy predictions by holter monitoring and electrophysiological study in the ESVEM Trial.
Authors	a.+b. The ESVEM Investigators.
	c.+d. Mason JW, for the ESVEM Investigators.
	e. Omioigui NA, Marcus FI, Mason JW, et al.
	f. Reiter MJ, Mann DE, Reiffel JE, et al.
Reference	a. Circulation 1989;79:1354-1360.
	b. Circulation 1993;87:323-329.
	c. N Engl J Med 1993;329:445-451.
	d. N Engl J Med 1993;329:452-458.
	e. Circulation 1995;91:1070-1076.
	f. Circulation 1995;91:1988-1995.
Disease	Ventricular tachyarrhythmias.
Purpose	To compare the efficacy and accuracy of electrophysiologic study (EPS) vs ambulatory electrocardiographic holter monitoring (HM) for prediction of antiarrhythmic drug efficacy in patients with aborted sudden death or sustained ventricular tachyarrhythmias.
Design	Randomized, open label, multicenter.

The Electrophysiologic Study Vs Electrocardiographic Monitoring
(continued)

Patients	486 patients who had been resuscitated from sudden death, or had documented sustained ventricular tachycardia or unmonitored syncope (with subsequent EPS demonstration inducible sustained monomorphic ventricular tachycardia) were screened. Only patients with ≥10 PVCs/h during 48 h HM and reproducibly inducible sustained ventricular tachyarrhythmias at EPS were included.
Follow-up	6.2 years.
Treatment regimen	Patients were randomized to serial drug evaluation by HM and exercise test or by EPS. Patients underwent testing of up to 6 drugs until one or none was predicted to be effective: imipramine, mexiletine, procainamide, quinidine, sotalol, pirmenol, and propafenone. Drugs were tested in random order. Patients were discharged from the hospital with a predicted effective drug. Subjects in whom no drug was effective were withdrawn from the study.
Results	Efficacy predictions were achieved in 45% of the EPS and 77% in the HM arms (p<0.001). Ejection fraction of <0.25 and presence of coronary artery disease were negative correlates (p<0.10) of drug efficacy prediction in the EPS arm. In the HM arm, only ejection fraction correlated with efficacy, although with only marginal significance (p=0.11). A multivariate model selected assessment by HM and higher ejection fraction as independent predictors (p<0.05) of drug efficacy. The drug evaluation process required an actuarial median time of 25 days in the EPS vs 10 days in the HM arms (p<0.0001). There was no significant difference between the EPS and HM arms in the actuarial probabilities of either death or recurrence of arrhythmia. Patients randomized to EPS had higher mean charge for evaluation ($42,002 vs $29,970, p=0.0015) and more drug trials (3.0 vs 2.1, p=0.0001). In the EPS group, the percentage of patients who had predictions of drug efficacy was higher with sotalol (35%) than with any other drugs (26%-10%, p<0.001). There was no significant difference among the drugs in the HM group. The least adverse effects was noted with sotalol (16% vs 23%-43% with the other drugs). The patients that received sotalol

had the lowest actuarial probability of recurrence of ventricular arrhythmia (RR 0.43, 95% CI 0.29-0.62, p<0.001), death from any cause (RR 0.50, 95% CI 0.30-0.80, p=0.004), cardiac death (RR 0.50, 95% CI 0.28-0.90, p=0.02), or arrhythmic death (RR 0.50, 95% CI 0.26-0.96, p=0.04). At the time of the first drug trial in the EPS group, HM and EPS were concordant in predicting efficacy in 23% and in predicting inefficiency in 23%. In 54% of the patients there was discordance between HP and EPS. At the time EPS predicted efficacy, 68 of the 100 patients also had suppression of arrhythmias in HM. Rates of arrhythmia recurrence or mortality were similar among patients with suppression of arrhythmias on both HM and EPS, compared with those who had suppression on EPS alone. There was no significant difference in outcome between the patients with suppression on both HM and EPS and those with suppression on the HM arm.

Conclusions

Drug efficacy predictions are achieved more frequently and faster with HM than EPS strategy. However, there was no significant difference in the success of drug therapy as selected by either EPS or HM. Sotalol was more effective than the other 6 drugs in preventing death and recurrence of ventricular arrhythmia, and was associated with less adverse effects than the other medications. There is frequent discordance in prediction of drug efficacy between HM and EPS. However, suppression of ventricular arrhythmias on both tests did not predict better outcome.

MADIT

The Multicenter Automatic Defibrillator Implantation Trial

Title	Improved survival with an implanted defibrillator in patients with coronary disease at high risk for ventricular arrhythmia.
Authors	Moss AJ, Hall WJ, Cannom DS, et al.
Reference	N Engl J Med 1996;335:1933-1940.
Disease	Coronary artery disease, arrhythmia.
Purpose	To assess whether prophylactic implantation of cardioverter-defibrillator, as compared with conventional medical therapy, would decrease mortality in patients with prior myocardial infarction, low ejection fraction, and episodes of asymptomatic unsustained ventricular tachycardia.
Design	Randomized, multicenter.
Patients	196 patients of either sex, 25–80 years old, with myocardial infarction >3 weeks before entry, documented episode of asymptomatic, nonsustained ventricular tachycardia (3–30 ventricular ectopic beats at a rate >120 per min), and left ventricular ejection fraction ≤0.35. Patients in NYHA class IV, indication for revascularization, previous cardiac arrest or symptomatic ventricular tachycardia, CABG within 2 months or PTCA within 3 months, advanced cerebrovascular disease, and serious noncardiac medical condition were not included. Eligible patients underwent electrophysiologic study, and only patients with reproducibly induced ventricular tachycardia or fibrillation that was not suppressed by procainamide or an equivalent drug were included.
Follow-up	Average follow-up 27 months (range <1 month to 61 months).

MADIT

The Multicenter Automatic Defibrillator Implantation Trial

(continued)

Treatment regimen	Within 30 days after the electrophysiologic study, patients were randomized to implantation of defibrillator or conventional medical therapy. The choice of medical therapy, including whether to use antiarrhythmic agents, was made by the patient's physician. The first 98 patients were randomized to medical therapy (n=53) or transthoracic defibrillator (n=45), and the last 98 patients to medical therapy (n=48) or nonthoracotomy defibrillator implantation with transvenous leads (n=50).
Results	The baseline characteristics of the defibrillator and medical therapy groups were similar. 11 patients in the medical therapy group received a defibrillator during the follow-up period and 5 patients assigned to defibrillator never received a defibrillator. There were no operative deaths. There were 15 deaths in the defibrillator group and 39 deaths in the medical therapy group (hazard ratio 0.46; 95% CI 0.26–0.82; p=0.009). There were 11 deaths from cardiac causes in the defibrillator group vs 27 in the medical therapy group. Both defibrillator types, with transthoracic and with intravenous leads were equally effective (ratio of the hazard ratios 0.86; p=0.78). There was no evidence that ß blockers, amiodarone, or other antiarrhythmic drugs had an influence on the hazard ratio. However, the power of the analysis for the drug interactions with hazard ratio is limited, due to small number of treated patients.
Conclusions	In patients with prior myocardial infarction, reduced left ventricular ejection fraction, and asymptomatic nonsustained ventricular tachycardia, who had reproducible sustained ventricular arrhythmia during electrophysiologic study that was not suppressible by intravenous antiarrhythmic drug, prophylactic implantation of defibrillator improved survival as compared with conventional medical therapy.

AVID

Antiarrhythmics Vs Implantable Defibrillators

Title	A comparison of antiarrhythmic drug therapy with implantable defibrillators in patients resuscitated from near-fatal ventricular arrhythmias.
Author	The Antiarrhythmics Vs Implantable Defibrillator (AVID) investigators.
Reference	N Engl J Med 1997; 337:1576-1583.
Disease	Ventricular fibrillation (VF), sustained ventricular tachycardia (VT).
Purpose	To determine survival of initial therapy of an implantable defibrillator vs amiodarone or sotalol in patients who were resuscitated from near fatal VF; or patients with symptomatic, sustained, and hemodynamically compromising VT.
Design	Randomized, multicenter, VT patients had to have sustained VT with syncope or an ejection fraction <.40 and symptoms suggesting severe hemodynamic compromise (near syncope, heart failure, angina).
Patients	1016 patients; mean age 65 years; 79% male. 455 had VF; 561 had VT.
Follow-up	3 years plus.
Treatment regimen	Implantable cardioverter-defibrillator vs anti-arrhythmic drug treatment (most took amiodarone followed by sotalol).

Results

There were fewer deaths among patients assigned to the implantable defibrillator (80) than antiarrhythmic drug group (122). Death rates at 18.2 months were 15.8% in the defibrillator group vs 24% in the anti-arrhythmic group. There was a decrease in death rate at 1, 2, and 3 years of 39, 27, 31%, respectively, in patients receiving the device vs drug; hence patients receiving the defibrillator had a better survival throughout the course of the study (p<0.02). Automatic pacing or shocks were more common among patients who entered the study with VT compared to those that entered with VF.

Conclusions

For survivors of VF or sustained, severely symptomatic VT, the implantable cardioverter defibrillator is superior to antiarrhythmic drugs regarding survival.

CABG - PATCH

Coronary Artery Bypass Graft (CABG) Patch

Title	Prophylactic use of implanted cardiac defibrillators in patients at high risk for ventricular arrhythmias after coronary artery bypass graft surgery.
Author	Bigger JT for the CABG patch trial investigators.
Reference	N Engl J Med 1997; 337:1569-1575.
Disease	Sudden death by sustained ventricular tachyarrhythmias in patients with coronary artery disease, left ventricular dysfunction, and abnormalities on signal-averaged electrocardiograms.
Purpose	To determine the effect of prophylactic implantation of cardioverter-defibrillators at the time of coronary artery bypass surgery on survival in patients with coronary artery disease, left ventricular dysfunction, and abnormalities in signal-averaged electrocardiograms.
Design	Randomized, multicenter.
Patients	1422 eligible, 1055 enrolled; 900 randomized (446-device; 454-no device). Patients had to be less than 80 (average ages were 64 and 63 in treated and untreated groups, respectively); had to have a left ventricular ejection fraction of <0.36; and had to have abnormalities on signal-averaged electrocardiogram.
Follow-up	Average follow-up was 32±16 months.
Treatment regimen	Implantable cardioverter-defibrillator or no device therapy at time of CABG. Trial prohibited use of anti-arrhythmic drugs for asymptomatic ventricular arrhythmias.

CABG - PATCH

Coronary Artery Bypass Graft (CABG) Patch

(continued)

Results
: At 32 months there were 101 deaths in the defibrillator group and 95 in the control group. There were 71 deaths due to cardiac causes in the defibrillator group and 72 in the control group (p = NS).

Conclusions
: Survival was not improved by prophylactic implantation of automatic cardioverter-defibrillator at the time of CABG in high risk patients.

D,l-Sotalol in Patients with Ventricular Tachycardia and in Survivors of Cardiac Arrest

Title	Efficacy and safety of d,l-Sotalol in patients with ventricular tachycardia and in survivors of cardiac arrest.
Authors	Haverkamp W, Martinez-Rubio A, Hief C, et al.
Reference	J Am Coll Cardiol 1997;30:487-495.
Disease	Ventricular tachycardia, ventricular fibrillation.
Purpose	To evaluate the safety and efficacy of d,l-sotalol in patients with ventricular tachycardia or ventricular fibrillation undergoing programmed ventricular stimulation.
Patients	396 patients, 56±14 years old, with inducible sustained ventricular tachycardia, ventricular fibrillation, or aborted sudden cardiac death who underwent programmed electrophysiologic ventricular stimulation. Patients within 48 h of acute myocardial infarction, unresponsive congestive heart failure, asthma or chronic obstructive pulmonary disease, previous adverse reaction to β-blockers, renal failure, and the need for concomitant medications that prolong the QT interval were excluded.
Follow-up	Mean follow-up 34±18 months.
Treatment regimen	d,l-sotalol 80 mg BID for 48 h. Dosage was increased gradually up to 480 mg/d. Programmed ventricular stimulation was repeated after reaching the target dose. If ventricular tachyarrhythmia was not suppressed, the dose was increased, if tolerated, up to 640 mg/d and programmed ventricular stimulation was repeated. Patients with non-inducible or more difficult to induce arrhythmia were discharged with d,l-sotalol.

Results

d,l-sotalol at an average dose of 465±90 mg/d suppressed inducible ventricular tachyarrhythmia in 151 patients (38.1%). In additional 76 patients (19.2%) induction of arrhythmia became more difficult. Side effects demanding discontinuation of d,l-sotalol during the short-term treatment phase occurred in 28 patients (7.1%). Proarrhythmic effects were detected in 10 patients (2.5%) and Torsade de pointes ventricular tachycardia occurred in 7 patients (1.8%). Only 210 patients (53%) were discharged receiving d,l-sotalol. During the follow-up period, symptomatic ventricular arrhythmia occurred in 41 patients (19.5%). Actuarial rates for patients free of arrhythmic event were 89% at 1 year and 77% at 3 years. Actuarial total survival rates were 94% at 1 year and 86% at 3 years. Actuarial sudden death rates at one year were 8% and at 3 years 11% for patients with coronary artery disease and 6% and 25% for patients with dilated cardiomyopathy. Ventricular tachyarrhythmia suppression during programmed stimulation by d,l-sotalol was an independent predictor of arrhythmia recurrence. However, noninducible ventricular arrhythmia did not predict freedom from sudden death.

Conclusions

Oral d,l-sotalol is safe and effective in suppression of ventricular tachyarrhythmias. However, sudden cardiac death occurred in a considerable proportion of patients despite d,l-sotalol therapy, and electrophysiologic studies did not discriminate between patients who developed sudden cardiac death during therapy.

Preoperative amiodarone as prophylaxis against atrial fibrillation after heart surgery.

Title	Preoperative amiodarone as prophylaxis against atrial fibrillation after heart surgery.
Author	Daoud EG, Strickberger A, Man KC
Reference	N Engl J Med 1997; 337:1785-1791.
Disease	Atrial fibrillation.
Purpose	To determine the effectiveness of preoperative amiodarone as prophylaxis against atrial fibrillation following cardiac surgery.
Design	Double blind, randomized study.
Patients	124 patients scheduled for cardiac surgery, average ages 57–61 years.
Follow-up	~ 7 days post hospital discharge.
Treatment regimen	64 patients received amiodarone; and 60 received placebo for a minimum of 7 days prior to surgery. Amiodarone was given as 600 mg per day x 7 days, then 200 mg per day until hospital discharge.
Results	Atrial fibrillation occurred in 25% of patients in the amiodarone group and 53% of patients in the placebo group following surgery (p=.003). Duration of hospitalization was shorter in the amiodarone patients (6.5±2.6 days) compared to placebo patients (7.9±4.3 days, p = 0.04). Hospitalization costs were lower in the amiodarone group.

Conclusions   Administration of oral amiodarone prior to cardiac surgery reduces the incidence of postoperative atrial fibrillation and duration and cost of hospitalization.

THEOPACE

Title	Effects of Permanent Pacemaker and Oral Theophylline in Sick Sinus Syndrome. The THEOPACE Study: A randomized controlled trial.
Author	Alboni P, Menozzi C, Brignole M, et al.
Reference	Circulation 1997; 96:260-266.
Disease	Sick sinus syndrome (arrhythmias).
Purpose	To determine the effects of oral theophylline vs permanent pacing on the symptoms and complications of sick sinus syndrome.
Design	Randomized, controlled, prospective trial.
Patients	170 patients with symptomatic sick sinus syndrome.
Follow-up	48 months.
Treatment regimen	No treatment (35 patients); oral theophylline (n = 36) or dual chamber rate responsive pacemaker therapy (n = 36).
Results	Frequency of syncope was lower in the pacemaker (6%) compared to control group (23%, p = .02) and tended to be lower than in the group receiving theophylline (17%, p = .07). Development of clinical heart failure was lower in the pacemaker (3%) and theophylline groups (3%) compared to no treatment (17%, p = .05). The frequency of sustained paroxysmal tachycardias, permanent atrial fibrillation, and thromboembolic events did not show any difference among the 3 groups.

Conclusions	In patients with symptomatic sick sinus syndrome, the frequency of syncope was lowered with pacemaker therapy. Both pacemaker therapy and theophylline reduce heart failure.

SWORD

Survival With ORal D-sotalol

Title	a. The SWORD trial. Survival with oral d-sotalol in patients with left ventricular dysfunction after myocardial infarction: rationale, design, and methods. b. Effect of d-sotalol on mortality in patients with left ventricular dysfunction after recent and remote myocardial infarction. c. Mortality in the Survival with ORAL D-Sotalol (SWORD) Trial: Why did patients die?
Authors	Waldo AL, Camm AJ, deRuyter H, et al. c. Pratt CM, Camm AJC, Cooper W, et al.
Reference	a. Am J Cardiol 1995;75:1023-1027. b. Lancet 1996;348:7-12. c. Am J Cardiol 1998; 81:869-876.
Disease	Congestive heart failure.
Purpose	To evaluate the effectiveness of d-sotalol, an antiarrhythmic agent with a pure potassium-channel-blocking effect, and to reduce mortality in patients with previous myocardial infarction and left ventricular dysfunction.
Design	Randomized, double blind, placebo-controlled, multicenter.
Patients	3121 patients, age ≥18 years, with left ventricular ejection fraction of ≤40% and a recent (6-42 days) or a remote (>42 days) myocardial infarction and class II-III heart failure. Patients with unstable angina, class IV heart failure, history of life-threatening arrhythmia unrelated to a myocardial infarction, sick sinus syndrome or high-grade atrioventricular block, recent (<14 days) coronary angioplasty or coronary artery bypass surgery, electrolyte abnormalities, prolonged QT, renal failure, or concomitant use of antiarrhythmic drugs were excluded.
Follow-up	Mean follow-up 148 days.

SWORD

Survival With ORal D-sotalol
(continued)

Treatment regimen	Randomization to oral d-sotalol 100 mg X2/d or placebo for 1 week. If the dose was tolerated and QTc <520 msec, the dose was increased to 200 mg X2/d. If QTc was >560 msec, the dose was reduced.
Additional therapy	β-blockers, calcium channel blockers, digoxin, diuretics, nitrates, and angiotensin-converting enzyme inhibitors were permitted.
Results	The trial was stopped prematurely after 3121 patients had been enrolled because of excess in mortality in the d-sotalol group. All causes mortality was 5.0% vs 3.1% in the d-sotalol and placebo group, respectively (relative risk (RR) 1.65; 95% CI 1.15-2.36; p=0.006), cardiac mortality was 4.7% vs 2.9%, respectively (RR 1.65; 95% CI 1.14-2.39; p=0.008), and presumed arrhythmic deaths 3.6% vs 2.0% (RR 1.77; 95% CI 1.15-2.74; p=0.008). Rates of non-fatal cardiac events were similar between the groups. The adverse effect associated with d-sotalol therapy was greater in patients with left ventricular ejection fraction of 31%-40% than in those with ≤30% (RR 4.0 vs 1.2; p=0.007).
	c. The mortality associated with d-sotalol was greatest in patients with remote myocardial infarction and LV ejection fractions of 31%-40%. Comparable placebo patients in this group had a very low mortality. Most variables associated with torsades de pointes were not predictive of d-sotalol risk of death, except female gender.
Conclusions	D-sotalol therapy in patients after myocardial infarction and a reduced left ventricular ejection fraction were associated with increased total and cardiac mortality, which was presumed primarily to be due to arrhythmic deaths.

9. Anticoagulation for Atrial Fibrillation

AFASAK

Aspirin vs Warfarin in Atrial Fibrillation

Title	Placebo-controlled, randomized trial of warfarin and aspirin for prevention of thromboembolic complications in chronic atrial fibrillation. The Copenhagen AFASAK study.
Authors	Petersen P, Boysen G, Godtfredsen J, et al.
Reference	Lancet 1989;I:175-179.
Disease	Atrial fibrillation.
Purpose	To evaluate the effects of low dose aspirin and warfarin anticoagulation on the incidence of thromboembolic events in patients with chronic nonrheumatic atrial fibrillation.
Design	Randomized, open label (warfarin vs no-warfarin), double blind in the group of no-warfarin (aspirin vs placebo), 2 centers.
Patients	1007 patients, ≥18 years old with chronic atrial fibrillation. Patients with previous anticoagulation therapy >6 months, cerebrovascular event within 1 month, severe hypertension, alcoholism, valve replacement, rheumatic heart disease, or with contraindication to aspirin or warfarin were excluded.
Follow-up	2 years.
Treatment regimen	Warfarin (open label), target INR was 2.8-4.2. Aspirin 75 mg/d or placebo.

AFASAK

Aspirin vs Warfarin in Atrial Fibrillation

(continued)

Results
Patients on warfarin were within INR 2.8-4.2 for 42% of the time. 26% of the time the INR was <2.4. Thromboembolic complications occurred in 1.5% of the warfarin, 6.0% in the aspirin, and 6.3% of the control group (p<0.05). The yearly incidence of thromboembolic events was 2.0% on warfarin and 5.5% on either aspirin or placebo. Vascular death occurred in 0.9%, 3.6%, and 4.5% of the warfarin, aspirin and placebo groups (p<0.02). 6.3% of the warfarin patients had nonfatal bleeding, while only 0.6% and 0 of the aspirin and placebo patients had bleeding.

Conclusions
Chronic anticoagulation with warfarin, but not with low dose aspirin, reduced vascular mortality and thromboembolic complications in patients with chronic non-rheumatic atrial fibrillation.

SPAF

Stroke Prevention in Atrial Fibrillation

Title	a. Preliminary report of the stroke prevention in atrial fibrillation study. b. Stroke prevention in atrial fibrillation study. Final results.
Authors	SPAF Investigators.
Reference	a. N Engl J Med 1990;322:863-868. b. Circulation 1991;84:527-539.
Disease	Atrial fibrillation.
Purpose	To determine the efficacy of warfarin and aspirin for primary prevention of ischemic stroke and systemic embolism in patients with nonrheumatic atrial fibrillation.
Design	Randomized, open label (warfarin), double blind (aspirin vs placebo), multicenter.
Patients	1330 patients with chronic or paroxysmal atrial fibrillation, without prosthetic heart valve or rheumatic mitral stenosis. Patients with congestive heart failure were excluded. 627 patients were eligible to receive warfarin (group 1) and 703 patients were not eligible (group 2).
Follow-up	a. An average of 1.13 years. b. An average of 1.3 years.
Treatment regimen	Group 1. warfarin vs aspirin 325 mg/d or placebo. Target INR for warfarin 2.0-4.5. Group 2. aspirin 325 mg/d vs placebo.

Results

a. The overall primary events (ischemic stroke and embolism) rate was 1.6% per year in the patients who received either aspirin or warfarin, and 8.3% per year in the placebo treated patients in group 1 (risk reduction 81%, 95% CI 56-91%, p<0.00005). Total primary end points occurred in 3.2% and 6.3% of the aspirin and placebo treated patients (group 1+2)(risk reduction 49% (15-69%), p=0.014). On the basis of these results, the placebo arm was discontinued by the safety committee.

b. Warfarin reduced the risk of primary events by 67% (2.3% vs 7.4% per year, 95% CI 27-85%, p=0.01). Aspirin reduced the risk of primary events by 42% (3.6% vs 6.3%, 95% CI 9-63%, p=0.02). Primary events or death were reduced by 58% (95% CI 20-78%, p=0.01) by warfarin and 32% (95% CI 7-50%, p=0.02) by aspirin. The risk of significant bleeding was 1.5%, 1.4%, and 1.6% per year in the warfarin, aspirin, and placebo, respectively.

Conclusions

Aspirin and warfarin are both effective in prevention of ischemic stroke and systemic embolism in patients with nonrheumatic atrial fibrillation.

BAATAF

Boston Area Anticoagulation Trial for Atrial Fibrillation

Title	The effect of low dose warfarin on the risk of stroke in patients with nonrheumatic atrial fibrillation.
Authors	The Boston Area Anticoagulation Trial for Atrial Fibrillation Investigators.
Reference	N Engl J Med 1990;323:1505-1511.
Disease	Atrial fibrillation.
Purpose	To assess the efficacy of low dose warfarin therapy in preventing stroke in patients with nonrheumatic atrial fibrillation.
Design	Randomized, open label, multicenter.
Patients	420 patients with chronic or paroxysmal atrial fibrillation without mitral stenosis. Patients with left ventricular thrombus, aneurysm, prosthetic heart valve, severe heart failure, transient ischemic attack or stroke within 6 months, or clear indication or contraindications to anti-coagulant therapy were excluded.
Follow-up	Clinical follow-up up to 4.5 years (mean 2.2 years).
Treatment regimen	Warfarin (target range for prothrombin-time ratio 1.2-1.5X control value [INR 1.5-2.7]) or no treatment.
Additional therapy	Aspirin therapy was not allowed in the anticoagulation group. Aspirin was permitted in the control group.

BAATAF

Boston Area Anticoagulation Trial for Atrial Fibrillation

(continued)

Results   Prothrombin time in the warfarin group was in the target
                  range 83% of the time. Only 10% of the patients discon-
                  tinued warfarin permanently. There were 2 strokes in the
                  warfarin and 13 in the control groups (p=0.0022);(inci-
                  dence of 0.41%/year vs 2.98%/year (incidence ratio 0.14,
                  95% CI 0.04-0.49. 2 and 1 patients in the warfarin and con-
                  trol group had major bleeding. There was no statistical sig-
                  nificant difference in the occurrence of minor bleeding.
                  Total mortality was 11 and 26 patients in the warfarin and
                  control patients (RR 0.38, 95% CI 0.17-0.82, p=0.005). The
                  same trend was seen for cardiac and noncardiac mortali-
                  ty. Patients with paroxysmal and chronic atrial fibrillation
                  had similar risk of stroke.

Conclusions   Long-term low dose warfarin therapy was associated with
                  reduced mortality and prevention of stroke in patients
                  with atrial fibrillation not associated with mitral stenosis.

CAFA

Canadian Atrial Fibrillation Anticoagulation

Title	Canadian Atrial Fibrillation Anticoagulation (CAFA) study.
Authors	Connolly SJ, Laupacis A, Gent M, et al.
Reference	J Am Coll Cardiol 1991;18:349-355.
Disease	Atrial fibrillation.
Purpose	To assess the efficacy and safety of warfarin therapy for nonrheumatic atrial fibrillation.
Design	Randomized, double blind, placebo-controlled, multicenter.
Patients	378 patients, ≥19 years of age, with paroxysmal recurrent or chronic atrial fibrillation, without mitral stenosis or mitral or aortic prosthetic valves. Patients with clear indications or contraindications to anticoagulation therapy, stroke or transient ischemic attack within 1 year, myocardial infarction within 1 month, uncontrolled hypertension, or antiplatelet therapy were excluded.
Follow-up	Clinical follow-up for up to 2.75 years (mean 15.2 months).
Treatment regimen	Warfarin or placebo. Target INR for warfarin was 2-3.
Additional therapy	Aspirin or antiplatelet therapy was not advised.

CAFA

Canadian Atrial Fibrillation Anticoagulation

(continued)

Results

Early permanent discontinuation of the therapy, not due to primary outcome event, occurred in 26.2% of the warfarin and 22.5% of the placebo group. The estimated percent of days during which the INR was 2-3 was 43.7%. The ratio was below the target in 39.6% of the days. The annual rate of major bleeding was 0.5% in the placebo and 2.5% in the warfarin group. Minor bleeding occurred in 9.4% and 16% of the patients, respectively. The annual rate of ischemic nonlacunar stroke, systemic embolization, or intracranial or fatal hemorrhage was 3.5% and 5.2% in the warfarin and placebo groups (risk reduction 37%, 95% CI -63.5%-75.5%, p=0.17).

Conclusions

Chronic anticoagulation therapy is relatively safe and effective therapy for reducing the risks of stroke and death in patients with nonrheumatic atrial fibrillation. This study was stopped prematurely due to the results of the AFASAK and SPAF studies.

SPINAF

Stroke Prevention in Nonrheumatic Atrial Fibrillation

Title	Warfarin in the prevention of stroke associated with non-rheumatic atrial fibrillation.
Authors	Ezekowitz MD, Bridgers SL, James KE, et al.
Reference	N Engl J Med 1992;327:1406-1412.
Disease	Atrial fibrillation.
Purpose	To evaluate whether low intensity anticoagulation will reduce the risk of stroke among patients with non-rheumatic atrial fibrillation.
Design	Randomized, double blind, placebo-controlled, multicenter.
Patients	525 males, no age limitation, with atrial fibrillation and no echocardiographic evidence of rheumatic heart disease.
Follow-up	Up to 3 years (an average of 1.7 years).
Treatment regimen	Sodium warfarin or placebo. Target INR 1.4-2.8.
Additional therapy	Aspirin and other anti-inflammatory drugs were not permitted.

SPINAF

Stroke Prevention in Nonrheumatic Atrial Fibrillation

(continued)

Results	Patients assigned to warfarin had their INR within the target range 56% of the time. Among patients with no previous stroke, cerebral infarction occurred at a rate of 4.3% per year in the placebo vs 0.9% per year in the warfarin group (risk reduction of 0.79, 95% CI 0.52-0.90, p=0.001). The annual event rate among the 228 patients over 70 years of age was 4.8% vs 0.9%, respectively (risk reduction 0.79, 95% CI 0.34-0.93, p=0.02). Only 1 nonfatal cerebral hemorrhage occurred in a patient that received warfarin. Major hemorrhages occurred in 0.9% vs 1.3% in the placebo and warfarin no previous stroke groups (risk reduction -0.53, 95% CI -4.22-0.55, p=0.54). Mortality of patients without prior stroke was 5.0% in the placebo vs 3.3% in the warfarin group (risk reduction 0.31, 95% CI -0.29-0.63, p=0.19). In patients with prior stroke, cerebral infarction occurred in 4 of the 25 patients in the placebo and in 2 of the 21 patients in the warfarin group (risk reduction 0.40, 95% CI -1.66-0.87, p=0.63).
Conclusions	Low intensity anticoagulation with warfarin reduced the rate of cerebral infarction in patients with nonrheumatic atrial fibrillation, without association with excess risk of bleeding.

EAFT

The European Atrial Fibrillation Trial

Title	a. Secondary prevention in nonrheumatic atrial fibrillation after transient ischaemic attack or minor stroke. b. Optimal oral anticoagulant therapy in patients with nonrheumatic atrial fibrillation and recent cerebral ischemia.
Authors	The European Atrial Fibrillation Trial Study Group.
Reference	a. Lancet 1993;342:1255-1262. b. N Engl J Med 1995;333:5-10.
Disease	Atrial fibrillation.
Purpose	a. To evaluate the effectiveness of oral anticoagulant therapy and oral aspirin for secondary prevention in patients with nonrheumatic atrial fibrillation and recent transient ischemic attack or minor ischemic stroke. b. To determine the optimal intensity of anticoagulation for secondary prevention in patients with nonrheumatic atrial fibrillation and recent transient ischemic attack or minor ischemic stroke.
Design	Randomized, open label (oral anticoagulant), double blind (aspirin vs placebo), multicenter.
Patients	a. Group 1: 669 patients, >25 years old, with chronic or paroxysmal nonrheumatic atrial fibrillation and recent (<3 months) minor ischemic stroke or transient ischemic attack randomized to anticoagulant, aspirin or placebo. Group 2: 338 patients with the same clinical characteristics but with contraindication to oral anticoagulants randomized to aspirin or placebo. b. 214 patients with nonrheumatic atrial fibrillation and a recent episode of minor cerebral ischemia who received anticoagulant therapy.
Follow-up	Mean follow-up 2.3 years.

The European Atrial Fibrillation Trial
(continued)

Treatment regimen	1. Oral anticoagulant (open label). 2. Aspirin 300 mg/d or placebo (double blind).
Results	a. Group 1. The annual rate of events (vascular death, stroke, myocardial infarction, and embolism) was 8% in patients assigned to anticoagulants and 17% in the placebo treated (Hazard ratio 0.53, 95% CI 0.36-0.79). The risk of stroke was reduced from 12%–4% per year (hazard ratio 0.34, 95% CI 0.20-0.57). Group 1+2: The annual incidence of outcome events was 15% in the aspirin vs 19% in the placebo (hazard ratio 0.83, 95% CI 0.65-1.05). The hazard ratio for stroke of aspirin vs placebo was 0.86 (95% CI 0.64-1.15). Anticoagulation was better than aspirin (hazard ratio 0.60, 95% CI 0.41-0.87; p=0.008). b. The optimal anticoagulation that results in the lower rate of bleeding and ischemic episodes was of INR 2.0-3.9. Most major bleedings occurred when INR was ≥5.0.
Conclusions	a. Oral anticoagulant is a safe and effective therapy for secondary prevention. Aspirin is less effective than anticoagulants. b. The target value for INR should be 3.0. Values <2.0 and >5.0 should be avoided.

SPAF-2

Stroke in Atrial Fibrillation II Study

Authors	Stroke Prevention in Atrial Fibrillation Investigators.
Title	Warfarin vs aspirin for prevention of thromboembolism in atrial fibrillation: stroke prevention in atrial fibrillation II study.
Reference	Lancet 1994;343:687-691.
Disease	Atrial fibrillation.
Purpose	To compare the efficacy of aspirin and warfarin for prevention of stroke and systemic embolism in patients with nonrheumatic atrial fibrillation.
Design	Randomized, multicenter.
Follow-up	Mean 2.3 years.
Treatment regimen	Warfarin (target prothrombin time ratio 1.3-1.8; INR 2.0-4.5) or aspirin 325 mg/d.
Patients	1100 patients (715 patients ≤75 years old and 385 patients >75 years old) with atrial fibrillation in the previous 12 months. Patients with prosthetic valves, mitral stenosis, or indication or contraindications to aspirin or warfarin were excluded. Patients <60 years old with lone atrial fibrillation and those with ischemic stroke or transient ischemic attack within 2 years were excluded.

SPAF-2

Stroke in Atrial Fibrillation II Study

(continued)

Results   In patients ≤75 years old primary events (ischemic stroke
               or systemic embolism) occurred at a rate of 1.3% per year
               in the warfarin group vs 1.9% in the aspirin group (RR
               0.67, 95% CI 0.34-1.3, p=0.24). The absolute rate of pri-
               mary events in low risk younger patients (without hyper-
               tension, heart failure, or previous thromboembolism) was
               0.5% on aspirin vs 1.0% on warfarin. Among older
               patients, the primary event rate was 3.6% per year with
               warfarin vs 4.8% with aspirin (RR 0.73, 95% CI 0.37-1.5,
               p=0.39). There was no statistically significant difference
               in mortality, or occurrence of all strokes with residual
               deficit between the aspirin and warfarin treated patients
               in both the ≤75 and >75 years old cohorts. In patients ≤75
               years old rates of major hemorrhage were 0.9% per year
               with aspirin vs 1.7% per year with warfarin (p=0.17). For
               older patients the rates were 1.6% vs 4.2%, respectively
               (p=0.04).

Conclusions   Warfarin may be more effective than aspirin for preven-
               tion of ischemic stroke or systemic embolism in patients
               with nonrheumatic atrial fibrillation. However, the
               absolute reduction in total stroke rate is small. Younger
               patients without risk factors had a low rate of stroke
               when treated with aspirin. The risk was higher for older
               patients, irrespective of which agent was used.

Optimal Oral Anticoagulant Therapy in Patients
With Mechanical Heart Valves

Title	Optimal oral anticoagulant therapy in patients with mechanical heart valves.
Authors	Cannegieter SC, Rosendaal FR, Wintzen AR, et al.
Reference	N Engl J Med 1995;333:11-17.
Disease	Mechanical heart valves.
Purpose	To determine the optimal intensity of anticoagulation in patients with mechanical heart valves.
Design	Events that occurred during a period of endocarditis were excluded.
Patients	1608 patients with mechanical valves.
Follow-up	Up to 6 years (6475 patient-years).
Treatment regimen	Phenprocoumon or acenocoumarol.
Results	The optimal intensity of anticoagulant therapy is that associated with the lowest incidence of both thromboembolic and bleeding events. This level has been achieved with an INR values of 2.5-4.9. At this level of INR the incidence of all adverse events was 2 per 100 patient-years (95% CI 1.0-3.8). The incidence rose sharply to 7.5 per 100 patient-year when INR was 2.0-2.4 (95% CI 3.6-12.6), and to 4.8 per 100 patient-year (95% CI 2.6-7.7) when the INR rose to 5.0-5.5. When INR was ≥6.5, the incidence was 75 per 100 patient-year (95% CI 54-101).
Conclusions	The intensity of anticoagulation for patients with prosthetic mechanical valves is optimal when the INR is 2.5-4.9. A target INR of 3.0-4.0 is recommended.

SPAF III

Stroke Prevention in Atrial Fibrillation III

Title	Adjusted dose warfarin vs low intensity, fixed dose warfarin plus aspirin for high risk patients with atrial fibrillation: Stroke Prevention in Atrial Fibrillation III randomized clinical trial.
Authors	Stroke Prevention in Atrial Fibrillation Investigators.
Reference	Lancet 1996;348:633-638.
Disease	Atrial fibrillation.
Purpose	To compare the efficacy of low intensity fixed dose warfarin plus aspirin with conventional adjusted dose warfarin in patients with atrial fibrillation at high risk of stroke.
Design	Randomized, multicenter.
Patients	1044 patients with atrial fibrillation. In addition, patients had to have at least 1 of the following 4 risk factors: 1. Recent congestive heart failure or left ventricular systolic dysfunction, 2. Systolic blood pressure >160 mmHg, 3. Prior ischemic stroke, transient ischemic attack or systemic embolism >30 days prior to entry, or 4. Being a women >75 years old. Patients with prosthetic heart valves, mitral stenosis, recent pulmonary embolism, other conditions that needed anticoagulation therapy, contraindication to aspirin or warfarin, or regular use of nonsteroidal anti-inflammatory drugs were excluded.
Follow-up	The trial was terminated prematurely after a mean follow-up of 1.1 years (range 0 to 2.5 years).

SPAF III

Stroke Prevention in Atrial Fibrillation III
(continued)

Treatment regimen	Randomization to either the combination therapy (warfarin 0.5–3.0 mg/d to raise INR to 1.2-1.5 on 2 successive measurements and aspirin 325 mg/d) or adjusted-dose warfarin (target INR 2.0-3.0).
Results	Withdrawal of assigned therapy unrelated to primary or secondary events occurred at a rate of 8.2% per year in the combination therapy group and 5.6% in the adjusted dose group (p=0.13). The mean INR was 1.3 vs 2.4 in the combination therapy and adjusted-dose groups . During the study period, 54% of the INRs in the combination therapy treated patients were 1.2-1.5 and 34% were <1.2. Among patients treated with adjusted dose warfarin, 61% of the INRs were within the therapeutic range 2.0-3.0, 25% were below this range. Ischemic stroke and systemic embolism occurred at a rate of 7.9% per year vs 1.9% per year in the combination therapy and adjusted dose group, respectively (absolute rate difference 6.0%; 95% CI 3.4 % to 8.6%; p<0.0001). The annual rates of disabling or fatal stroke (5.6% vs 1.7%; p=0.0007) and of stroke, systemic embolism, or vascular death (11.8% vs 6.4%; p=0.002) were higher in the combination therapy group. By analysis restricted to patients taking assigned therapy, the relative risk reduction by adjusted dose vs combination therapy was 77% for stroke or systemic embolism (p<0.0001) and 48% for stroke, systemic embolism, or vascular death (p=0.002). Rates of major bleeding were comparable (2.4% per year vs 2.1% per year in the combination therapy and adjusted dose group, respectively).
Conclusions	The efficacy of low intensity fixed dose warfarin plus aspirin in preventing stroke, systemic embolism or vascular death in patients with atrial fibrillation at high risk for thromboembolism is inferior to the conventional adjusted dose warfarin therapy.

10. Deep Vein Thrombosis/ Pulmonary Embolism

A clinical trial of vena caval filters in the prevention of pulmonary embolism in patients with proximal deep vein thrombosis.

Title	A clinical trial of vena caval filters in the prevention of pulmonary embolism in patients with proximal deep vein thrombosis.
Author	Decousus H, Leizorovicz A, Parent F, et al.
Reference	N Engl J Med 1998; 338:409-415.
Disease	Deep vein thrombosis, pulmonary embolism.
Purpose	To determine the efficacy and risks of prophylactic placement of vena caval filters in addition to anticoagulant therapy in patients with deep vein thrombosis at high risk for pulmonary embolism.
Design	Randomized, multicenter.
Patients	400 patients with proximal deep vein thrombosis at risk for pulmonary embolism randomized to vena caval filter (200 patients) vs no filter (200 patients) and low molecular weight heparin (enoxaparin, 195 patients) vs unfractionated heparin (205 patients).
Follow-up	12 days and 2 years.
Treatment regimen	Unfractionated heparin 5000 IU bolus followed by a continuous infusion of 500 IU/kg per day for 8-12 days with aPTT at 1.5-2.5 controls or subcutaneous enoxaparin 1 mg every 12 h for 8-12 days. Permanent vena caval filters vs no vena caval filters, warfarin, or acenocourmarol was started on day 4 and continued for 3 months.

A clinical trial of vena caval filters in the prevention of pulmonary embolism in patients with proximal deep vein thrombosis.

(continued)

Results

At day 12 1.1% of patients who received filters had pulmonary embolism vs 4.8% of those not receiving filters (odds ratio 0.22, 95% CI = .05–.90). At 2 years 20.8% of filter group vs 11.6% of no filter group had recurrent deep vein thrombosis (odds ratio 1.87; 95% CI = 1.10 - 3.20) There was no significant difference in mortality between groups. At 2 years symptomatic pulmonary embolism occurred in 6 patients in the filter group and 12 in the no filter group (p = 0.16). At day 12, 3 (1.6%) patients receiving low molecular weight heparin had pulmonary embolism vs 8 patients receiving unfractionated heparin (4.2%, odds ratio .38; 95% CI = 0.10 - 1.38).

Conclusions

An initial benefit of vena caval filters for prevention of pulmonary embolism was offset by an excess of recurrent deep vein thrombosis with no improvement in mortality. Low molecular-weight heparin was as effective and safe as unfractionated heparin for prevention of pulmonary embolism.

DURAC II

Duration of Anticoagulation Trial Study

Title	The duration of oral anticoagulant therapy after a second episode of venous thromboembolism.
Author	Schulman S, Granqvist S, Holmstrom M, et al.
Reference	N Engl J Med 1997; 336:393-398.
Disease	Second episode of venous thromboembolism.
Purpose	To determine the optimal duration of oral anticoagulation therapy after a second episode of venous thromboembolism.
Design	Randomized, open label trial, multicenter.
Patients	227 patients with second episode of venous thromboembolism (diagnoses included venography for deep vein thrombosis; angiography or combination of chest x-ray and ventilation-perfusion lung scan for pulmonary embolism).
Follow-up	4 years.
Treatment regimen	Initial therapy was unfractionated or low molecular weight heparin given I.V. or S.C. for at least 5 days. Oral anticoagulation with warfarin sodium or dicumarol started at same time as heparin in order to achieve an INR of 2.0 - 2.85. 111 patients were randomized to 6 months of anticoagulation therapy and 116 were assigned to indefinite anticoagulation.

DURAC II

Duration of Anticoagulation Trial Study

(continued)

Results
At 4 years there were 23 (20.7%) recurrences of venous thromboembolism in the group assigned to 6 months of therapy and 3 (2.6%) in the group assigned to continuing therapy. Relative risk of thromboembolic recurrence in 6 month vs indefinite group was 8.0 (95% CI = 2.5-25.9). There were 3 major hemorrhages in the 6 month group (2.7%) and 10 in the indefinite treatment group (8.6%). There were no significant differences in mortality between the groups.

Conclusions
Indefinite oral anticoagulation following a second episode of venous thromboembolism was associated with a lower recurrence of venous thromboembolism compared to only 6 months of therapy. However major hemorrhage tended to be higher when anticoagulation was continued indefinitely.

Low molecular weight heparin in the treatment of patients with venous thromboembolism.

Title	Low molecular weight heparin in the treatment of patients with venous thromboembolism.
Author	The Columbus Investigators.
Reference	N Engl J Med 1997;337:657-662.
Disease	Venous thromboembolism.
Purpose	To determine whether fixed dose, subcutaneous, low molecular weight heparin and adjusted dose, IV, unfractionated heparin infusion have equivalent efficacy in patients with symptomatic venous thromboembolism.
Design	Randomized, open-label, multicenter.
Patients	1021 patients with acute symptomatic deep vein thrombosis, pulmonary embolism, or both. Diagnosis had to be documented by ultrasonography or venography, lung scanning, or pulmonary angiography.
Follow-up	12 weeks.
Treatment regimen	Reviparin sodium (low molecular weight heparin) given subcutaneously at various fixed doses by range of weight: 6300 U x2/d for patients > 60 kg; 4200 U x2/d for patients 46-60 kg; and 3500 U x2/d for patients 35-45kg. Unfractionated heparin was given as IV bolus 5000 IU, followed by infusion of 1250 IU per hour and adjusted as needed. Study drug was continued for at least 5 days. Oral anticoagulant was started in the first or second day and continued for 12 weeks.

Results

510 patients assigned to low molecular weight heparin reviparin and 511 patients to unfractionated heparin. 5.3% of patients receiving reviparin had recurrent thromboembolic events vs 4.9% of patients receiving unfractionated heparin. Major bleeding occurred in 3.1% of reviparin and 2.3% of unfractionated heparin group. Mortality rates were similar in the 2 groups at 7.1 and 7.6%, respectively.

Conclusions

Fixed dose, subcutaneous, low molecular weight heparin was as effective and safe as infusion of unfractionated heparin in patients with venous thromboembolism with or without pulmonary embolus.

THESEE

Tinzaparin ou Heparine Standard: Evaluations dans 1' Embolic Pulmonaire

Title	A comparison of low molecular weight heparin with unfractionated heparin for acute pulmonary embolism.
Author	Simonneau G, Sors H, Charbonnier B, et al.
Reference	N Engl J Med 1997; 337:663-669.
Disease	Pulmonary embolism.
Purpose	To determine whether low molecular weight heparin (tinzaparin) is safe and effective in treating acute pulmonary embolism.
Design	Randomized, multicenter.
Patients	612 patients with symptomatic pulmonary embolism not requiring thrombolytic therapy or embolectomy. Objective evidence of pulmonary embolism required by lung scanning of if lung scanning was indeterminant evidence of deep vein thrombosis was confirmed by venography or ultrasonography.
Follow-up	90 days.
Treatment regimen	175 IU/kg of tinzaparin, a low molecular weight heparin, given subcutaneously once daily or unfractionated heparin, given as an initial bolus of 50 IU/kg, followed by a continues IV infusion at an initial rate of 500 IU per kg/day, with adjustments based on aPTT. Oral anticoagulants begun within 1–3 days and continued for 3 months.

THESEE

Tinzaparin ou Heparine Standard: Evaluations dans l' Embolic Pulmonaire

(continued)

Results   Primary end point was combined outcome event of
                 death, symptomatic recurrent thromboembolism, or
                 major bleeding assessed on day 8 and 90. At day 8, 9 of
                 308 (2.9%) in the unfractionated heparin group reached
                 at least 1 endpoint vs 9 of 304 (3.0%) assigned to low mol-
                 ecular weight heparin. At day 90 7.1% and 5.9% had
                 reached 1 endpoint, respectively. Risk of major bleeding
                 was similar between the 2 groups. In patients receiving
                 follow-up lung scan the percentage of scintigraphically
                 detectable vascular obstruction was similar in the 2
                 groups.

Conclusions   In patients with symptomatic pulmonary embolism, ini-
                 tial subcutaneous therapy with low molecular weight
                 heparin was as effective and safe as IV infusions of unfrac-
                 tionated heparin.

11. Coronary Artery Disease, Atherosclerosis- Prevention of Progression

INTACT

International Nifedipine Trial on Antiatherosclerotic Therapy

Title	Retardation of angiographic progression of coronary artery disease by nifedipine. Results of the International Nifedipine Trial on Antiatherosclerotic Therapy (INTACT).
Authors	Lichtlen PR, Hugenholtz PG, Rafflenbeul W, et al.
Reference	Lancet 1990;335:1109-1113.
Disease	Coronary artery disease.
Purpose	To evaluate the effects of 3 years of nifedipine therapy on progression of coronary artery disease and formation of new lesions.
Design	Randomized, double blind, placebo-controlled, multicenter.
Patients	348 patients, <65 years old, with mild or single vessel coronary artery disease. Patients with multivessel disease, ejection fraction <40%, mandatory therapy with calcium channel blockers, or prior therapy with calcium channel blockers >6 months were excluded.
Follow-up	Clinical follow-up and repeated angiography after 36 months.
Treatment regimen	Placebo or nifedipine 5 mg X3/d , with gradual increments to 20 mg X4/d.
Additional therapy	Oral nitrates, ß blockers, aspirin, anticoagulants, and lipid lowering drugs were permitted.

INTACT

International Nifedipine Trial on Antiatherosclerotic Therapy

(continued)

Results
There were 16 side effects in the placebo and 55 in the nifedipine group (p=0.003), and 44 vs 52 critical cardiac events (p=0.60). Cardiac mortality was 0.8% vs 2.4%, in the placebo and nifedipine groups, respectively. On the repeated angiography, ≥20% progression of stenosis in pre-existing lesions was found in 9% vs 12%, respectively, while regression of ≥20% was found in 4% and 3%, respectively. 87% vs 85% of the lesions remained unchanged (p=NS). However, new lesions in previously angiographic normal sites were found more in the placebo than nifedipine treated patients (0.82 vs 0.59 new lesions per patient, 28% reduction, p=0.034). In contrast, the mean degree of stenosis did not differ between the groups.

Conclusions
Nifedipine was associated with mild reduction of the formation of new angiographic coronary lesions. However, nifedipine was associated with more side effects and a trend towards more critical cardiac events and death.

SCRIP

The Stanford Coronary Risk Intervention Project

Title	a. Effects of intensive multiple risk factor reduction on coronary atherosclerosis and clinical cardiac events in men and women with coronary artery disease. The Stanford Coronary Risk Intervention Project (SCRIP). b. Development of new coronary atherosclerotic lesions during a 4 year multifactor risk reduction program: the Stanford Coronary Risk Intervention Project (SCRIP).
Authors	a. Haskell WL, Alderman EL, Fair JM, et al. b. Quinn TG, Alderman EL, McMillan A, et al.
Reference	a. Circulation 1994;89:975-990. b. J Am Coll Cardiol 1994;24:900-908.
Disease	Coronary artery disease.
Purpose	To determine whether an intensive multifactor risk reduction program over 4 years would reduce the rate of progression of atherosclerosis.
Design	Randomized, 4 centers.
Patients	300 patients, age <75 years, with coronary artery disease (≥ 1 major coronary artery with 5-69% luminal stenosis that was unaffected by revascularization procedures). Patients with heart failure, pulmonary, or peripheral vascular disease were excluded.
Follow-up	4 years clinical follow-up. Coronary angiography at baseline and after 4 years.

SCRIP

The Stanford Coronary Risk Intervention Project

(continued)

Treatment regimen	Usual care by the patients' own physician or individualized, multifactor, risk reduction program including low fat low cholesterol diet, exercise, weight loss, smoking cessation, and medications for altering lipid profile. A major goal was to decrease LDL cholesterol to <110 mg/dl and triglyceride to <100 mg/dl and to increase HDL cholesterol to >55 mg/dl.

Results	274 patients (91.3%) completed a follow-up angiogram and 246 (82%) had comparative measurements of segments with visible disease at baseline and follow-up. Intensive risk reduction resulted in highly significant improvements in various risk factors, including the lipid profile, body weight, and exercise capacity, compared with the usual care group. No change was observed in lipoprotein (a). The change in minimal luminal diameter between the 4 years and baseline angiograms was -0.024±0.066 mm/y in the risk reduction group vs -0.045±0.073 mm/y in the usual care (p<0.02). Mortality rates were similar. However, there were 25 hospitalizations in the risk reduction vs 44 in the usual care group (RR 0.61, 95% CI 0.4-0.9, p=0.05). There were 7.6% segments with new lesions in the usual care group vs 4.7% in the risk reduction group (p=0.05). New lesions were detected in 31% vs 23%, respectively (p=0.16). The mean number of new lesions/patient was 0.47 vs 0.30, respectively (p=0.06).

Conclusions	Intensive risk reduction reduced the rate of progression of luminal narrowing in coronary arteries of patients with atherosclerosis and reduced the hospitalization rate for clinical cardiac causes.

CAPRIE

Clopidogrel vs Aspirin in Patients at Risk of Ischemic Events

Title	A randomized, blinded, trial of clopidogrel vs aspirin in patients at risk of ischaemic events (CAPRIE).
Authors	CAPRIE Steering Committee.
Reference	Lancet 1996;348:1329-1339.
Disease	Atherosclerotic cardiovascular disease
Purpose	To compare the effect of clopidogrel, a new thienopyridine derivative that inhibits platelet aggregation induced by adenosine diphosphate, and aspirin in reducing the risk of ischemic stroke, myocardial infarction, or cardiovascular death in patients with atherosclerotic cardiovascular disease.
Design	Randomized, blind, multicenter.
Patients	19,185 patients with recent ischemic stroke (≤6 months), recent myocardial infarction (≤35 days), or symptomatic atherosclerotic peripheral arterial disease.
Follow-up	Average follow-up of 1.9 years (1-3 years).
Treatment regimen	Clopidogrel 75 mg X1/d or aspirin 325 mg X1/d.
Additional therapy	Use of anticoagulation or anti-platelet drugs was prohibited.

Results   21.1% vs 21.3% of the aspirin and clopidogrel-treated groups discontinued the drug early for reasons other than the occurrence of an outcome event. The rate of adverse effects was similar: rash (0.10% vs 0.26%, respectively), diarrhea (0.11% vs 0.23%), intracranial hemorrhage (0.47% vs 0.33%), and gastrointestinal hemorrhage (0.72% vs 0.52%). Neutropenia occurred in 0.10% of the clopidogrel vs 0.17% of the aspirin group, respectively. By intention to treat analysis, the clopidogrel-treated patients had an annual 5.32% risk of ischemic stroke, myocardial infarction, or vascular death compared with 5.83% among the aspirin-treated patients (relative-risk reduction of 8.7%; 95% CI 0.3-16.5; p=0.043). For patients with stroke as the inclusion criterion, the average annual event rate was 7.15% vs 7.71 with clopidegrel and aspirin, respectively (relative-risk reduction of 7.3% in favor of clopidogrel; p=0.26). For patients with myocardial infarction, annual event rates were 5.03% vs 4.84%, respectively (relative-risk increase of 3.7%; p=0.66), whereas for patients with peripheral arterial disease, the annual event rates were 3.71% vs 4.86%, respectively (a relative-risk reduction of 23.8%; 95% CI 8.9 to 36.2%; p=0.0028).

Conclusions   Long-term clopidogrel therapy was more effective than aspirin in reducing the combined risk of ischemic stroke, myocardial infarction, or vascular death, especially in patients with peripheral arterial disease. Clopidogrel is as safe as medium dose aspirin and is probably safer than ticlopidine.

The Physician's Health Study
(The Beta Carotene Component)

Title	Lack of effect of long-term supplementation with beta carotene on the incidence of malignant neoplasms and cardiovascular disease.
Authors	Hennekens CH, Buring JE, Manson JE, et al.
Reference	N Engl J Med 1996;334:1145-1149.
Disease	Coronary artery disease.
Purpose	To evaluate the long-term effect of beta carotene supplementation on mortality and morbidity.
Design	Randomized, double blind, placebo-controlled, multicenter.
Patients	22,071 US male physicians, 40–84 years old at entry, with no history of cancer, myocardial infarction, stroke, or transient cerebral ischemia.
Follow-up	An average of 12 years (11.6–14.2 years).
Treatment regimen	Randomization to 1 of 4 groups: 1. Aspirin 325 mg on alternate days + β carotene 50 mg on alternate days; 2. Aspirin + β carotene placebo; 3. Aspirin placebo + β carotene; 4. Both placebo.

Results

The randomized aspirin component of the study was terminated early in 1988 because there was a statistically significant 44% reduction in the risk of first myocardial infarction with aspirin (p<0.001). The β carotene component continued as planned. By the end of 11 years of follow-up, 80% of the participants were still taking the drug medication, 78% of the study drugs were still being taken by the β carotene patients, whereas 6% of the placebo group were taking supplemental β carotene. There were no early or late differences in overall mortality, the incidence of malignancy or cardiovascular disease between the groups. Myocardial infarction occurred in 468 vs 489 patients in the β carotene and placebo groups, respectively (p=0.50), stroke in 367 vs 382 patients (p=0.60), death from cardiovascular disease in 338 vs 313 patients (p=0.28), and the number of any of the major cardiovascular endpoints 967 vs 972 patients (p=0.90). There were no major side effects associated with β carotene supplementation.

Conclusions

Supplementation with β carotene for 12 years was not associated with either benefit or harm concerning mortality, incidence of malignancy, or cardiovascular morbidity.

CARET

The Beta Carotene and Retinol Efficacy Trial

Title	Effects of a combination of beta carotene and vitamin A on lung cancer and cardiovascular disease.
Authors	Omenn GS, Goodman GE, Thornquist MD, et al.
Reference	N Engl J Med 1996;334:1150-1155.
Disease	Cardiovascular disease.
Purpose	To assess the efficacy of beta carotene and retinol (Vitamin A) supplementation to reduce incidence of cancer and mortality rate from cancer and cardiovascular disease.
Design	Randomized, double blind, placebo-controlled, multicenter.
Patients	18,314 men and women, 45-74 years of age, who were smokers, former smokers, or workers exposed to asbestos.
Follow-up	mean length of follow-up, 4.0 years.
Treatment regimen	Patients were randomized to a combination of 30 mg/d β carotene and retinyl palmitate 25,000 IU/d, or placebo.
Additional therapy	Supplemental intake of vitamin A was restricted to <5500 IU/d. Beta carotene supplementation was prohibited.

CARET

The Beta Carotene and Retinol Efficacy Trial

(continued)

Results
The β carotene retinol treated patients had higher incidence of lung cancer than the placebo group (5.92 vs 4.62 cases/1000 person-year; a relative risk 1.28; 95% CI 1.04–1.57; p=0.02). Total mortality was 14.45 vs 11.91 deaths per 1000 person-year, respectively; relative risk 1.17; 95% CI 1.03–1.33; p=0.02). The β carotene retinol group had a relative risk of cardiovascular mortality of 1.26 (95% CI 0.99–1.61). On the basis of these findings, the randomized trial was terminated prematurely.

Conclusions
Supplementation of β carotene and retinol for an average of 4 years in high risk patients (smokers and workers exposed to asbestos) had no benefit on the incidence of cancer and on mortality from cardiovascular causes and cancer. Supplementation of β carotene and retinol may have had an adverse effect on the incidence of lung cancer and mortality.

The Iowa Women's Health Study

Title	Dietary antioxidant vitamins and death from coronary heart disease in postmenopausal women.
Authors	Kushi LH, Folsom AR, Prineas RJ, et al.
Reference	N Engl J Med 1996;334:1156-1162.
Disease	Coronary artery disease.
Purpose	To asses whether dietary intake of antioxidants is related to mortality from coronary artery disease.
Design	Prospective cohort study.
Patients	34,386 postmenopausal women, 55-69 years of age.
Follow-up	7 years.
Treatment regimen	The study evaluated the intake of vitamins A, E, and C from diet and supplements.
Results	In analyses adjusted for age and dietary calorie intake, an inverse correlation was found between vitamin E consumption and cardiovascular mortality. This association was especially significant in the subgroup of women who did not consume vitamin supplements (n=21,809; relative risks from lowest to highest quintile of vitamin E intake, 1.0, 0.68, 0.71, 0.42, and 0.42; p for trend=0.008). After adjustment for confounding variables, this association remained significant (relative risks 1.0, 0.70, 0.76, 0.32, and 0.38; p for trend=0.004). Multivariate analysis suggested no association between supplemental vitamin E intake and risk of death from coronary artery disease. Intake of vitamins A and C was not associated with the risk of mortality from coronary heart disease.

Conclusions   In postmenopausal women the intake of vitamin E from food, but not from supplements, is inversely associated with mortality rate from coronary heart disease. This may suggest that vitamin E consumed in food is a marker for other dietary factors associated with the risk of coronary heart disease. By contrast, intake of vitamins A and C, either from diet or from supplements, was not associated with lower mortality from coronary disease.

CHAOS

Cambridge Heart Antioxidant Study

Title	Randomized controlled trial of vitamin E in patients with coronary disease: Cambridge Heart Antioxidant Study (CHAOS).
Authors	Stephens NG, Parsons A, Schofield PM, et al.
Reference	Lancet 1996;347:781-786.
Disease	Coronary artery disease.
Purpose	To determine whether treatment with high dose α-tocopherol (Vitamin E) would reduce the incidence of myocardial infarction and cardiovascular death in patients with ischemic heart disease.
Design	Randomized, double blind, placebo-controlled, single center.
Patients	2002 patients with angiographically proven coronary artery disease. Patients with prior use of vitamin supplements containing vitamin E were excluded.
Follow-up	Median follow-up 510 days (range 3 to 981 days).
Treatment regimen	α-tocopherol (Vitamin E) 400 or 800 IU/d or placebo.

CHAOS

Cambridge Heart Antioxidant Study

(continued)

Results   Plasma α-tocopherol levels were increased in the active-ly treated group (from baseline mean 34.2 μmol/L-51.1 μmol/L with 400 IU/d and to 64.5 μmol/L in the 800 IU/d), but remained the same in the placebo group (32.4 μmol/L). Treatment with α-tocopherol did not affect serum cholesterol. α-tocopherol therapy significantly reduced the risk of cardiovascular death and myocardial infarction. Nonfatal myocardial infarction occurred in 1.4% vs 4.2% of the α-tocopherol and placebo group, respectively (relative risk (RR) 0.23; 95% CI 0.11-0.47; $p<0.001$). However, cardiovascular mortality was similar (2.6% vs 2.4%, respectively; RR 1.18; 95% CI 0.62-2.27; $p=0.61$). Treatment was well tolerated. All cause mortality was 3.5% vs 2.7% ($p=0.31$). Only 0.55% of the patients discontinued therapy because of side effects. There was no significant difference between the placebo and α-tocopherol groups in occurrence of side effects.

Conclusions   α-tocopherol therapy in patients with coronary artery disease reduced the rate of nonfatal myocardial infarction. However, there was no effect on total or cardiovascular mortality.

***Effect of vitamin E and β carotene on the incidence of
primary nonfatal myocardial infarction and fatal coronary
heart disease.***

Title	Effect of vitamin E and β carotene on the incidence of primary nonfatal myocardial infarction and fatal coronary heart disease.
Author	Virtamo J, Rapola JM, Ripatti S, et al.
Reference	Arch Intern Med 1998; 158:668-675.
Disease	Prevention of coronary events. Coronary artery disease, myocardial infarction.
Purpose	To determine the primary preventive effect of vitamin E (alpha tocopherol) and beta carotene supplements on the development of major coronary events in the Alpha-tocopherol, beta carotene cancer prevention study.
Design	Randomized, double blind, placebo-controlled trial.
Patients	Male smokers, ages 50–69, (N = 27,271) with no history of myocardial infarction.
Follow-up	5–8 years; median 61 years.
Treatment regimen	Patients were randomized to receive Vitamin E (50 mg), beta carotene (20 mg), both agents, or placebo.

Effect of vitamin E and β carotene on the incidence of primary nonfatal myocardial infarction and fatal coronary heart disease.

(continued)

Results

The incidence of the primary major coronary events end-point (nonfatal myocardial infarction or fatal coronary heart disease) was decreased 4% (95% CI = -12% to 4%) among patients receiving Vitamin E and increased by 1% (95% CI = -7% to 10%) among patients on beta carotene. Vitamin E decreased the incidence of fatal coronary heart disease by 8% (95% CI = -19% to 5%); beta carotene had no effect on this endpoint. Neither agent influenced the incidence of nonfatal myocardial infarction.

Conclusions

Small doses of vitamin E have only marginal effects on the incidence of fatal coronary heart disease in male smokers and have no influence on nonfatal myocardial infarction. Beta carotene supplements had no effect on coronary events.

Title	Thrombosis Prevention Trial: Randomized trial of low intensity oral anticoagulation with warfarin and low dose aspirin in the primary prevention of ischaemic heart disease in men at increased risk
Authors	The Medical Research Council's General Practice Research Framework.
Reference	Lancet 1998;351:233-241.
Disease	Coronary artery disease.
Purpose	To assess the effects of low dose aspirin, low dose warfarin, and their combination in the primary prevention of coronary artery disease.
Design	Randomized, double blind, placebo-controlled, multicenter.
Patients	5499 men, aged 45-69 years, at high risk of coronary artery disease.
Follow-up	Up to 8-10 years.
Treatment regimen	Randomization to: 1. active warfarin and placebo aspirin (n=1268); 2. active warfarin and active aspirin (n=1277); 3. placebo warfarin and active aspirin (n=1268); and 4. placebo warfarin and placebo aspirin (n=1272). The initial dose of warfarin was 2.5 mg/d. The dose was adjusted to achieve INR 1.5.

Results
With a mean dose of 4.1 mg/d (range 0.5 mg-12.5 mg), the mean INR of the patients treated with active warfarin was 1.47 (INR 1.41-1.54). Warfarin (with or without aspirin) reduced ischemic heart disease events by 21% (95% CI 4-35%; p=0.02). Warfarin therapy resulted in a reduction of coronary mortality and fatal myocardial infarction by 39% (95% CI 15-57%; p=0.003), and all causes mortality by 17% (95% CI 1-30%; p=0.04). Stroke occurred in 3.1 per 1000 person years of the active warfarin groups vs 2.7 in the placebo-warfarin groups (% proportional reduction -15%; 95% CI -68-22%). Aspirin therapy (with or without warfarin) resulted in a decrease in all ischemic heart disease events by 20% (95% CI 1-35%; p=0.04). However, aspirin reduced mainly nonfatal events (by 32%; 95% CI 12-48%; p=0.004). Aspirin therapy was associated with increased risk for fatal ischemic heart disease events (% proportional reduction -12% (95% CI -63-22%). All causes mortality was 13.0 per 1000 person years in the aspirin treated patients vs 12.2 in the no-aspirin groups (% proportional reduction -6%; 95% CI -28-12%). Aspirin therapy resulted in increased risk of hemorrhagic stroke (0.6 per 1000 person years vs 0.1; p=0.01). Total ischemic heart disease events were 13.3 per 1000 person years in the placebo-aspirin and placebo warfarin group vs only 8.7 in the active aspirin and active warfarin group (proportional reduction by 34%; 95% CI 11-51%; p=0.006). Total ischemic heart disease events per 1000 person years was 10.3 in the warfarin alone group and 10.2 in the aspirin alone group (the difference vs the placebo aspirin and placebo warfarin group was not significant). Fatal ischemic heart disease event rate was 3.0 per 1000 person years in the aspirin and warfarin group; 2.4 in the warfarin alone group; 4.4 in the aspirin alone group; and 4.2 in the placebo aspirin and placebo warfarin group. All causes mortality rates were 12.4, 11.4, 13.6, and 13.1 per 1000 person years, respectively.

Conclusions
Aspirin reduces mainly nonfatal ischemic heart disease events, whereas warfarin reduces mainly fatal events. Combined therapy with low dose warfarin and aspirin was more effective in reducing all ischemic heart disease events, mainly due to a reduction of nonfatal events, as compared to warfarin alone. However, all causes mortality with warfarin alone tended to be lower than with the combination therapy.

12. Ongoing Clinical Trials

During the last years numerous studies have been conducted on various cardiovascular subjects. In the previous chapters we described some of the major studies that have already been completed and published in the medical literature. Nevertheless, several other important studies are still ongoing, or their preliminary results have been published as abstracts.

In this chapter we shall review some of these ongoing studies:

a. Acute Myocardial Infarction

GRAMI TRIAL

Coronary stents improved hospital results during coronary angioplasty in acute myocardial infarction: Preliminary results of a randomized controlled study (GRAMI Trial)

Reference	J Am Coll Cardiol 1997; 29 (Suppl A); 221A.
Disease	Acute myocardial infarction.
Purpose	To determine if GRII (Cook Inc) stents can improve outcome in patients undergoing angioplasty during acute myocardial infarction.
Design	Randomized.
Patients	Preliminary report of 65 patients randomized to primary PTCA (n=25) vs stent (n=40) for acute myocardial infarction. Patients underwent angiography predischarge. No difference in age, sex, previous MI, Killip class.
Follow-up	In-hospital, ongoing.
Treatment	Primary PTCA vs stent. Stent patients received IV heparin for 48 h, aspirin, ticlopidine.
Remarks	Technical failure or death occurred in 24% of PTCA patients and 0% of stent patients. Authors conclude that stents as a primary therapy of myocardial infarction improved this composite endpoint.

AMI

The Argatroban in Myocardial Infarction Trial

Reference	J Am Coll Cardiol 1997;30:1-7.
Disease	Acute myocardial infarction.
Purpose	To assess the effect of adding argatroban, a direct thrombin inhibitor, to streptokinase thrombolysis in patients with acute myocardial infarction.
Design	Randomized, double blind, placebo-controlled, multicenter, phase II.
Patients	910 patients with acute myocardial infarction.
Treatment regimen	Intravenous streptokinase. Randomization to low or high dose argatroban or placebo.
Remarks	Death, shock, congestive heart failure, or recurrent myocardial infarction at 30 days occurred in 16.1% of the placebo group, in 19.9% of the low dose argatroban group, and in 18.8% of the high dose argatroban group (p=NS). The individual components of the composite end point occurred in similar rates among the 3 groups. In patients treated ≤3 h of onset of symptoms, the high dose argatroban was associated with a significant risk reduction. Argatroban was not associated with increased major bleeding rate. The safety profile of argatroban was good.

AMISTAD

Acute Myocardial Infarction Study of Adenosine

Title	Kenneth W. Mahaffey, et al. for the presentation at the 70th Scientific Sessions of the American Heart Association, Orlando Florida, November 10–13, 1997.
Disease	Acute myocardial infarction.
Purpose	To determine the effects of adenosine given to patients with acute myocardial infarction treated with thrombolytic therapy. Primary end-point was myocardial infarct size determined by 99m-sestamibi SPECT imaging.
Design	Randomized, placebo-controlled, multicenter.
Patients	236 patients with acute myocardial infarction.
Follow-up	4–6 weeks.
Preliminary results	At 6 days adenosine treatment was associated with a 33% relative reduction in infarct size (p=0.03). This was primarily due to reduction in infarct size of 67% in patients with anterior infarcts. However, there was a tendency for more adverse clinical events in the adenosine group.

ASSENT-1

Phase II Trial of TNK-TPA in Acute Myocardial Infarction

Reference	Clin Cardiol 1997;20:1031
Disease	Acute myocardial infarction.
Purpose	To estimate safety and efficacy of intracranial hemorrhage with escalating doses of TNK-TPA in patients with acute myocardial infarction.
Design	Randomized.
Patients	3,325 patients with acute myocardial infarction associated with ST segment elevation, presenting ≤12 h of symptom onset.
Follow-up	Coronary angiography 60, 75, and 90 min following initiation of therapy.
Treatment regimen	TNK-TPA (30, 40, or 50 mg) or front loaded tPA.
Remarks	Data were presented at the XIX congress of the European Society of Cardiology, Stockholm, Sweden, 1997. Intracranial hemorrhages were reported in 0 of the TNK-TPA 50 mg, 0.76% of the TNK-TPA 40 mg, and in 0.94% of the TNK-TPA 30 mg groups.

ASSENT-2

Assessment of the Safety and Efficacy of a New Thrombolytic Agent

Disease	Acute myocardial infarction.
Purpose	To show therapeutic equivalence in 30 day mortality between TNK-TPA, administered as a single bolus, and front loaded tPA in patients with acute myocardial infarction.
Design	Randomized, double blind, double dummy, controlled, multicenter, phase III.
Patients	16,500 patients, ≥18 years old, with suspected acute myocardial infarction, presenting within 6 hours of onset of symptoms and without contraindications to thrombolytic therapy.
Follow-up	30 days clinical follow-up.
Treatment regimen	Randomization to active tPA (Alteplase, Activase) and placebo TNK-TPA, or placebo tPA and TNK-TPA. The dose of TNK-TPA will be weight-adjusted (30-50 mg). TPA will be given as follows: 15 mg as a bolus, followed by 0.75 mg/kg (maximum 50 mg) over 30 min, and then 0.5 mg/kg (maximum 35 mg) over 60 min. All patients receive oral aspirin and intravenous heparin.
Remarks	Results are not available yet.

GIK

Glucose-Insulin-Potassium Pilot Trial

Reference	Clin Cardiol 1997;20:1031
Disease	Acute myocardial infarction.
Purpose	To assess the efficacy of adding glucose-insulin-potassium (GIK) solution to standard therapy in patients with acute myocardial infarction (treated with or without thrombolytic therapy).
Design	Randomized, multicenter.
Patients	407 patients with suspected acute myocardial infarction presented within 24 h of symptom onset.
Treatment regimen	Randomization to: 1. high dose GIK (25% glucose 500 ml, 25 IU insulin and 40 mEq KCL at a 1.5 mg/kg/h infusion over 24 h). 2. low dose GIK (10% glucose 500 ml, 10 IU insulin and 20 mEq KCL at a 1.0 mg/kg/h infusion over 24 h. 3. control.
Remarks	Data were presented at the XIX congress of the European Society of Cardiology, Stockholm, Sweden, 1997. 252 (60%) of the patients received reperfusion therapy. GIK infusion was associated with lower rate of electro-mechanical dissociation (1.5%) than the control group (5.8%)(p=0.0161). There was a nonsignificant trend toward fewer events (death, severe heart failure, severe arrhythmias) with GIK compared with control. Among patients who received reperfusion therapy, GIK infusion was associated with a 66% reduction in mortality (5.2% vs 15.2%; p=0.008). GIK infusion was well tolerated and side effects were few and minor. GIK infusion is feasible and safe and is beneficial in patients undergoing reperfusion therapy.

IN TIME TRIAL

Intravenous nPA for Treatment of Infarcting Myocardium Early

Reference	Peter den Heijer, et al. for the presentation at the 46th Annual Scientific Sessions of the American College of Cardiology March 16–19, 1997, Anaheim, CA.
Disease	Acute myocardial infarction.
Purpose	To compare TIMI flow grade in patients treated with lanoteplase, variant of TPA with a half life that is 10 times greater than TPA to TPA.
Design	Randomized, multicenter.
Patients	602 patients with acute myocardial infarction randomized to 1 of 4 doses of lanoteplase vs standard front loaded TPA.
Preliminary results	The highest dose group of lanoteplase (120 KU/Kg) achieved patency defined as TIMI 2 or 3 in 83% of patients vs 71.4% in the TPA group (p=.05). TIMI 3 was achieved in 57.1% of lanoteplase vs 46.4% of the TPA group. There was a trend for fewer adverse cardiac events to occur in the lanoteplase group (11% vs 24%). Lanoteplase is effective for achieving rapid and effective clot lysis.

Reference	Ik-Kyung Jang for the XIXth Congress of the European Society of Cardiology, 1997.
Disease	Acute myocardial infarction.
Purpose	To determine whether the direct thrombin inhibitor Argatroban as an adjunct to t-PA improves angiographic patency at 90 min.
Design	Randomized, controlled, dose ranging trial.
Patients	120 patients with acute myocardial infarction randomized to heparin, low dose Argatroban or high dose Argatroban. All patients received aspirin and t-PA.
Follow-up	90 min angiogram.
Preliminary results	The Argatroban group showed more frequent TIMI grade 3 flow at 57.8% vs heparin alone at 43.2%. Argatroban was not associated with increased bleeding.

PACT

Plasminogen Activator Angioplasty Compatibility Trial (PACT)

Title	Plasminogen Activator Angioplasty Compatibility Trial (PACT).
Reference	Internal Medicine News, February 15, 1998 Volume 4, page 1. Presentation at the meeting in Snowmass, Colorado, by the American College of Cardiology by Dr. Allan M. Ross, and Annual Meeting of the American College of Cardiology, March 1998, Atlanta, Georgia.
Disease	Myocardial infarction.
Purpose	To determine the effects of acute angioplasty with or without initial thrombolysis with tissue plasminogen activator (TPA).
Design	Double blind, randomized study.
Patients	606 patients with acute myocardial infarction, eligible for thrombolysis.
Follow-up	30 days, 1 year.
Treatment regimen	Patients randomized to 50 mg bolus of TPA vs placebo and then went to the cardiac catheterization laboratory. If coronary angiography revealed TIMI-3 flow in the infarct artery patient received second bolus of TPA, was managed conservatively and had repeat angiogram at 5–7 days. If TIMI 3 not initially seen, then coronary angioplasty performed.

PACT

Plasminogen Activator Angioplasty Compatibility Trial (PACT)
(continued)

Preliminary
results

Initial angiography 1 h after bolus showed that 32% of patients on TPA had TIMI-3 flow vs 15% on placebo. Reperfusion was achieved by 1.7 h in patients who required angioplasty. In hospital outcomes including mortality, complications, and technical outcome did not differ between patients who had angioplasty with TPA vs those who had angioplasty with placebo. LV ejection fraction was 62% in patients with TIMI 3 flow rates on catheterization, 58% in those who achieved TIMI 3 only after PTCA, and 55% for those with TIMI grades less than 3. 1 year results are pending.

Stent PAMI Trial

Title	Stent PAMI Trial
Reference	Cindy L. Grines for the presentation at the Annual American College of Cardiology Meetings, March 1998, Atlanta, Georgia.
Disease	Acute myocardial infarction.
Purpose	To compare the use of primary PTCA to implantation of heparin-coated Palmaz-Schatz stent for acute myocardial infarction.
Design	Randomized, multicenter.
Patients	910 patients with acute myocardial infarction entered within 12 h of onset of acute myocardial infarction symptoms.
Follow-up	90 day data reported.
Preliminary results	Use of heparin-coated stents resulted in greater angiographically determined lumen size (2.55mm) vs PTCA (2.11 mm). Procedural success occurred in 98.7% stent patients vs 84.9% of those receiving PTCA. There was reduced early ischemia-driven target-vessel revascularization (0.6%) with stenting than with PTCA (2.5%), and overall reduced target vessel revascularization (0.9%) for stenting vs PTCA (3.5%); recurrent chest pain with ST-segment elevation was less common in stented patients (1.2%) vs PTCA patients (3.5%) and hospital stay was shorter at 4 days for stented vs PTCA patients. However primary combined endpoint of death, recurrent myocardial infarction, disabling stroke, or ischemia-driven target-vessel revascularization did not significantly differ between groups at 30 days (4.2% for stenting; 5.4% for PTCA).

Stent PAMI Trial

Conclusions   Palmaz-Schatz heparin-coated stents caused greater lumen size and reduced early target vessel revascularization. 6 month data are pending.

TIMI 10B

Phase II Trial of TNK-TPA in Acute Myocardial Infarction

Reference	Clin Cardiol 1997;20:1031.
Disease	Acute myocardial infarction.
Purpose	To compare TNK-TPA with tPA in patients with acute myocardial infarction.
Design	Randomized.
Patients	886 patients with acute myocardial infarction associated with ST segment elevation, presenting ≤12 h of symptom onset.
Follow-up	Coronary angiography 60, 75, and 90 min following initiation of therapy.
Treatment regimen	TNK-TPA (30 or 50 mg) or front loaded tPA.
Remarks	Data were presented at the XIX congress of the European Society of Cardiology, Stockholm, Sweden, 1997. TNK-TPA at 50 mg was associated with increased bleeding (intracranial hemorrhages were reported in 3.8% of the patients). Therefore the dose was reduced to 40 mg. 90 min TIMI flow 3 was achieved by 55% of the TNK 30 mg, by 63% of the TNK 40 mg, and by 63% of the tPA treated patients. At 60, 75, and 90 min post treatment, TNK-TPA 40 mg was associated with faster blood flow than front-loaded tPA. TNK-TPA, given as a single intravenous bolus appears to be a promising thrombolytic agent.

TIMI 14

Title	Elliott Antman, et al. for the presentation at the 70th Scientific Sessions of the American Heart Association.
Disease	Acute myocardial infarction.
Purpose	To determine the incidence of TIMI Grade III flow at 90 minutes of angiography comparing standard front loaded tPA (100 mg); low dose tPA (20, 35, or 50 mg) plus abciximab; low dose streptokinase (500,000–1,250,000 U) plus abciximab; or abciximab alone.
Design	Randomized, prospective, multicenter.
Patients	444 patients with acute myocardial infarction.
Follow-up	90 min angiography.
Treatment regimen	As above.
Preliminary results	TIMI III flow - achieved in 52% of patients with standard tPA alone, 32% in abciximab - alone group, 53% - 61% in low dose tPA plus abciximab; and 42% - 49% in streptokinase plus abciximab group. Thrombolytic therapy plus abciximab resulted in better thrombolysis. Abciximab was not as effective as thrombolysis alone. At higher doses of streptokinase plus abciximab the incidence of bleeding was increased (12%) compared to other groups (0 - 8%).

b. Unstable Angina
Non Q wave myocardial infarction

GUSTO IV Unstable Angina

Global Utilization of Strategies To Open Occluded Coronary Arteries IV

Disease	Unstable angina.
Purpose	To assess the effects of abciximab infusion on the composite endpoint of 30 day death and myocardial infarction in patients with acute coronary syndromes without ST elevation.
Design	Randomized, double blind, placebo-controlled, multicenter, phase III.
Patients	~7800 patients, ≥21 years old, with anginal syndrome at rest, ≤24 h of the last episode, associated with ST segment depression and/or positive troponin T/I test. Patients who receive thrombolytic therapy, have ST segment elevation, or are scheduled for coronary revascularization within 30 days of enrollment will be excluded.
Follow-up	6 months.
Treatment regimen	Randomization to: 1. Abciximab bolus + infusion for 48 h. 2. Abciximab bolus + infusion for 24 h and placebo infusion for additional 24 h. 3. Placebo bolus + placebo infusion for 48 h.
Remarks	Results are not available yet.

OPUS

Orbofiban in Patients with Unstable Coronary Syndromes

Disease	Unstable angina, acute myocardial infarction.
Purpose	To assess the efficacy and safety of adding orbofiban, a novel antiplatelet agent that blocks the binding of fibrinogen to GPIIb/IIIa integrin receptors, to aspirin in reducing major cardiovascular events in patients with unstable coronary syndromes.
Design	Randomized, double blind, placebo-controlled, multicenter.
Patients	~12,000 patients, >18 years old, with unstable coronary syndromes.
Follow-up	Mean 1 year, minimum 6 months.
Treatment regimen	Randomization to placebo or orbofiban 50 mg BID, or 50 mg BID for 30 days and then, 30 mg BID. All patients will receive aspirin 150-162 mg/d. Intravenous heparin, thrombolysis, other medications, angiography and revascularizations are performed at the discretion of the treating physician. In patients who experience unprovoked minor bleeding, the orbofiban dose will be reduced.
Remarks	Results are not available yet.

PURSUIT

Platelet Glycoprotein IIb-IIIa in Unstable Angina: Receptor Suppression Using Integrilin Therapy

Title	Design and methodology of the PURSUIT Trial: Evaluating eptifibatide for acute ischemic coronary syndromes.
Author	Harrington RA.
Reference	Am J Cardiol 1997; 80 (4A):34B-38B.
Disease	Coronary artery disease, unstable angina, non Q wave myocardial infarction.
Purpose	To determine whether the GPIIb/IIIa inhibitor eptifibatide (Integrilin) reduced cardiac events following unstable angina or non Q wave myocardial infarction. Primary endpoints are death or acute myocardial infarction at 30 days.
Design	Randomized, multicenter.
Patients	10,948 patients with unstable angina or non Q wave myocardial infarction.
Follow-up	30 day.
Treatment regimen	Initially placebo vs 1 of 2 doses. Low dose dropped and randomization changed to placebo vs bolus (180 µg kg) plus infusion.

PURSUIT

Platelet Glycoprotein IIb-IIIa in Unstable Angina: Receptor Suppression Using Integrilin Therapy

(continued)

Results Preliminary results were presented at the XIXth Congress of the European Society of Cardiology, 1997 by Robert M. Califf et al. Integrilin caused a significant reduction in combined endpoints of death, myocardial infarction (14.2%) vs placebo (15.7%). There was some increase in major bleeding with Integrilin. Integrilin may be a useful drug in patients with unstable angina and non Q wave myocardial infarction.

PARAGON

Delaying and Preventing Ischemic Events in Patients with Acute Coronary Syndromes using the Platelet Glycoprotein IIb/IIIa Inhibitor Lamifiban

Reference	J Am Coll Cardiol 1997; 29 (Suppl A); 409A.
Disease	Unstable angina, non Q wave myocardial infarction.
Purpose	To determine the incidence and timing of 30 day reinfarction or infarction and in-hospital refractory ischemia in patients receiving low or high dose lamifiban with or without heparin vs standard therapy.
Design	Randomized, multicenter.
Patients	2282 patients with unstable angina or non Q wave myocardial infarction.
Follow-up	30 days.
Treatment regimen	Low dose lamifiban vs high dose lamifiban, with or without heparin, vs standard therapy - heparin alone.
Remarks	Low dose lamifiban with and without heparin delayed and prevented infarction/reinfarction and ischemic events compared to other groups.

c. Hypertension

ALLHAT

Antihypertensive and Lipid Lowering Treatment to Prevent Heart Attack Trial

Reference	J Natl Med Assoc 1995;87:627-629.
Disease	Hypertension.
Purpose	1. To assess whether antihypertensive therapy with amlodipine, lisinopril, doxazosin, or chlorthalidone is associated with reduced incidence of fatal coronary heart disease or nonfatal myocardial infarction. 2. To determine whether pravastatin therapy for moderately hypercholesterolemic patients ≥60 years old will reduce mortality.
Design	Randomized, open label, multicenter.
Patients	40000 patients, ≥60 years old, with hypertension are expected to be recruited. Patients with fasting LDL cholesterol 120-189 mg/dl and triglyceride <350 mg/dl will be eligible for the cholesterol lowering substudy.
Follow-up	7 years.

LIFE STUDY

Losartan Intervention for Endpoint Reduction in Hypertension

Disease	Hypertension.
Purpose	To compare the effects of losartan and atenolol on cardiovascular mortality and morbidity in patients with hypertension.
Design	Randomized, triple blind, controlled.
Patients	8300 patients, aged 55-88 years, with hypertension and ECG documented LVH. Patients with prior myocardial infarction, heart failure, or stroke will be excluded.
Follow-up	4 years or more.
Treatment regimen	2 week placebo initiation period. Active therapy for 4 years. Randomization to losartan + placebo or placebo + atenolol in daily 50 mg doses. Hydrochlorothiazide and additional agents may be added to provide blood pressure control.

HOT

The Hypertension Optimal Treatment

Reference	1. Blood Press 1993;2:62-68. 2. Blood Press 1994;3:322-327. 3. Blood Press 1995;4:313-319.
Disease	Hypertension.
Purpose	1. To determine what is the optimal therapeutic goal for diastolic blood pressure (≤90, ≤85 or ≤80 mmHg) for patients with hypertension in order to prevent cardiovascular morbidity and mortality. 2. To assess the efficacy of low dose aspirin in reduction of cardiovascular mortality and morbidity in hypertensive patients.
Design	Randomized, open label, multicenter.
Patients	19,196 patients, 50-80 years old, with diastolic blood pressure 101-115 mmHg.
Follow-up	>2 years.
Treatment regimen	1. Felodipine 5 mg/d. If blood pressure is not controlled, additional therapy according to 4 more steps is given: low dose ACE inhibitor or ß blocker; the felodipine dose is increased to 10 mg; the dose of the additional drug is increased; an alternative drug or hydrochlorothiazide is added. 2. Aspirin 75 mg/d or placebo.

HOT

The Hypertension Optimal Treatment

(continued)

Preliminary
results

4. Preliminary results were presented in June 1998 at the International Society of Hypertension. Patients whose blood pressure was reduced to a target of 80 mmHg (diastolic) had 61 myocardial infarcts; those whose blood pressure was reduced to 85 had 64 myocardial infarcts, while those whose blood pressure was reduced to only 90 mmHg had 84 myocardial infarcts. The results were more dramatic in hypertensive patients with diabetes; in these patients cardiovascular risk was reduced in half when blood pressure was decreased to 80 mmHg.

5. Data on a substudy presented at a satellite symposium of the 70th Scientific Sessions of the American Heart Association revealed information on a Psychological General Well - Being Index. This was an analysis of 610 patients from the US and Scandinavia who participated in HOT. There was a linear relationship between lower diastolic blood pressure and improvement in quality in life. For patients with blood pressures of 86–90 mmHg, there was an improvement in perceived quality of life. Mood improved as blood pressure was lowered. Patients with diastolic blood pressures of 90 mmHg noted some deterioration in quality of life. In general, side effects of the drugs were minor and did not impede quality of life.

Update

At about the time this publication went to press the HOT study was published in *Lancet* 1998; 356(June 13): 1755–1762. The investigators observed that the lowest frequency of cardiovascular events was achieved at a diastolic pressure of 82.6 and lowest risk of cardiovascular mortality at 86.5 mmHg. In diabetics, there was a 51% reduction in major cardiovascular events in patients in the ≤80 mmHg target group vs the ≤90 mmHg target group (p=0.005).

CAPPP

The Captopril Prevention Project

Reference	1. J Hypertens 1990;8:985-990. 2. Am J Hypertens 1994;7:82S-83S.
Disease	Hypertension.
Purpose	To compare the effectiveness of conventional therapy with diuretics and or ß blockers vs captopril in patients with hypertension regarding cardiovascular mortality.
Design	Randomized, open label, placebo-controlled, multicenter.
Patients	10800 patients, 25-66 years old, with diastolic blood pressure >100 mmHg.
Follow-up	5 years.
Treatment regimen	Captopril 50 mg/d or conventional therapy (ß blockers or diuretics).

PRESERVE

Prospective Randomized Enalapril Study Evaluating Regression of Ventricular Enlargement

Reference	Am J Cardiol 1996;78:61-65.
Disease	Hypertension.
Purpose	To compare the efficacy of enalapril and nifedipine GITs to reduce left ventricular mass and to normalize the Doppler echocardiographic ratio of early to late mitral inflow flow velocities in hypertensive patients.
Design	Randomized, double blind, parallel group, multicenter.
Patients	480 patients, ≥50 years old, with ≥140 mmHg systolic blood pressure if on anti-hypertensive therapy, or ≥150 systolic blood pressure if unmedicated, and/or ≥90 mmHg diastolic blood pressure, and echocardiographic LV mass >116 g/m2 in men and >104 g/m2 in women. Patients with left ventricular ejection fraction <0.40 or evidence of severe valvular heart disease or coexisting cardiomyopathy will be excluded.
Follow-up	1 year with clinical follow-up and repeated echocardiogram at baseline, 6 and 12 months.
Treatment regimen	Enalapril 10-20 mg/d or nifedipine GITs 30-60 mg/d. In cases where maximum dose is reached and further blood pressure control is needed, hydrochlorothiazide 25 mg, and then atenolol 25 mg will be added.

STOP Hypertension 2

Swedish Trial in Old Patients with Hypertension 2

Reference	Blood Press 1993;2:136-141.
Disease	Hypertension.
Purpose	A prospective interventional trial of "newer" vs "older" treatment alternatives in old patients with hypertension. STOP Hypertension 1 showed that among elderly men and women (aged 70-84) treated for hypertension (with a beta blocker - atenolol, metroprolol or pindolol - and diuretic hydrochlorothlazide plus amiloride) compared to placebo, that there was a 47% reduction in stroke morbidity and mortality, 40% reduction in all cardiovascular endpoints and 43% reduction in total mortality with therapy (Lancet 1991;338:1281-1285). STOP Hypertension 2 will compare the effect of older drugs (β blockers and diuretics) to the newer alternative (calcium channel blockers-isradipine and felodipine) and ACE-inhibitors (enalapril and lisinopril) on cardiovascular mortality.
Design	Prospective, randomized, open, blinded endpoint evaluation.
Patients	Over 6600 hypertensive patients ages 70-84 years with supine BP> or = 180/105 mmHg.
Follow-up	4 years.
Treatment regimen	Diuretic-β blocker regimen against either ACE-inhibitor (enalapril. lisinopril) or calcium blockers (isradipine, felodipine).

AASK

African American Study of Kidney Disease

Reference	Journal of Controlled Clinical Trials, August 1996.
Disease	Hypertension, hypertensive nephrosclerosis.
Purpose	Evaluate the efficacy of different antihypertensive treatment regimens and different levels of blood pressure control in slowing the progression of renal artery disease in African American hypertensive patients with chronic renal insufficiency.
Design	Prospective, blinded, randomized, controlled study.
Patients	~ 1000 African American patients with hypertension and established renal insufficiency.
Follow-up	~ 5 years.
Treatment regimen	Amlodipine, ramipril, and metoprolol XL with 2 levels of blood pressure control on progression of hypertensive nephrosclerosis. One group will have goal mean arterial pressure (MAP) ≤92 mmHg and the other group will have a MAP between 102–107 mmHg. BP will also be treated to <160/90 in all participants. There will be 3 drug regimens, each initiated by a different agent.
Remarks	Endpoints include measurement of GFR (glomerular filtration rate) and end stage renal disease. The study is expected to be completed in 2001.

d. Congestive Heart Failure

PRAISE - 2

Prospective Randomized Amlodipine Survival Evaluation - 2

Reference	Ongoing study (Packer M et al.)
Disease	Congestive heart failure.
Purpose	To determine the effect of amlodipine on mortality in patients with severe heart failure of nonischemic origin.
Design	Prospective, randomized, double-blind, multicenter study.
Patients	1800 patients with New York Heart Association Class III - IV heart failure; ejection fraction ≤29%.
Follow-up	First patient enrolled on 12/27/95, expected to complete in mid 1999.
Treatment regimen	Amlodipine 10 mg or placebo added to background therapy of digoxin, diuretics, and angiotensin-converting enzyme inhibitors.
Remarks	The primary end-point is all cause mortality. Substudies will investigate the effects of amlodipine on echocardiography, positron emission tomography, right ventriculography, and neurohormones.

Note: Amlodipine is not indicated for CHF.

RESOLVED Pilot Study

Randomized Evaluation of Strategies for Left Ventricular Dysfunction

Reference	a. Can J Cardiol 1997;13:1166-1174. b. Circulation 1997;96(Suppl I):I-452.
Disease	Congestive heart failure.
Purpose	Stage I: to compare the efficacy and safety of candesartan (an angiotensin II receptor antagonist), enalapril (an angiotensin-converting enzyme inhibitor), and their combination in patients with congestive heart failure. In a second stage the effect of adding metoprolol or placebo to the above regimens was assessed.
Design	Randomized, two stage trial, multicenter.
Patients	769 patients with congestive heart failure (NYHA class II-IV), left ventricular ejection fraction <40%, and 6 min walk distance of ≤500 m.
Follow-up	Stage I: 20 weeks. Stage II: 46 weeks.
Treatment regimen	Stage I: randomization to candesartan alone (4 mg/d [n=111] 8 mg/d [n=108], and 16 mg/d [n=109]), enalapril alone (10 mg BID [n=109]), or their combination (enalapril 10 mg/d and candesartan 4 mg/d [n=165] or enalapril 10 mg/d and candesartan 8 mg/day [n = 167]) for 5 months. Stage II: randomization to addition of metoprolol (200 mg/d) or placebo to their study medications for additional 6 months.

RESOLVED Pilot Study

Randomized Evaluation of Strategies for Left Ventricular Dysfunction

(continued)

Remarks | All 3 regimens were well tolerated, withdrawal because of adverse effects occurred in only 8.6%. Candesartan and enalapril had similar effects on 6 min walking distance, left ventricular ejection fraction, and neurohormone levels. The combination group had a decrease in systolic and diastolic blood pressure, improvement in left ventricular ejection fraction and a decrease in left ventricular volumes (week 43) compared with enalapril alone and candesartan alone. The combination therapy had an improvement in 6 min walk distance after 18 weeks. However, subsequently the difference was less apparent. Brain natiuretic peptide (BNP) and aldosterone levels decreased in the combination group, but increased in the enalapril alone and candesartan alone. Metoprolol was associated with decreased heart rate, but systolic and diastolic pressure were not changed. Metoprolol did not alter quality of life, NYHA class, and 6 min walk distance. Metoprolol caused an increase in BNP levels.

ATLAS

The Assessment of Treatment with Lisinopril and Surviva.
(ATLAS)

Title	The Assessment of Treatment with Lisinopril and Survival.
Reference	Milton Packer et al. for the presentation at the annual meeting of the American College of Cardiology, March 1998, Atlanta, Georgia.
Disease	Congestive heart failure.
Purpose	To determine outcome of lower dose vs higher dose angiotensin-converting enzyme (ACE) inhibitor in patients with congestive heart failure. It was noted that most physicians prescribe ACE inhibitors in doses equivalent to the low dose arm, for heart failure.
Design	Randomized, double blind, multicenter.
Patients	3164 patients with moderate to severe congestive heart failure.
Follow-up	Median 4 years.
Treatment regimen	2.5-5 mg/day of lisinopril vs 32.5 -35 mg/day of lisinopril.

The Assessment of Treatment with Lisinopril and Survival (ATLAS)

(continued)

Preliminary results	There was a highly significant (p=.002) reduction in combined endpoint of all cause death or hospitalization in patients on high dose (1,251 events) vs low dose (1,339) representing a 12% reduction. In addition, there were 717 deaths in low dose group vs 666 in high dose group indicating an 8% reduction in mortality when high dose was used (p = NS). High dose lisinopril reduced cardiovascular mortality by 10% (p=NS) and the number of hospitalizations for congestive heart failure by 24% compared to lower dose. Adverse events secondary to drugs was not markedly different between groups. Cough was less common in high dose group.
Conclusions	High dose ACE inhibitors with lisinopril was more effective than lower dose for treating congestive heart failure. High dose ACE inhibitor was associated with better outcomes.

e. Prevention of Progression of Coronary Artery Disease

QUIET

The Quinapril Ischemic Event Trial

Reference	Blood Press 1992;1(Suppl 4):11-12.
Disease	Coronary artery disease.
Purpose	To evaluate the role of quinapril, an ACE inhibitor, on the development of ischemic events and progression of atherosclerosis in patients with coronary artery disease.
Design	Randomized, placebo-controlled, multicenter.
Patients	1900 patients with coronary artery disease, <75 years old, with left ventricular ejection fraction ≥40%, a serum LDL cholesterol ≤165 mg/dl, a blood pressure <160/95 mmHg.
Follow-up	3 year clinical follow-up. In 500 patients- repeated coronary angiography.
Treatment regimen	Quinapril 20 mg/d or placebo.

ACADEMIC

Azithromycin in Coronary Artery Disease Elimination of Myocardial Infection with Chlamydia

Title	Azithromycin in Coronary Artery Disease Elimination of Myocardial Infection with Chlamydia.
Reference	Joseph B. Muhlestein for the presentation at the 1998 American College of Cardiology Meetings, Atlanta, Georgia.
Disease	Coronary artery disease.
Purpose	To determine whether the antibiotic azithromycin could reduce coronary events in patients with coronary artery disease and positive antichlamydial antibody titers.
Design	Randomized, double blind.
Patients	302 patients with coronary artery disease and positive antichlamydial antibody titers.
Follow-up	Scheduled for 2 years. Interim report was for 6 months.
Treatment regimen	3 month course of azithromycin vs placebo.
Preliminary results	At 6 months there were 9 adverse cardiovascular events in the treated group and 7 in the placebo group. C-reactive protein and interleukin:6 were significantly reduced with therapy at 6 months. Serologic tests for antibodies to C pneumoniae were not changed throughout the 6 months.

BANFF

Brachial Artery ultrasound Normalization of Forearm Flow

Title	A comparative study of 4 anti-hypertensive agents on endothelial function agents on endothelial function in patients with coronary disease. (Brachial Artery Ultrasound Normalization of Forearm Flow).
Author	Anderson TJ, et al.
Reference	47th Scientific Session of the American College of Cardiology, Atlanta, Georgia 1998.
Disease	Coronary artery disease.
Purpose	To compare the chronic effects of 4 anti-hypertensives on brachial artery flow-mediated vasodilation in patients with documented coronary artery disease.
Design	Partial block, cross-over design trial, and randomized in 1 of 4 different, open label drug sequences. High resolution ultrasound to compare flow-mediated vasodilator and nitroglycerin dilation before and after 8 weeks of study drug.
Patients	80 patients with coronary artery disease.
Preliminary results	Of quinapril, enalapril, losartan, and amlodipine, only quinapril improved flow mediated dilatation.

PREVENT

Prospective, Randomized, Evaluation of Vascular Effects of Norvasc

Reference	Ongoing study (Furburg CD, Pitt B et al.).
Disease	Coronary artery disease, atherosclerosis.
Purpose	To evaluate the effectiveness of amlodipine relative to placebo on the development and progression of atherosclerotic lesions in coronary and carotid arteries of patients with coronary artery disease. To correlate rates of progression in these 2 vascular beds.
Design	Multicenter, double blind, randomized, placebo-controlled.
Patients	683 patients with paired angiograms (of 828 patients that completed the trial).
Follow-up	3 years.
Treatment regimen	Placebo vs amlodipine.
Remarks	Patients have angiographic documentation of coronary artery disease. All entry patients have quantitative coronary angiography and B- mode carotid arterial compliance. Baseline and post-treatment angiograms and sequential 6 month carotid artery B mode ultrasonograms are evaluated for new lesions or progression of existing atherosclerotic lesion. Primary endpoint is change in average minimal diameter of the early atherosclerotic lesions.

f. Arrhythmia

ALIVE

The Azimilide Post-Infarct Survival Evaluation

Reference	Am J Cardiol 1998;81:35D-39D.
Disease	Arrhythmia.
Purpose	To assess the effects of azimilide dihydrochloride, a novel type of antiarrhythmic agent that blocks both the rapid (I_{Kr}) and slow (I_{Ks}) components of the delayed rectifier K+ currents, on survival of patients after myocardial infarction who are at high risk for sudden cardiac death.
Design	Randomized, double blind, placebo-controlled, multicenter.
Patients	Will enroll 5,900 patients, 18-75 years old, who had a recent (within 6-21 days) acute myocardial infarction, with left ventricular ejection fraction 15-35%, and a low heart rate variability. Patients with a history of torsade de pointes; ventricular tachycardia; decompensated congestive heart failure at the time of enrollment or chronic NYHA class IV; unstable angina; syncope or aborted sudden death after the qualifying myocardial infarction; severe valvular disease; AV block or bradycardia; scheduled for revascularization; AICD; long QTc; stroke; Wolff-Parkinson-White syndrome; concomitant severe illness; renal or hepatic failure; uncontrolled hypertension; prior amiodarone therapy; on current antiarrhythmic therapy or are alcohol or drug abusers will be excluded.
Follow-up	1 year.
Treatment regimen	Randomization to: 1. azimilide 75 mg/d; 2. azimilide 100 mg/d; and 3. placebo.
Remarks	Results are not available yet.

ARCH

Amiodarone Reduces CABG Hospitalization

Reference	Thomas Guarnieri for the presentation at the American College of Cardiology 47th Award Scientific Sessions, March, 1998.
Disease	Atrial fibrillation following open heart surgery.
Purpose	To determine the effect of amiodarone on the incidence of atrial fibrillation following open heart procedures.
Design	Randomized, single center.
Patients	300 patients undergoing open heart surgery. (80% received CABG).
Follow-up	In hospital.
Preliminary results	Patients received 1 gm of amiodarone every 24 h or placebo through a central catheter over 2 days, beginning immediately following surgery. Amiodarone decreased the incidence of atrial fibrillation (47.2% in placebo group vs 35.4% in treated). Amiodarone delayed onset of atrial fibrillation in those that developed it and decreased hospital stay form 8.2–7.5 days.

ARREST

Amiodarone in the Out-of-Hospital Resuscitation of Refractory Sustained Ventricular Tachyarrhythmia

Reference	Clin Cardiol 1998;21:52-54.
Disease	Out-of-hospital cardiac arrest.
Purpose	To assess the efficacy of intravenous amiodarone added to the Advanced Cardiac Life Support (ACLS) guidelines treatment in patients with out-of-hospital cardiac arrest due to ventricular tachyarrhythmia refractory to electrical cardioversion.
Design	Randomized, double blind, placebo-controlled.
Patients	504 patients (75% men), >18 years old, with out-of-hospital cardiac arrest, and ongoing ventricular tachycardia or fibrillation after ≥3 electrical shocks.
Follow-up	Admission alive to the hospital.
Treatment regimen	Randomization to intravenous amiodarone 300 mg or placebo. Medication was injected rapidly as a bolus via peripheral infusion. All patients received standard ACLS care by paramedics.
Remarks	Preliminary data were presented at the 70th Scientific Sessions of the American Heart Association, Orlando, Florida. The percent of patients admitted alive to the hospital was 26% greater in the amiodarone treated patients. However, there was no significant effect on patients with asystole/pulsless electrical activity converting to ventricular fibrillation during the course of resuscitation. There was 56% improvement in the proportion of patients admitted to the hospital whose pulses could be temporarily restored but not maintained after electrical defibrillation prior to intravenous administration of amiodarone. More than half of the patients were discharged from hospital without significant neurologic sequela.

CIDS

Canadian Implantable Defibrillator Study

Reference	Am J Cardiol 1993;72:103F-108F.
Disease	Ventricular arrhythmia.
Purpose	To compare implantable cardioverter-defibrillator (ICD) to amiodarone in patients at high risk for arrhythmic death because of ventricular tachyarrhythmia.
Design	Randomized, multicenter.
Patients	659 patients with documented ventricular fibrillation, out-of-hospital cardiac arrest requiring defibrillation or cardioversion, sustained ventricular tachycardia causing syncope, sustained ventricular tachycardia ≥150 beats/min causing presyncope or angina in a patient with ejection fraction ≤35%, or syncope with subsequent documentation of either spontaneous or programmed ventricular stimulation induced ventricular tachycardia.
Follow-up	The primary end points were arrhythmic death and total mortality occurring within 30 days of initiation of therapy. Secondary end points were clinical outcome during long follow-up (4 years).
Treatment regimen	Randomization to ICD (n=328) or amiodarone therapy (n=331). Amiodarone was given ≥1200 mg/d for ≥1 week, then ≥400 mg/d for ≥10 weeks, and thereafter ≥300 mg/d. Dose could be lowered to 200 mg/d in patients who were not able to tolerate 300 mg/d. Patients who could not tolerate the amiodarone 200 mg/d, or had recurrent arrhythmia while on amiodarone, could receive another form of therapy, including ICD.
Remarks	Preliminary data were reported at the American College of Cardiology Meeting, 1998. By intention to treat analysis, risk of all cause mortality was 19.6% lower in the ICD group (p=0.072). 22% of the patients assigned to amiodarone received ICD within 4 years.

Diamond

Danish Investigators of Arrhythmia and Mortality ON Dofetilide

(continued)

Reference	a. Clin Cardiol 1997;20:704-710. b. Clin Cardiol 1998;21:53-54.
Disease	Acute myocardial infarction, arrhythmia.
Purpose	To assess whether dofetilide, a class III, highly-selective potassium channel blocker, will reduce mortality and morbidity in patients with congestive heart failure and with LV dysfunction after myocardial infarction.
Design	Randomized, placebo-controlled, multicenter.
Patients	First study: 1518 patients admitted to the hospital with congestive heart failure and LVEF≤35%. Second study: 1510 patients within 7 d of acute myocardial infarction and LVEF ≤35%.
Follow-up	Minimum of 12 months.
Treatment regimen	Randomization to dofetilide 0.5 mg BID or placebo. Dose was adjusted to 0.25 mg BID for patients with renal failure, QTc prolongation, or atrial fibrillation. Patients were monitored by telemetry during the first 3 d of therapy.
Remarks	Preliminary data of the myocardial infarction study were presented at the 70th Scientific Sessions of the American Heart Association, Orlando, Florida. Patients were randomized within 2.7 d after onset of symptoms. Mortality rate was comparable between the groups (230 in the dofetilide group and 243 in the placebo group). Secondary end points occurred in similar rates. More patients receiving dofetilide than placebo who had atrial fibrillation converted to sinus rhythm. Dofetilide did not alter mortality in patients with LV dysfunction following myocardial infarction. However, when initiated in hospital using telemetry monitoring, this drug seems to be effective and safe for atrial fibrillation in patients with impaired left ventricular function after myocardial infarction.

g. Interventional Cardiology

ASCENT

ACS Multilink Clinical Equivalence Trial

(continued)

Reference	Clin Cardiol 1997;20:1030-1031.
Disease	Coronary artery disease.
Purpose	To compare the ACS Multilink stent with Palmaz-Schatz stent.
Design	Randomized.
Patients	1040 patients with de novo coronary artery lesions. 538 patients were assigned to repeated angiography at 6 months.
Follow-up	6 months.
Treatment regimen	Randomization to 15 mm ACS or Palmaz-Schatz stents.
Remarks	Preliminary data were presented at the XIX congress of the European Society of Cardiology, Stockholm, Sweden, 1997. Successful stent delivery was obtained in 95.8% of the Palmaz-Schatz assigned patients and in 97.5% of the ACS assigned group. Immediately post-procedure residual stenosis was 8% in the ACS vs 10% in the Palmaz-Schatz group. There was a trend towards less major events (death, myocardial infarction, or target vessel revascularization) at 30 days in the ACS group (4.4% vs 6.5%). #0-day mortality was 0 in the ACS vs 1.2% in the Palmaz-Schatz group. Restenosis rates were comparable. Cumulative rates at 6 months of target vessel failure or need for revascularization were comparable (16.5% vs 18.3%, respectively). Mortality was higher in the Palmaz-Schatz group (3.1% vs 1.5%). The data shows that the ACS stent is equivalent or superior to the Palmaz-Schatz stent in treatment of de novo coronary lesions.

EPISTENT

Evaluation of IIb/IIIa Platelet Inhibitor for Stenting

Reference	Eric G. Topol, MD, for the presentation at the American College of Cardiology 47th Annual Scientific Session, Atlanta, Georgia, March 1998.
Disease	Coronary artery disease.
Purpose	To compare outcomes of stent plus placebo plus standard heparin dose; to abciximab plus stent plus low dose heparin; to abciximab/PTCA plus low dose heparin.
Design	Randomized, multicenter.
Patients	2,400 patients with coronary artery disease with a > 60% stenosis of target vessel, eligible for PTCA, or stent.
Follow-up	Report of 30 day outcomes.
Preliminary results	Primary endpoint was the composite of death, myocardial infarction, or target vessel revascularization. It occurred in 5.3% of abciximab/stent patients; 6.9% of abciximab/PTCA patients and 10.8% of stent/placebo patients. The majority of benefit was in patients with large non Q wave infarcts. Abciximab plus stent resulted in a 51% reduction in primary endpoint vs stent/placebo (p=0001); abciximab/PTCA resulted in a 36% reduction in primary endpoint compared to stent/placebo. There was no incidence of intracerebral hemorrhage.

ERASER

Evaluation of Reopro and Stenting to Eliminate Restenosis

Title	Evaluation of Reopro and Stenting to Eliminate Restenosis.
Reference	Presentation at the 70th Scientific Sessions of the American Heart Association. November 10-13, 1997, Orlando, Florida, Stephen Ellis et al.
Disease	Coronary artery disease.
Purpose	To determine whether the platelet GP IIb/IIIa receptor antagonist abciximab reduced percent volume obstruction at 6 months assessed by intravascular ultrasound (IVUS).
Design	Prospective, randomized, placebo-controlled, multicenter.
Patients	225 patients randomized to receive either placebo, bolus and 12 h infusion of abciximab, or bolus plus 24 h infusion of abciximab.
Follow-up	6 months.
Preliminary results	The mean IVUS % obstruction was 32.4% with placebo, 32.7% in the 12 h abciximab infusion group, and 34.2% in the 24 h abciximab group. Thus abciximab did not decrease intimal hyperplasia associated with stent deployment.

FLARE

Fluvastatin Angioplasty Restenosis

Reference	a. Am J Cardiol 1994;26:50D-61D. b. J Am Clin Cardiol 1997;30:5.
Disease	Coronary artery disease.
Purpose	To determine the effect of fluvastatin, a 3-hydroxy-3-methyulglutaryl-coenzyme A reductase inhibitor, on outcome after percutaneous transluminal coronary angioplasty.
Design	Randomized, double blind, placebo-controlled, multicenter.
Patients	1054 patients with native primary coronary artery lesions who were scheduled for elective coronary angioplasty.
Follow-up	Coronary angiography at baseline and after 26±2 weeks. Clinical follow-up for 9 months.
Treatment regimen	Randomization to fluvastatin 40 mg BID or placebo. Patients started study medication 2 weeks before scheduled procedure and continued therapy for 26±2 weeks after angioplasty.

FLARE

Fluvastatin Angioplasty Restenosis

Remarks   In the fluvastatin group, LDL cholesterol decreased by 37% within the first 2 weeks of therapy before angioplasty was performed. At 6 months, serum LDL cholesterol was 33% lower than at baseline in the fluvastatin group, whereas in the placebo group there was no change in LDL cholesterol. Fluvastatin had no effect on minimum lumen diameter after 26 weeks. The combined incidence of death and myocardial infarction was 1.5% in the fluvastatin group vs 4% in the placebo group. Death, myocardial infarction, coronary artery bypass surgery, or repeated angioplasty within 9 months occurred in 92 patients in the fluvastatin group vs 99 patients in the placebo group. Fluvastatin 80 mg/d, started 2 weeks before elective coronary angioplasty did not reduce the rate of restenosis, however, it reduced the incidence of death and myocardial infarction.

REST

Stent Implantation and Restenosis Study

Reference	Clin Cardiol 1997;20:1030-1031.
Disease	Coronary artery disease, restenosis.
Purpose	To compare stenting vs conventional PTCA for restenosis after PTCA.
Design	Randomized.
Patients	400 patients with restenosis after initially successful PTCA.
Follow-up	Coronary angiography at baseline and after 6 months. Clinical follow-up for 6 months.
Treatment regimen	PTCA with or without 15 mm Palmaz-Schatz stent implantation. Intravenous heparin during procedure and aspirin and coumadin for 3 months for the patients who underwent stent implantation. The PTCA assigned group received aspirin 100 mg/d.

REST

Stent Implantation and Restenosis Study

(continued)

Remarks   Data were presented at the XIX congress of the European Society of Cardiology, Stockholm, Sweden, 1997. Procedure was technically successful in 98.9% of the stent group vs only 93.2% of the PTCA alone group. Of the PTCA assigned group, 12 patients crossed over to bailout stenting. Mortality was similar (2 patients in each group). Q wave myocardial infarction occurred more frequently in the stent group (2.8%) than in the PTCA group (0.6%)(p=NS). Thrombotic complications (3.9% vs 0) and bleeding (6.3% vs 1.4%) were more prevalent in the stent group. Hospitalization was longer in the stent group. Post-procedure minimum lumen diameter was larger for the stent group (3.02 mm) than the PTCA group (2.23 mm). Minimum lumen diameter at 6 months was 2.23 mm in the stent group vs 1.85 mm for the PTCA group (p=0.01). Restenosis at 6 months occurred in 18% of the stent group vs 32% of the PTCA group. 10% of the stent group vs 24% of the PTCA group underwent repeated revascularization procedures. The anticoagulation regimen was associated with increased risk of bleeding and thrombotic events. Stenting restenotic coronary lesions was associated with better technical success, larger post-procedure and 6 months minimum lumen diameter, less restenosis, and less need for revascularization.

h. Lipid Lowering Studies

AVERT

Atorvastatin Vs Revascularization Treatment

Reference	Am J Cardiol 1997;80:1130-1133.
Disease	Coronary artery disease.
Purpose	To compare the efficacy and safety of aggressive lipid lowering therapy with atorvastatin to catheter-based revascularization followed by conventional care in patients with stable angina pectoris and documented coronary artery disease.
Design	Randomized, open label, multicenter.
Patients	341 patients, 18-80 years old, with moderate angina (Canadian Cardiovascular Society Class I-II), with serum LDL cholesterol ≥115 mg/dl and serum triglycerides ≤500 mg/dl, who have ≥1 angiographically proven native coronary artery lesion ≥50% diameter stenosis. Only patients who were being able to complete ≥4 min of Bruce treadmill protocol or a 20 W/min bicycle exercise test without developing marked ischemic ECG changes were included. Patients with left main coronary disease, 3 vessel disease, unstable angina or myocardial infarction within 2 weeks of randomization, left ventricular ejection fraction <40%, NYHA Class III-IV congestive heart failure, catheter based revascularization within 6 months prior to enrollment, coronary artery bypass surgery, renal or hepatic dysfunction, elevated levels of serum creatine kinase, or hypersensitivity of HMG coenzyme A reductase inhibitors were excluded.
Follow-up	18 months of clinical follow-up. Cardiovascular mortality and nonfatal events (including the need for revascularization), all-cause mortality, quality of life, economic outcomes, and occurrence of adverse effects will be monitored.

AVERT

Atorvastatin Vs Revascularization Treatment

(continued)

Treatment regimen	Randomization to atorvastatin 80 mg/d or to undergo a catheter-based revascularization followed by conventional therapy. Lipid lowering agents, diet, and behavior modification are permitted for the intervention group. All patients are advised to take aspirin.
Remarks	Randomization was completed on December 31, 1996. The study is expected to be completed in June 1998.

LIPID

Long-Term Intervention with Pravastatin in Ischemic Disease

Reference	a. Am J Cardiol 1995;76:474-479. b. Control Clin Trials 1997;18:464-476. c. Clin Cardiol 1998;21:54.
Disease	Coronary artery disease.
Purpose	To assess the long-term effects of pravastatin in patients with average cholesterol levels and a history of myocardial infarction or unstable angina.
Design	Randomized, double blind, placebo-controlled, multicenter.
Patients	9,014 patients (7,503 men), 31-75 years old, with a serum total cholesterol level 155-271 mg/dl, and a history of acute myocardial infarction or unstable angina.
Follow-up	> 5 years.
Treatment regimen	Dietary advice according to National Heart Foundation guidelines. Randomization to pravastatin 40 mg/d or placebo.

Long-Term Intervention with Pravastatin in Ischemic Disease

(continued)

Remarks   Preliminary data of the myocardial infarction study were presented at the 70th Scientific Sessions of the American Heart Association, Orlando, Florida. Serum total cholesterol was reduced by 18% in the pravastatin compared with the placebo group. LDL cholesterol was reduced by 25%, triglycerides were reduced by 12%, and HDL cholesterol was increased by 6% in the pravastatin group. All cause mortality was 23% lower, and coronary heart disease mortality was 24% lower in the pravastatin group, compared with the placebo group. Combined fatal coronary heart disease and nonfatal myocardial infarction were reduced by 23% with pravastatin, and stroke rate was reduced by 20%. Patients with serum total cholesterol <250 mg/dl had significant reductions in the combined end-points. Among every 20 patients treated with pravastatin for 6 years, one fatal or serious event was prevented. Mortality due to cancer was comparable between the groups. Pravastatin was well tolerated.

MIRACL

Myocardial Ischemia Reduction With Aggressive Cholesterol Lowering

Reference	Am J Cardiol 1998;81:578-581.
Disease	Non Q wave myocardial infarction, unstable angina, hyper-cholesterolemia.
Purpose	To assess whether early intensive reduction in serum total and LDL cholesterol will reduce subsequent recurrent ischemia in patients presenting with unstable angina or non Q wave myocardial infarction.
Design	Randomized, double blind, placebo-controlled, multicenter.
Patients	2100 patients, ≥18 years old, with unstable angina or non Q wave myocardial infarction. Patients are randomized 24-96 h after admission. Patients with serum total cholesterol >270 mg/dl; those who are scheduled for coronary intervention during the index hospitalization; CABG within 3 months; PTCA within 6 months; Q wave myocardial infarction within 4 weeks; left bundle branch block; life threatening arrhythmias; severe heart failure; hepatic dysfunction or renal failure requiring dialysis; uncontrolled diabetes; concurrent therapy with lipid altering drugs, immunosuppressive agents, erythromycin, or azole antifungals; pregnancy or lactation are excluded.
Follow-up	16 weeks.
Treatment regimen	Randomization to atorvastatin 80 mg/d or placebo.
Remarks	Results are not available yet.

INDEX

(continued)

INDEX

(continued)

(continued)

INDEX

(continued)

INDEX

(continued)

(continued)

INDEX

(continued)